DENTAL TERMINOLOGY

Calista Kindle | 4ᵗʰ Edition
Charline Dofka

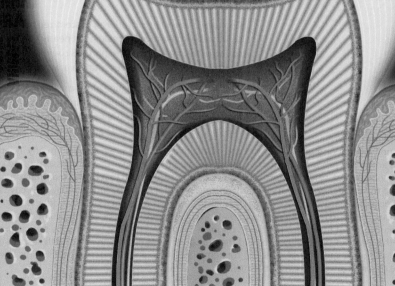
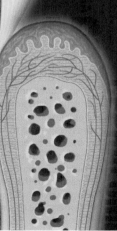

 CENGAGE

Australia • Brazil • Canada • Mexico • Singapore • United Kingdom • United States

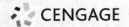
CENGAGE

Dental Terminology, **Fourth Edition**
Calista Kindle, Charline Dofka

SVP, Higher Education & Skills Product:
Erin Joyner

VP, Content and Learning: Julia Callabero

Product Director: Jason Fremder

Product Manager: Lauren Whalen

Product Assistant: Dallas Wilkes

Content Manager: Anubhav Kaushal,
MPS Limited

Digital Delivery Lead: David O'Connor

Marketing Manager: Courtney Cozzy

IP Analyst: Ashley Maynard

IP Project Manager: Nick Barrows

Production Service: MPS Limited

Designer: Angela Sheehan

Cover Image Source: anatomy of the tooth -
shutterstock.com/ilusmedical

For product information and technology assistance,
contact us at **Cengage Customer & Sales Support,**
1-800-354-9706 or **support.cengage.com.**

For permission to use material from this text or product,
submit all requests online at
www.cengage.com/permissions.

Library of Congress Control Number: 2021935988

Student Edition:
ISBN: 978-0-357-45682-8

Loose-leaf Edition:
ISBN: 978-0-357-45684-2

Cengage
200 Pier 4 Boulevard
Boston, MA 02210
USA

Cengage is a leading provider of customized learning
solutions with employees residing in nearly 40 different
countries and sales in more than 125 countries around the
world. Find your local representative at **www.cengage.com.**

To learn more about Cengage platforms and services,
register or access your online learning solution, or purchase
materials for your course, visit **www.cengage.com.**

Notice to the Reader
Publisher does not warrant or guarantee any of the products described herein or perform any independent analysis in
connection with any of the product information contained herein. Publisher does not assume, and expressly disclaims,
any obligation to obtain and include information other than that provided to it by the manufacturer. The reader is
expressly warned to consider and adopt all safety precautions that might be indicated by the activities described herein
and to avoid all potential hazards. By following the instructions contained herein, the reader willingly assumes all risks in
connection with such instructions. The publisher makes no representations or warranties of any kind, including but not
limited to, the warranties of fitness for particular purpose or merchantability, nor are any such representations implied
with respect to the material set forth herein, and the publisher takes no responsibility with respect to such material.
The publisher shall not be liable for any special, consequential, or exemplary damages resulting, in whole or part, from
the readers' use of, or reliance upon, this material.

Printed at CLDPC, USA, 01-25

CONTENTS

PREFACE

DENTAL TERMINOLOGY, Fourth Edition, is a valuable tool to introduce the dental field to an individual interested in starting their dental career. This text is meant to lay the foundation needed to advance in dental assistant studies. As an instructor, you will be delighted to use this text as a tool to teach your students how to break down, use, and pronounce dental terminology. This edition takes a word-building approach to help dental assistants understand and remember dental terminology better than ever before. DENTAL TERMINOLOGY is not a strict dictionary of dental terms, but rather a word bank with pronunciation guides and definitions applied to practice areas. It's the resource that dental professionals can use for years to come. The chapters are organized by specialty area, so readers can always find the information quickly. Whether learning in the classroom or on the job, DENTAL TERMINOLOGY, Fourth Edition, is the easy-to-use reference that comes in handy again and again.

The book language is plain, common, and easy to understand. When large words are introduced, they are broken down into syllables and shown in a "sounds like" manner to help the student learn how to speak the term. Further, this edition includes a Spanish translation to many of the words listed in the glossary to assist the student or to transfer information in working with patients with a limited knowledge of English terms.

Although the mission and practice of dentistry with its healing arts do not change, technology does. DENTAL TERMINOLOGY, Fourth Edition, has updated information, including new equipment, materials, and techniques. More graphic and enhanced visual aids with color have been added to make the book more attractive and more informative, as well as to serve as an aid to the learning process.

The direct, clear, and useful word-building approach will instruct students about the origins and proper use of dental terminology. This text leaves students with a clear understanding of how to use dental words and gives them a cut above the rest when going forward with their dental studies throughout each course. When students begin with DENTAL TERMINOLOGY, they will have the tools to be successful in all their dental courses, having the capabilities to grasp and understand complex procedures and dental scenarios because of their solid background using DENTAL TERMINOLOGY, Fourth Edition.

NEW TO THIS EDITION

Chapter 1
- New tests and examples have been added throughout the chapter for more enforcement and understanding of the lesson.

Chapter 2
- More information has been introduced on palate structure, palatine areas, and sensory divisions and branches of the trigeminal nerve.

Chapter 3
- Tooth eruption and exfoliation information is given, along with added timetables for deciduous and permanent teeth.

Chapter 4
- Updating of duties, services, and employment concerns are discussed.
- New instrument information is included.

Chapter 5
- Concern and care for disease prevention has been expanded.
- New CDC classifications of risk categories for instruments and equipment have been added.

Chapter 6
- New guidelines for cardiopulmonary resuscitation and the use of automated external defibrillation are included.

Chapter 7

- The importance of proper and thorough patient health information data is discussed.
- More information is included about additional oral examination concerns and diagnostic testing.

Chapter 8

- Additional descriptions of anxiety abatement controls as a method of pain reduction are introduced.

Chapter 9

- Digital radiography with recovery and enhancement has been added.
- Cone beam 3D radiography and tomography information is given.
- Revised discussions concerning measurement of radiation energy, biological effects, and safety are included.

Chapter 10

- Information regarding new isolation of restorative sites methods with new matrix placement and dry field illuminators is introduced.

Chapter 11

- Smile makeover with tooth reconstruction, gingival reductions and augmentation, implant placement, and other cosmetic procedures are explained.

Chapter 12

- Material combinations, makeup, and uses are reviewed as well as a look at the requirements for practice in this specialty.

Chapter 13

- Charting and diagnosis of pulpal conditions have been added.
- New instruments, such as flowmeters, loupes, microscopic surgical instruments, and methods, are discussed.

Chapter 14

- Various surgical procedures for maxillofacial treatment of TMJ, bone reconstruction, implant placement, and other disorders are given. There is a discussion regarding the surgical participation in aesthetic dentistry.

Chapter 15

- Expanded review is included of corrective orthodontic procedures involving direct or indirect banding or brackets, lingual or Invisalign braces, and Class II corrective and anchor devices.
- Involvement of orthodontic practices in orthognathic procedures is introduced.

Chapter 16

- Expanded information related to the measurement and recording of periodontal conditions is given.
- A new section describing periodontic treatment in cosmetic dentistry is included.

Chapter 17

- Development and growth concerns of the child patient are described, as well as control and sedation of the child.

Chapter 18

- Digital impression methods and the uses in prosthetic procedures are explained. Use of dental materials and metal information is enlarged.

Chapter 19

- Additional discussion of computer-assisted systems in the CAD/CAM area of dental restoration and appliances is included.

Chapter 20

- HIPAA regulations are discussed. Expansion of the dental insurance, legal, and ethical terms is provided.

End-of-chapter exercises have been revised for each chapter. A new glossary approach is prepared with the addition of legal, insurance, and ethical words. Spanish translations of many words are given at the end of the word listing.

ACCOMPANYING TEACHING AND LEARNING RESOURCES

Spend less time planning and more time teaching with Delmar Cengage Learning's Instructor Resources to Accompany DENTAL TERMINOLOGY, Fourth Edition. All Instructor Resources can be accessed by going to www.cengagebrain.com and creating a unique user log-in. The password-protected Instructor Resources include the following.

Online Instructor's Manual

An Instructor Manual accompanies this book. It includes answers to the core textbook assessments for access at any time.

PowerPoint® Lecture Slides

These vibrant, customizable Microsoft® PowerPoint lecture slides for each chapter assist you with your lecture by providing concept coverage using images, figures, and tables directly from the textbook!

Cengage Learning Testing Powered by Cognero

Cengage Learning Testing Powered by Cognero is a flexible online system that allows you to author, edit, and manage test bank content from multiple Cengage Learning solutions; create multiple test versions in an instant; and deliver tests from your LMS, your classroom, or wherever you want.

Audio Library

The Audio Library is a reference that includes audio pronunciations and definitions for many dental terms! Use the audio library to practice pronunciation and review definitions for dental terms.

ABOUT THE AUTHORS

Calista Kindle, EFDA, CDA, was a staff writer at a local newspaper in Ashtabula, Ohio, for five years. She has been in the dental field for over 15 years. She was employed as a dental assistant and oral surgical assistant before she became a dental assistant instructor for Great Lakes Institute of Technology, in Erie, Pennsylvania. Soon after employment as an instructor, she was promoted as the program director of the Dental Assistant program. She devotes her time and effort to each individual student, making sure they are the best in the field. Her students maintain high DANB Certificate pass rates, along with high successful job placement immediately after graduating the dental program. While being the program director, she attended Westmoreland Community College to become an expanded function dental assistant. She has a current license in the state of Pennsylvania as an expanded function assistant and works part time at a local dental office, while performing her duties as a program director/instructor for the dental program at Great Lakes Institute of Technology. She continues her education at Clarion University to elevate the dental program at Great Lakes and to expand her career.

Charline M. Dofka received an MS from the University of Dayton. She has taken postgraduate studies at Ohio State, West Virginia University, Kent State, and Ohio University. She was employed as a dental assistant/hygienist in oral surgery, orthodontics, and general practices before she became a dental assisting instructor and Diversified Cooperative Health Occupations coordinator at Belmont Career Center in St. Clairsville, Ohio. Along with teaching duties, she chartered the National Honor Society participation of the vocational school and was advisor for the VICA opening and closing ceremony team to national competition representing the state of Ohio. Mrs. Dofka has retired from active teaching but maintains life membership in the Iota Lambda Sigma, professional vocational teaching fraternity, DANB dental assisting certification, and maintains retired status as a dental hygienist in West Virginia.

FEEDBACK

The authors hope that *Dental Terminology* will aid in understanding and using dental terms. Comments, viewpoints, or input regarding this book will be appreciated.

Reviewers of the Current and Past Editions

Barbara Bennett, CDA, RDH, MS,
Texas State Technical College,
Harlingen, Texas

Robert Bennett, DMD,
Texas State Technical College,
Harlingen, Texas

Cindy Bradley, CDA, CDPMA, EFDA,
Orlando Tech,
Orlando, Florida

Sharilyn Eldredge, CDA, COA,
Mountainland Technical College,
Orem, Utah

Patricia Frese, RDH, Med,
Raymond Walters College,
Cincinnati, Ohio

Terri Heintz, CDA, RDA,
Des Moines Area Community College,
Ankeny, Iowa

Vivian Koistinen, CDA, RDA, BS,
Anthem Education Group,
Phoenix, Arizona

Kathryn Mosley, RDA, BS, MS,
Silicon Valley College,
Fremont, California

Denise Murphy, CDA, CDPMA, EFDA,
Orland Tech,
Orlando, Florida

Yolanda Ortiz, RDA, MBA,
Vista College,
El Paso, Texas

Gloria Pacheco,
Luna Community College,
Las Vegas, New Mexico

Juanita Robinson, CDA, EFDA, LDH, MSEd,
Indiana University Northeast,
Gary, Indiana

Lori Scribner, CDA, PhD, ATA
Career Education,
Spring Hill, Florida

Kelly Svanda, CDA,
Southeast Community College,
Nehawka, Nebraska

Janet Wilburn, BS, CDA,
Phoenix College,
Phoenix, Arizona

CHAPTER 1

INTRODUCTION TO DENTAL TERMINOLOGY

✔ Learning Objectives

On completion of this chapter, you should be able to:

1. Identify the roles of the four types of word parts used in forming dental terms.

2. Use your knowledge of word parts to analyze unfamiliar dental terms.

3. Define the commonly used word roots, combining forms, suffixes, and prefixes introduced in this chapter.

4. Use the "sounds-like" pronunciation system and audio files to correctly pronounce the primary terms introduced in this chapter.

5. Recognize the importance of spelling dental terms correctly.

6. State why caution is important when using abbreviations.

7. Recognize, define, spell, pronounce, and correctly use the dental words introduced in this chapter.

LOCATE THE DENTAL WORD

Learning dental terminology is easy once you understand what word parts are and how they work together to form a dental word. This text will assist you on your path to expert word-building skills.

Dental words are arranged and listed alphabetically in dictionaries, reference works, or glossary listings. A few terms, such as AIDS (acquired immune deficiency syndrome) and HVE (high volume evacuator), are commonly listed in an abbreviated form made up of the first letters of several words. These **acronyms** (**ACK**-roh-nims) are listed along with other abbreviations representing a combination of word pieces or initials that can indicate an occupation, specialty, procedure, condition, or chemical. In filling prescriptions and writing labels, the science of pharmacology uses many abbreviations, such as *b.i.d.* (twice a day). Radiology and dental

Vocabulary Related to the Introduction to Dental Terminology

This list contains essential word parts and dental terms for this chapter. These and the other important **primary terms** are shown in boldface, and *secondary terms* appear in italics throughout the chapter. You may use the list to review these terms and to practice pronouncing them correctly. When you work with the audio for this chapter, listen to the word, repeat it, and then place a checkmark in the box. Proceed to the next boxed word, and repeat the process.

(hyphen before word means it's a suffix, hyphen after word means prefix, no hyphen means root word.)

Word Part	Meaning	Word Part	Meaning
furca	branch	occlus	shut, close-up
-tion	condition of	-ion	action, condition
trans-	through, across	sub-	below
illumina	give light	mandibul	mandible jaw
vas/o	vessel	-ar	pertaining to
constrict	bind or tie tightly	bio-	life
-or	agent	degrad	break down
inter-	between, among	-able	capable of
dent	tooth	myo	muscle
-al	pertaining to	card	heart
peri-	around	-ium	small, tissue
o/dont	tooth	ortho-	straight
mal-	bad	-ist	specialist

charting procedures also use many acronyms and abbreviations.

Care must be taken when looking for or using acronyms or abbreviations to shorten words because many abbreviations are not universal. For example, the abbreviation *imp* in general dentistry charting may indicate an impression, but an oral surgeon's office may use *imp* to designate an impaction. Some dental facilities develop a specific code or method of designating conditions and procedures. When in doubt about the spelling or meaning of an abbreviation or an acronym, it is best to spell out the word or look it up in a dictionary, glossary, or office manual.

Here are some examples of abbreviations or acronyms that may be found in reference works:

- **ALARA:** as low as reasonably achievable
- **ANUG:** acute necrotic ulcerative gingivitis
- **CDA:** Certified Dental Assistant
- **CCD:** charge coupled device
- **CAT:** computer assisted tomography
- **CEREC:** ceramic reconstruction

CAUTION!

Homonyms are similar in sound and spelling, but they have different meanings. Common homonyms used in dentistry are:

Die: tooth or bridge pattern used in prosthodontic dentistry
Dye: coloring material; may be used to indicate plaque

Auxiliary: dental assistant
Axillary: armpit site for taking body temperature

Palpation: examination method using fingers
Palpitation: increased heartbeat

Suture: area where two bones join together
Suture: stitches for wound closure

- **DDS/DMD:** Doctor of Dental Surgery or Doctor of Dental Medicine
- **FFD:** film focus distance or focal film distance
- **HIPAA:** Health Insurance Portability and Accountability Act
- **HIV:** human immunodeficiency virus
- **HVE:** high volume evacuation
- **MPD:** maximum permissible dose
- **MRSA:** methicillin-resistant *Staphylococcus aureus*

Vocabulary Related to the Introduction to Dental Terminology *continued*

Key Terms

- ❏ -algia (**AL**-jee-ah)
- ❏ ante- (**AN**-tea)
- ❏ anti- (**AN**-tie)
- ❏ Bi- (**BYE**)
- ❏ dys- (**DIS**)
- ❏ -ectomy (**ECK**-toh-me)
- ❏ endo- (**EN**-doe)
- ❏ hyper- (**HIGH**-per)
- ❏ hypo- (**HIGH**-poh)
- ❏ infra- (**INN**-frah)
- ❏ intra- (**INN**-trah)
- ❏ -itis (**EYE**-tiss)
- ❏ -oid (**OYD**)
- ❏ -ologist (**AH**-logh-jist)
- ❏ -otomy (**AH**-toh-mee)
- ❏ peri- (**PEAR**-ee)
- ❏ -plasty (**PLAS**-tee)
- ❏ poly- (**PAHL**-ee)
- ❏ retro- (**REH**-troh)
- ❏ supra (**SOO**-prah)
- ❏ -trophy (**TROH**-fee)
- ❏ Acronyms
- ❏ Homonyms
- ❏ Eponyms
- ❏ Prefix
- ❏ combining form
- ❏ suffix
- ❏ root word
- ❏ syncope
- ❏ xerostomia

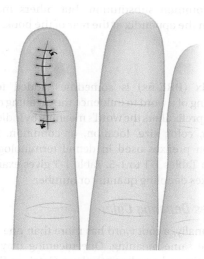

Wound Sutures

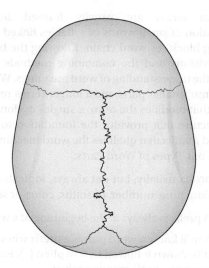

Skull Sutures

- **MSDS:** Material Safety Data Sheet
- **PID:** Position Indicating Device
- **PDR:** *Physician's Desk Reference*
- **PPE:** personal protection equipment
- **RDH:** Registered Dental Hygienist
- **ZOE:** zinc-oxide eugenol

Sometimes dental terminology denotes the person who developed the procedure, discovered the anatomical area, designed the instrument, named the disease, and the like. Examples are *Nasmyth membrane, Sharpey's fibers,* or *Bass Technique.* These terms are called **eponyms** (**EP**-oh-nims).

PRONOUNCE THE DENTAL WORD

After locating the word, it has to be pronounced. In this book, each dental term is broken into "sounds-like" syllables or elements that appear in parentheses. **BOLD** uppercase letters are used to indicate the syllables that are to receive the most emphasis when pronouncing the word. If the word has a secondary syllable or element of stress, it is printed in **bold** lowercase letters. All other elements are printed in the phonetic "sounds-like" manner.

To pronounce a word, say it just as it is spelled out within the parentheses. For example, in *periodontitis* (**pear**-ee-oh-don-**TIE**-tis), the syllable **TIE** receives the most emphasis, and secondary, or lesser, stress is also placed on the first syllable, **pear**. In *gingivitis* (**jin**-jih-**VIE**-tis), the main emphasis is placed on **VIE**, with secondary stress on the first syllable, **jin**.

Pronunciation rules are standard. Some vocal accents, however, show regional/geographic differences or differences related to the school where the words are learned.

ANALYZE THE STRUCTURE OF THE DENTAL WORD

Dental terminology involves the study of words and terms related specifically to the dental sciences. Every science has its own unique terminology. Rules and conventions are standardized for formation, pronunciation, pluralization, and meaning of terms.

In medical terminology, many words refer to the proximity or nearness to anatomical structures. Many dental terms originate from the names of bones or structures, but more often, from the names of dental procedures or practical approaches.

3

Dental terms are usually formed by a combination of small words or syllables linked in a "building block" or word chain. Knowing the basic small divisions and the combining methods can assist in the understanding of word meanings. When broken into smaller parts, most longer terms reveal a prefix that modifies the term, a single- or double-root structure that provides the foundation to the term, and a suffix that qualifies the word meaning.

The Four Types of Word Parts:

1. A **prefix** usually, but not always, indicates location, time, number, or status, color, or size.

    -   A prefix is always at the beginning of a word.

    -   You'll know a word part is a prefix when it is shown followed by a hyphen (-). For example, **anti-** means against.

    -   A word may or may not have a prefix.

2. A **root word** provides the basic meaning for the word. In medical and dental terminology, this word part usually, but not always, indicates the involved body part. For example, the root word meaning tooth is **dent** or **o/dont**.

3. A **combining form** is a root word with a combining vowel added. A dental term may have more than one root. When two roots are combined, a *combining vowel* (usually o) is used to connect them. When a combining form appears alone, it is shown with a backslash (/) between the root word and the combining vowel. For example, the combining form of root word dont is o/dont.

4. A **suffix** usually, but not always, indicates the procedure, condition, disorder, or disease.

    -   A suffix is always at the end of the word.

    -   You'll know a word part is a suffix when it is shown with a hyphen (-) preceding it. For example, the suffix -itis means inflammation.

A word may be easier to analyze by beginning with the suffix and working toward the beginning of the word. Many word structures have multiple meanings, either from the Greek, Latin, or French languages. The exercises in this book will use the more common substitution, but others may be found in the appendix at the rear of the book.

Prefix

A **prefix** (**PRE**-fix) is sometimes added to the beginning of a word to influence the meaning of that term. A prefix alters the word's meaning by indicating number, color, size, location, or condition. Some common prefixes used in dental terminology are listed in Tables 1-1 to 1-5. Table 1-1 gives examples of prefixes denoting quantity or number.

Prefixes Denoting Color

Occasionally, a root word has more than one prefix with the same meaning. One meaning may stem from Latin and another may be a Greek or French version. For example, *alba*, from the Latin word *albus*, refers to white, such as in *albumen* and *albino*. *Leuko* is a Greek prefix meaning white and is used in *leukoplakia* (a white, precancerous patch found inside the cheek). Although *leuko* may be more popular, both prefixes are correct. Table 1-2 includes other prefixes denoting color.

Prefixes Denoting Size or Degree

Some prefixes are used to qualify the size or degree of development of the root term. Table 1-3 gives examples.

Prefixes Denoting Location or Direction

Some prefixes are used to specify the location or the position of the root term and the involvement occurring, such as treatment occurring inside (*endo*) the tooth or treatment around (*peri*) the gingiva. Table 1-4 contains some examples of prefixes referring to location and/or position.

Prefixes Denoting Condition

Some prefixes are used to denote the condition of the root element. These prefixes may indicate that the condition is new (*neo*) or that the root term is not in effect, as in the word *infertile* (not fertile). Some examples denoting the condition of the root are presented in Table 1-5.

Table 1-1 Examples of Prefixes Denoting Quantity or Number

Prefix	Meaning	Example	Sounds Like
a- an-	without	*an*emia	(ah-**NEE**-me-ah)
bi-	two, double	*bi*furcation	(bye-fur-**KAY**-shun)
hemi-	half	*hemi*section	(**HEM**-ih-seck-shun)
cent-	hundred	*centi*meter	(**SEN**-tah-mee-ter)
deca(i)-	ten	*deci*bel	(**DESS**-ih-bull)
holo-	all	*holi*stic	(ho-**LIS**-tick)
mon/o-	one	*mon*omer	(**MON**-oh-mer)
poly-	many	*poly*merization	(pol-ah-mer-ah-**ZAY**-shun)
prim-/i	first	*pri*mary	(**PRY**-mary)
quad-/quat-	four	*quad*rant	(**KWAH**-drant)
semi-	half	*semi*luminal	(sem-**EE**-lum-in-al)
tri-	three	*tri*geminal	(try-**JEM**-in-al)
uni-	one	*uni*lateral	(you-nah-**LAT**-er-ol)

Table 1-2 Examples of Prefixes Denoting Color

Prefix	Color	Example	Sounds Like
albus-	white	*albu*men	(al-**BU**-men)
chlor-/o-	green	*chlor*ophyll	(**CHLOR**-oh-fill)
cyan-/o-	blue	*cyan*osis	(sigh-ah-**NO**-sis)
erythr-/o-	red	*erythr*ocyte	(eh-**RITH**-row-site)
leuk-/o-	white	*leuk*oplakia	(loo-koh-**PLAY**-key-ah)
melan-/o-	black	*melan*oma	(mel-ah-**NO**-ma)
xanth-/o-	yellow	*xanth*oma	(zan-**THO**-ma)

Root Word

The main section or division of a term that provides the foundation or basic meaning is a root word. A word may have one or more root sections. When a root section is combined or connected with other word elements, it may take on a combining vowel and become a **combining form**. The most common combining vowel is *o*. For example, the word *temporal* relates to the temporal bone in the skull, and the word *mandible* is the lower jaw bone. Independently, these are two separate words, but they can be combined to form the word *temporomandibular*, as in temporomandibular

5

Table 1-3 Examples of Prefixes Denoting Size or Degree

Prefix	Meaning	Example	Sounds Like
hyper-	over/excess	*hyper*trophy	(high-**PER**-troh-fee)
hypo-	under/below	*hypo*plasia	(high-poh-**PLAY**-zee-ah)
iso-	equal	*iso*graft	(**I**-so-graft)
macro-	large	*macro*dontia	(mack-row-**DON**-she-ah)
micro-	small/minute	*micro*be	(**MY**-crobe)
pan-	all around	*pan*oramic	(**PAN**-oh-ram-ic)
ultra-	extreme/beyond	*ultra*sonic	(**UL**-trah-son-ic)

Table 1-4 Examples of Prefixes Denoting Location or Direction

Prefix	Meaning	Example	Sounds Like
ab-	away from	*ab*sent	(**AB**-sent)
ad-	toward/near	*ad*jacent	(ad-**JAY**-cent)
ambi-	both sides	*ambi*dextrous	(am-bah-**DECK**-strous)
ana-	apart	*ana*lysis	(ah-**NAL**-ah-sis)
ante-	in front	*ante*rior	(an-**TIER**-ee-or)
de-	down from	*de*hydration	(de-high-**DRAY**-shun)
dexi-	right side	*dex*ter	(**DECKS**-ter)
dia-	complete	*dia*lysis	(die-**AL**-ah-sis)
ecto-	outside	*ecto*pic	(eck-**TOP**-ic)
endo-	within	*endo*dontic	(en-dough-**DON**-tic)
epi-	upon/over	*epi*dermis	(ep-ah-**DER**-mis)
ex/o-	out from	*ex*cretion	(eeks-**KREE**-shun)
in-	into/in	*in*cision	(in-**SIZH**-shun)
infra-	below	*infra*orbital	(in-frah-**OR**-bih-tal)
inter-	in midst of	*inter*dental	(in-ter-**DEN**-tal)
im-	into/position	*im*plant	(**IM**-plant)
mes-/o-	mid, among	*mesio*clusion	(me-zee-oh-**CLUE**-shun)
para-	near/beside	*par*enteral	(**PARE**-en-ter-al)
peri-/o-	around	*perio*dontal	(pear-ee-oh-**DON**-tal)

(*Continues*)

Table 1-4 (*Continued*)

Prefix	Meaning	Example	Sounds Like
post-	after/later	*post*erior	(pahs-**TEE**-ree-or)
pre-/ante-	before	*pre*molar	(pree-**MOL**-ar)
retro-	behind/back	*retro*molar	(rhet-tro-**MOLE**-ar)
sub-	under, lesser	*sub*dermal	(sub-**DER**-mal)
supra-	above/over	*supra*orbital	(sue-pra-**OR**-bih-tal)
syn-	together	*syn*ergism	(**SIN**-er-jizm)
trans-	through	*trans*plant	(**TRANS**-plant)

Table 1-5 Examples of Prefixes Denoting Condition

Prefix	Meaning	Example	Sounds Like
a-, an-	without	anodontia	(an-oh-**DON**-she-ah)
anti-	opposite to	antiseptic	(an-tih-**SEP**-tick)
brady-	slow	bradycardia	(bray-dee-**KAR**-dee-ah)
con-	with	connective	(con-**NECK**-tive)
contra-	against	contrangle	(**CON**-tra-ang-el)
dis-	take away	disinfectant	(dis-inn-**FECK**-tant)
in-	not	insoluble	(in-**SOL**-you-bull)
mal-	bad	malocclusion	(mal-oh-**CLUE**-zhun)
malaco-	soft	malacosis	(mal-ah-**KO**-sis)
neo-	new	neoplasm	(**NEE**-oh-plazm)
pachy-	thick	pachyderma	(pack-ah-**DERM**-ah)
sclero-	hard	scleroma	(sklay-**ROW**-ma)
tachy-	fast	tachycardia	(tack-ee-**KAR**-dee-ah)
un-	non/not	unerupted	(un-ee-**RUPT**-ed)

joint (TMJ). Note that the combining vowel *o* is inserted in place of the *al* in *temporal*.

As another example, two roots are combined to designate specific areas of teeth. In referring to the back chewing surface of a tooth, the root term for back or distant is *distal* and the term *occlusal* refers to chewing or occluding area. When combining these two roots with the combining vowel *o*, we have *distocclusal*, the back chewing surface.

Table 1-6 Common Dental Root/Combining Forms

Root Word	Sounds Like	Combo Form	Pertains To
alveolar	(al-**VEE**-oh-lar)	alveo	alveolus
apical	(**AY**-pih-kahl)	apic-/o-	apex of a root
axis	(**ACK**-sis)	ax-/o-	axis/midline
buccal	(**BUCK**-ahl)	bucc-/o-	cheek
cheilo	(key-**LOH**)	cheil-/o-	lip
coronal	(kor-**OH**-nal)	coron-/o-	crown
dens	(denz)	dent-/o-	tooth
distal	(**DIS**-tal)	dist-/o-	farthest from center
enamel	(ee-**NAM**-el)	ename-/o- or amel-/o-	tooth, enamel tissue
fluoride	(**FLOOR**-eyed)	fluor-/o-	chemical, fluoride
frenum	(**FREE**-num)	frene-	frenum
front	(front)	front-/o-	forehead
gingiva	(**JIN**-jih-vah)	gingiv-/o-	gingiva, gum tissue
glossa	(**GLOSS**-ah)	gloss-/o- or gloss/a	tongue
gnatho	(nah-**TH**-oh)	gnath-/o-	jaw, cheek
incisor	(in-**SIGH**-zore)	incis-/o-	incisor tooth
labia	(**LAY**-bee-ah)	labi-/o-	lip area
lingua	(**LING**-wa)	lingu-/o-	tongue
mandible	(**MAN**-dih-bull)	mandibu-/a-	lower jaw
maxilla	(**MACK**-sih-lah)	maxilla-/o-	upper jaw
mesial	(**ME**-zee-al)	mesi-/o-	middle, midplane
mucosa	(myou-**KOH**-sah)	muc-/o-	tissue lining an orifice
occlude	(oh-**KLUDE**)	occlus-/o-	occluding, jaw close
odont	(oh-**DONT**)	odont-/o-	tooth
orthos	(**OR**-thohs)	orth-/o-	straight, proper order
stoma	(**STOW**-mah)	stoma-	mouth
temporal	(**TEM**-pore-al)	tempor-/o-	temporal bone

Other examples of terms with two roots are thermometer, cementoenamel junction, and radiograph. Table 1-6 gives examples of common root words and combining forms used in dental terminology. More examples of root words are provided in the appendix.

Suffix

An element added to the end of a root word or combining form to describe or qualify the word meaning is a **suffix** (**SUF**-icks). A suffix cannot stand alone and is usually united with a root element by inserting a combining vowel (*o*) unless the suffix begins with a vowel. In that case, the combining form or vowel is dropped. For example, the surgical removal of gum tissue is the meaning of *gingivectomy* from the root word *gingivo* (gum) and suffix *ectomy* (surgical excision). Dropping the ending vowel in *gingivo* and adding *ectomy* to make *gingivectomy* unite these two word elements. Suffixes have the ability to transform a noun or verb into an adjective, or verbs into nouns, by the addition of a word ending. Suffixes can also indicate time and size, condition, agents, or specialists. Some examples of common suffixes used in dental terminology are given in Tables 1-7 to 1-10. A more complete listing of common suffixes is contained in the appendix.

Suffixes Meaning "Pertaining to"

An adjective is a word that defines or describes. In dental terminology, many suffixes meaning "pertaining to" are used to change the meaning of a root word into an adjective. For example, the root word **gingiv** means tissue surrounding the teeth (gums), and the suffix -al means pertaining to. When these word elements are combined, they form the term *gingival*, an adjective that means pertaining to the gingiva tissue. Commonly used suffixes that mean *pertaining to* are show in Table 1-7.

Suffixes Meaning "Abnormal Condition or Disease"

A suffix added to a root may indicate the condition of the root word. It may denote that disease (*pathy*) or inflammation (*itis*) is occurring, or it may indicate that the condition exists (*tion*). Table 1-8 gives examples of suffixes that mean *condition*.

Suffixes Denoting Agent or Specialist

Some suffixes are added to the root element to indicate an agent involving an action, or a person concerned with or trained in that specialty. The suffixes in Table 1-9 are some of the more familiar ones, and many more are used to indicate specialization.

Table 1-7 Suffixes Meaning "Pertaining to"

• -a	• -al	• -ary
• -ial	• -ical	• -ior
• -tic	• -an	• -eal
• -ac	• -ic	• -ory
• -ile	• -ar	• -ia
• -um	• -ine	• -ous

Table 1-8 Suffixes Indicating Condition

• -ant	• -ion	• -oma
• -cle	• -ism	• -pathy
• -ule	• -itis	• -sion
• -ia	• -ity	• -tic
• -ible, ile	• -ium	• -tion
• -id	• -olus	• -y

Table 1-9 Suffixes Denoting Agent or Person Concerned

Suffix	Agent or Person
-ee	train*ee*, employ*ee*, leas*ee*
-ent	pati*ent*, recipi*ent*, resid*ent*
-eon	surg*eon*
-er	subscrib*er*, examin*er*, practition*er*
-ician	phys*ician*
-ist	dent*ist*, orthodont*ist*
-or	doct*or*, don*or*

Suffixes Related to Pathology and Procedures

Some suffixes are added to root elements to show processes, uses, or healing. When analyzing a long dental word, starting at the suffix may indicate something happening to the root word element, such as *ectomy* (surgical removal) or *trophy* (development). Other suffixes are added to indicate pain (*algia*) or bleeding (*rrhage*) and so on. Table 1-10 gives some examples.

DEFINE THE MEANING OF THE DENTAL WORD

After providing the word and its pronunciation, this text gives the meaning of the word, including

Table 1-10 Suffixes Expressing Medical Terms, Processes, Uses

Suffix	Meaning	Sample Words
-algia	pain	odont*algia*, neurol*algia*, my*algia*
-ate, -ize	use/action	vaccin*ate*, lux*ate*, palp*ate*, visual*ize*
-cide	kill	germi*cide*, homi*cide*
-cyte	cell	leuko*cyte*, osteo*cyte*
-ectomy	surgical removal	apico*ectomy*, append*ectomy*
-gnosis	knowledge	pro*gnosis*, dia*gnosis*
-ology	study of	hist*ology*, bi*ology*
-oma	tumor	carcin*oma*
-opsy	view	bi*opsy*, aut*opsy*
-phobia	dread fear	claustro*phobia*
-plasty	surgical repair	gingivo*plasty*
-plegia	paralysis	para*plegia*
-rrhea	discharge	hemmo*rrhea*, sialo*rrhea*
-scope	instrument	micro*scope* (micro), laryngo*scope* (larynx)
-tomy	incision	myo*tomy* (muscle)
-trophy	development	osteo*trophy* (bone development)

the definition and any relevant feature that occurs within or about the word. For example:

syncope (**SIN**-koh-pee): a temporary loss of consciousness resulting from an inadequate supply of blood to the brain; also known as swooning or fainting.

xerostomia (**zeer**-oh-**STOH**-me-ah; xeros = *dry*, stoma = *mouth*): dryness of the mouth caused by the lack of normal saliva secretion.

In the first example, synonyms (e.g., fainting) are provided for *syncope*. The second example contains information about the derivation of the word *xerostomia; xeros* is Greek for dry, and *stoma* is the word for mouth.

PLURALIZE THE DENTAL WORD

As the majority of dental terminology originates from Latin and Greek, the rules for changing terms

from singular to plural are predetermined by the conventions of those languages. The first step is to learn the basic rules for changing word endings, bearing in mind that a few terms will not conform to the rules given in Table 1-11. Look up terms in a dictionary or reference book to verify spelling on any terms in question.

USE THE DENTAL WORD

Read, pronounce, and determine the structure of the term. Breaking down the word parts and learning the meaning of the word parts will help determine if your structure analysis was correct and will reinforce word meanings. Strengthen your knowledge of the dental term when incorporating the dental term into a sentence or statement.

Table 1-11 Guideline for Plural Forms

Word Endings	Change To	Singular	Plural
a	*ae* (add *e* to end)	gingiva	gingivae
ex, ix	*ices* (drop *x*, add *ices*)	apex	apices
itis	*ides* (drop *s*, add *des*)	pulpitis	pulpitides
sis	*sis* (change *is* to *ses*)	cementosis	cementoses
nx	*nges* (change *nx* to *nges*)	larynx	larynges
on	*a* (change *on* to *a*)	ganglion	ganglia
oma	*omas* (add *s* to the end)	dentinoma	dentinomas
um	*a* (change *um* to *a*)	frenum	frena
us	*i* (change *us* to *i*)	sulcus	sulci
y	*ies* (drop *y*, add *ies*)	biopsy	biopsies

Test Your Knowledge

Complete the following practices to enforce your understanding of Chapter 1. The answers to the practice challenges can be found in the back of this textbook.

Practice 1

Underline the prefixes used in the following words and specify what number or amount each represents:

1. **anaerobic** _____oxygen/s
2. **hemisphere** _____sphere/s
3. **quaternary** _____element/s
4. **primordal** _____form/s
5. **anesthesia** _____feeling/s
6. **monocular** _____eyepiece/s
7. **anemia** _____hemoglobin/s
8. **bicuspid** _____cusp/s
9. **tripod** _____foot/feet
10. **polypnea** _____breath/s
11. **unilateral** _____side/s
12. **trifurcation** _____division/s
13. **semicoma** _____coma/s
14. **decimeter** _____meter/s
15. **monocell** _____cell/s

Practice 2

Match each prefix in Column A with the color it represents in Column B. (An answer in Column B may be used more than once.)

Column A		Column B	
1.	_____melan-/o-	**A.**	white
2.	_____cyan-/o-	**B.**	yellow
3.	_____chlor-/o-	**C.**	violet
4.	_____erythr-/o-	**D.**	blue
5.	_____leuk-/o-	**E.**	black
6.	_____alba-	**F.**	red
7.	_____xanth-/o-	**G.**	green

Practice 3

Give the meaning of the prefix underlined in the following words:

1. **macroglossia** = _____tongue
2. **isocoria** = _____pupil size
3. **hyperglycemia** = _____blood sugar
4. **hypocementosis** = _____cementum
5. **micrognathia** = _____jaw
6. **panoramic** = _____view
7. **ultrasonic** = _____sounds

Practice 4

Using the prefix list given, choose the prefix that best describes the meaning of the term:

ab-, ad-, ambi-, ana-, de-, dexi-, dia-, ecto-, endo-, ex-, in-, mes-, peri-, post-, pre-, retro-, sub-, supra-, syn-, trans-

1. **around** = _____
2. **outside** = _____
3. **behind** = _____
4. **under** = _____
5. **toward** = _____
6. **mid/among** = _____
7. **apart** = _____
8. **through** = _____
9. **together** = _____
10. **down** from = _____
11. **right** = _____
12. **after** = _____
13. **before** = _____
14. **both** sides = _____
15. **into** = _____
16. **away** from = _____
17. **out** from = _____
18. **within** = _____
19. **above** = _____
20. **complete** = _____

Practice 5

Match the prefix in Column A to the term it best describes in Column B:

Column A	Column B
1. neo-_____	A. soft
2. pachy-_____	B. bad
3. con-_____	C. without
4. sclero-_____	D. against
5. dis-_____	E. hard
6. a- or an-_____	F. fast
7. mal-_____	G. opposite to
8. anti-_____	H. not/non
9. un- or in-_____	I. new
10. tacky-_____	J. removal
11. contra-_____	K. with
12. malaco-_____	L. slow
13. brady-_____	M. thick

Practice 6

Place a root element for the given words in the blanks provided.

1. gum tissue _____
2. lip area _____
3. root apex _____
4. tongue _____
5. upper jaw _____
6. mouth opening _____
7. middle _____
8. orifice tissue lining_____
9. far from center _____
10. crown area _____

Practice 7

Underline the suffix indicating relationship in each given word, and write it in the blank next to the word.

1. filliform _____
2. chronic _____
3. kilogram _____
4. condyloid _____
5. endosteal _____
6. posterior _____
7. vascular _____
8. squamous _____
9. apical _____
10. cardiac _____
11. xenograph _____
12. intraligamentary _____

Practice 8

Insert the correct suffix to complete the root element.

1. condition of being acid = acid_____
2. surgical cut = inci_____
3. term for a germ = bacter_____
4. fatty tumor = lip_____
5. act of chewing = mastica_____
6. dead tissue = necro_____
7. muscle damage disease = myo_____
8. small bit of matter = a mole_____
9. tooth grinding = brux_____
10. air sac = alve_____

Practice 9

List six agents and/or persons concerned with a specialty area, and underline the suffix denoting their position.

1. _____
2. _____
3. _____
4. _____
5. _____
6. _____

Practice 10

Examine the boldfaced words in each sentence, and circle the suffix denoting a medical procedure, use, or condition of the root element. Then write the meaning of the word in the space below.

1. A **gingivoplasty** may be the correct treatment for an infected third molar area.

2. The patient's health history included drugs for her **fibromyalgia** condition.

3. The assistant prepares the **germicide** according to the manufacturer's instructions.

4. A **stethoscope** is used to determine blood flow sounds in a blood pressure examination.

5. Tissue **hemorrhea** may be an indicator of a serious blood disease.

6. The dentist will **cauterize** the patient's gingiva during the surgical procedure.

7. Jimmy will need a **frenectomy** before the central incisors can be moved into the area.

8. The patient was referred to an oral surgeon for the **apicoectomy**.

9. To avoid bone and tooth damage, the dentist will **rotate** the tooth before removal.

10. Some patients claim to suffer **claustrophobia** when visiting the dental office.

11. A complete dental exam includes inspection for oral **carcinoma** symptoms.

12. The patient was anxious to hear a good **prognosis** from the dentist.

13. The assistant prepared the **biopsy** slide for shipment to the laboratory.

14. An infection could be the cause of an elevated **leukocyte** count.

15. **Histology** is the study of microscopic structure of tissue.

Practice 11

Provide the plural form for each singular word listed here:

Singular	Plural
1. matrix	
2. mamelon	
3. frenum	
4. radius	
5. sulcus	
6. iris	
7. axillary	
8. diagnosis	
9. gingiva	
10. stoma	

Review Exercises

Complete the following Review Exercises to strengthen your knowledge of the dental terms introduced in this chapter.

Matching

Match the following word elements with their meanings:

1. _____ poly-   **A.** tongue
2. _____ supra-   **B.** from, away from
3. _____ peri-   **C.** many
4. _____ -trophy   **D.** mouth
5. _____ mesial   **E.** black
6. _____ ab-   **F.** tumor
7. _____ -oma   **G.** gum tissue
8. _____ melano-   **H.** middle, midplane
9. _____ retro-   **I.** around or about
10. _____ mini-   **J.** inflammation
11. _____ mal-   **K.** development, growth
12. _____ -itis   **L.** evil, sickness, disorder, poor
13. _____ pathy-   **M.** cutting into, incision into
14. _____ dens   **N.** backward
15. _____ -otomy   **O.** fear
16. _____ glossa   **P.** above
17. _____ stoma   **Q.** small
18. _____ neo-   **R.** disease
19. _____ gingiva   **S.** tooth
20. _____ phobia   **T.** new

Multiple Choice

Using the selection given for each sentence, choose the best term to complete the definition.

1. The root/combining word for lip is _____.
   a. labia
   b. glossa
   c. frenum
   d. buccal

2. Which suffix means pain or ache?
   a. -soma
   b. -oma
   c. -ous
   d. -algia

3. Which prefix means toward or increase?
   a. an-
   b. ad-
   c. ab-
   d. in-

4. The abbreviated form for high volume evacuation is:
   a. HIV
   b. HVE
   c. HEE
   d. HCC

5. Which prefix means together?
   a. con-
   b. bi-
   c. syn-
   d. retro-

6. The root or combining word for lower jaw is:
   a. maxilla
   b. mesial
   c. mandible
   d. megial

7. Which suffix means tissue death, decay?
   a. -plasty
   b. -pathogy
   c. -ectomy
   d. -necrosis

8. The combining form for straight or for proper order is:
   a. occlus/o
   b. anti/e
   c. oppos/o
   d. orth/o

9. Which suffix means graph or picture (especially in radiology)?
   a. -grate
   b. -photo
   c. -gram
   d. -trophy

10. Which prefixes determine the number to be two?
    a. bi- and semi-
    b. bi- and uni-
    c. tri- and bi-
    d. bi- and pan-

11. Which combining form means apex of the root?
    a. apix/o
    b. apic/o
    c. axi/o
    d. axium

12. A pattern used in prosthodontic dentistry is:
    a. dia-
    b. dye
    c. dys-
    d. die

13. What is the plural form of frenum?
    a. frenix
    b. freni
    c. frena
    d. frenia

14. Which prefix means less than, below, or under?
    a. hypo-
    b. hyper-
    c. trans-
    d. hydro-

15. Which suffix designates a specialist in a particular study?
    a. -ology
    b. -ier
    c. -ologist
    d. -teur

Building Skills

Locate and define the prefix, root/combining form, and suffix (if present) in the following words.

1. **bifurcation** (**bye**-fer-**KAY**-shun): branching into two parts.
   prefix _____ means:
   root or combining form _____ means:
   suffix _____ means:

2. **transillumination** (trans-ill-**lum**-mih-**NAY**-shun): passage of light through an object.
   prefix _____ means:
   root or combining form _____ means:
   suffix _____ means:

3. **vasoconstrictor** (vas-oh-kahn-**STRIK**-tore): chemical used to constrict blood vessels.
   prefix _____ means:
   root or combining form _____ means:
   suffix _____ means:

4. **interdental** (in-ter-**DENT**-al): between two teeth.
   prefix _____ means:
   root or combining form _____ means:
   suffix _____ means:

5. **periodontitis** (**pear**-ee-oh-don-**TIE**-tis): inflammation/degeneration of dental periosteum.
   prefix _____ means:
   root or combining form _____ means:
   suffix _____ means:

6. **malocclusion** (**mal**-oh-**KLOO**-shun): imperfect occlusion of the teeth, improper closure.
   prefix _____ means:
   root or combining form _____ means:
   suffix _____ means:

7. **submandibular** (sub-man-**DIB**-you-lar): beneath the lower jaw or mandible.
   prefix _____ means:
   root or combining form _____ means:
   suffix _____ means:

8. **biodegradable** (**bye**-oh-dee-**GRADE**-ah-bull): metabolic breakdown of protein matter.
    prefix _____ means:
    root or combining form _____ means:
    suffix _____ means:

9. **myocardium** (my-oh-**KAR**-dee-um): middle cardiac muscular layer.
    prefix _____ means:
    root or combining form _____ means:
    suffix _____ means:

10. **orthodontist** (**or**-thoh-**DON**-tist): a specialist dealing with tooth arrangement.
    prefix _____ means:
    root or combining form _____ means:
    suffix _____ means:

Plurals

Use the blank space to write in the plural form of each given word.

1. **ala** _____
2. **apex** _____
3. **calculus** _____
4. **diagnosis** _____
5. **larynx** _____
6. **dens** _____
7. **bacterium** _____
8. **carcinoma** _____
9. **bacillus** _____
10. **labium** _____
11. **therapy** _____
12. **focus** _____
13. **fossa** _____
14. **enema** _____
15. **appendix** _____

Word Use

Read the following sentences and define the word written in boldfaced letters.

1. The dentist suggested topical **anesthesia** for the treatment.
   _____
   _____

2. The hygienist explained that a **gingivectomy** is a common treatment for necrotic gingival tissue.
   _____
   _____

3. The dentist wrote a prescription for therapeutic vitamin B complex medicine for the patient suffering from **cheilosis**.
   _____
   _____

4. A calcium deposit in the **sublingual** salivary duct caused a large and uncomfortable swelling in the mouth.
   _____
   _____

5. An incorrect bite can be one of the causes of a **temporomandibular** joint disorder.
   _____
   _____

6. The assistant attached the **biopsy** report to the patient's records.
   _____
   _____

7. The dentist pointed out the patient's abscess on the enlarged digital **radiograph**.
   _____
   _____

8. During the dental examination, the patient is screened for the presence of an oral **carcinoma**.
   _____
   _____

9. Sometimes a **posterior** dental X-ray may be difficult to place in a small mouth.
   _____
   _____

10. All maxillary molars exhibited a **trifurcation** of the root, while mandibular molars showed a bifurcation.
    _____
    _____

Please note that the answers to this chapter's exercise may be found in Appendix B.

CHAPTER 2 | ANATOMY AND ORAL STRUCTURES

✓ Learning Objectives

On completion of this chapter, you should be able to:

1. Name and identify the major bones of the face and skull.

2. Locate the sinus cavities, sutures, processes, and foramina of the skull.

3. Locate the major structural points of the mandible, and explain their functions or purposes.

4. Identify the names and locations of the major muscles of mastication, and explain the function of each.

5. Describe the principal branches of the trigeminal nerve, and explain the functions of each division.

6. Locate and identify the major blood vessels to and from the cranium.

7. Describe the placement and functions of the major salivary glands.

8. Discuss the tissue bodies present in the cranium and their function in fighting infection and assisting with immunity.

9. Locate and explain features in the oral cavity, such as the labia, frena, tongue, and palate structures and miscellaneous tissues.

Vocabulary Related to Anatomy and Oral Structures

This list contains selected new and important word parts and terms from this chapter. Take the time to learn these word parts and their meanings. You may use the list to review these terms and practice pronouncing them correctly. When you work with the audio for this chapter, listen to the word, repeat it, and then place a checkmark in the box. Proceed to the next boxed word, and repeat the process.

(hyphen before word means it's a suffix, hyphen after word means prefix, no hyphen means root word.)

Word Parts	Meaning	Word Parts	Meaning
infra-	under, below	palat	hard palate in mouth
orbit	eye area	-ine	pertaining to
-al	pertaining to	sub-	under
peri-	around	mandibul	mandible jaw
oste	bone	-ar	pertaining to
-um	pertaining to	tempor/o	temporal bone
gloss/o	tongue	pariet	parietal bone

Key Terms

- ❏ **abducens (UHB**-doo-snz)
- ❏ **adenoid (A**-duh-noyd)
- ❏ **alveolar (al-VEE**-oh-lar)
- ❏ **alveolus (al-VEE**-oh-lus)
- ❏ **ankyloglossia** (ang-key-loh-**GLOSS**-ee-ah)
- ❏ **anopia (an-OH**-pee-ah)
- ❏ **anosmia (an-OZ**-mee-ah)
- ❏ **antibody (AN**-tie-bah-dee)
- ❏ **antigens (AN**-tih-jens)
- ❏ **articular eminence (ar-TICK-**you-lar **EM**-ih-nense)
- ❏ **Bell's palsy (PAUL**-zee)
- ❏ **buccinator (BUCK**-sin-ay-tor)
- ❏ **capillaries (KAP**-ih-lair-eez)
- ❏ **carotid (care-OT**-id)
- ❏ **cervical (SIR**-vih-kul)
- ❏ **circumvallate** (sir-kum-**VAL**-ate)
- ❏ **commissure (KOM**-ih-shur)
- ❏ **conchae (KONG**-kee) (pl. of concha)
- ❏ **condyle (KON**-dial)
- ❏ **condyloid (KON**-dih-loyd)

Vocabulary Related to The Introduction to Dental Terminology *continued*

Key Terms *continued*

- coronal (kor-**OH**-nal)
- coronoid (**KOR**-oh-noid)
- cranium (**KRAY**-nee-um)
- deglutition (dee-glue-**TISH**-un)
- diplopia (die-**PLOH**-pee-ah)
- ethmoid (**ETH**-moyd)
- expectorate (ex-**PECK**-tuh-rate)
- fauces (**FOH**-sez)
- filiform (**FIL**-ih-form)
- foliate (**FOH**-lee-ate)
- foramen (foh-**RAY**-men)
- frenum (**FREE**-num)
- frontal (**FRON**-tal)
- fungiform (**FUN**-jih-form)
- ganglion (**GANG**-lee-un)
- glenoid fossa (**GLEE**-noyd **FAH**-sah)
- glossa (**GLOSS**-ah)
- glossopalatine (gloss-oh-**PAL**-ah-tine)
- glossopharyngeal (gloss-oh-fair-an-**JEE**-al)
- hyoid (**HIGH**-oyd)
- hypoglossal (high-poh-**GLOSS**-al)
- immunoglobulin (im-you-no-**GLOB**-you-lin)
- incisive (in-**SIGH**-siv)
- incus (**IN**-kus)
- infraorbital (**IN**-frah-**OR**-bih-tal)
- interferon (in-ter-**FEAR**-on)
- jugular (**JUG**-you-lar)
- lacrimal (**LACK**-rih-mal)
- lambdoid (**LAM**-doyd)
- lymph (**LIMF**)
- lymphocytes (**LIM**-foe-sites)
- malleus (**MAL**-ee-us)
- mandible (**MAN**-dih-bull)
- masseter (mass-**EE**-ter)
- mastoid (**MASS**-toyd)
- maxillary (**MACK**-sih-lair-e)
- meatus (mee-**AY**-tus)
- meniscus (men-**IS**-kus)
- mentalis (men-**TAL**-is)
- mucin (**MYOU**-sin)
- mucoperiosteum (**myou**-koh-pear-ee-**AHS**-tee-um)
- mucosa (**MU**-co-sah)
- mylohyoid (my-loh-**HIGH**-oyd)
- nasal (**NAY**-zel)
- nasion (**NAY**-zhun)
- nasociallary (**nay**-zoh-**SIL**-ee-air-e)
- nasopalatine (**nay**-zoh-**PAL**-ah-tine)
- occipital (ock-**SIP**-ih-tal)
- oculomotor (ock-you-low-**MOE**-tor)
- olfactory (ol-**FACK**-toh-ree)
- ophthalmic (off-**THAL**-mick)
- orbicularis oris (or-**bick**-you-**LAIR**-iss **OR**-iss)
- palatine (**PAL**-ah-tine)
- papillae (pah-**PIH**-lie) (pl. of papilla)
- parietal (pah-**RYE**-eh-tal)
- parotid (pah-**ROT**-id)
- periosteum (pdh-ree-**OW**-stee-uhm)
- phagocytes (**FAG**-oh-sites)
- pharyngopalatine (fare-in-goh-**PAL**-ah-tine)
- philtrum (**FIL**-trum)
- posterior (pahs-**TEE**-ree-or)
- protuberance (proh-**TOO**-ber-an)
- pterygoid (**TER**-eh-goyd)
- ptosis (**TOE**-sis)
- ramus (**RAY**-mus)
- raphe (**RAH**-fay)
- retromolar (ret-trow-**MOLE**-a)
- rugae (**RUE**-guy)
- sagittal (**SAJ**-ih-tal)
- sigmoid (**SIG**-moyd)
- sphenoid (**SFEE**-noyd)
- sphenopalatine (sfee-no-**PAL**-ah-tine)
- squamous (**SKWAY**-mus)
- stapes (**STAY**-peez)
- strabismus (strah-**BIZ**-muss)
- styloid (**STY**-loyd)
- sulcus (**SULL**-kus)
- symphysis (**SIM**-fih-sis)
- synovial (sin-**OH**-vee-al)
- temporal (**TEM**-pore-al)
- temporomandibur (tem-poe-roe-man-**DIB**-you-lar)
- temporoparietal (tem-poe-roe-pah-**RYE**-eh-tal)
- tinnitus (tin-**EYE**-tuss)
- tonsil (**TAHN**-sill)
- trachlear (**TRAH**-klee-ur)
- trigeminal (try-**JEM**-in-al)
- umami (oo-**MAH**-me)
- uvula (**YOU**-view-lah)
- vagus (**VAY**-gus)
- vermillion border (ver-**MILL**-yon **BORE**-der)
- vertigo (**VER**-tih-go)
- vestibule (**VES**-tih-byul)
- vestibulocochlear (ves-**tib**-you-low-**COCK**-lee-ar)
- vomer (**VOH**-mer)
- zygomatic (zye-goh-**MAT**-ic)
- zygomaticofacial (zye-goh-**MAT**-ee-coe-fay-shal)

ANATOMY OF THE SKULL

Medical terminology deals with the entire body and all its systems. The terminology of dentistry is related mostly to the head region. The skull area is composed of two main bone divisions: the cranium and the facial section.

Cranium

The **cranium** (**KRAY**-nee-um) is the portion of the skull that encloses the brain. Eight bones make up this section of the skull (Figure 2-1):

- **temporal** (**TEM**-pore-al): two fan-shaped bones, one on each side of the skull, in the temporal area above each ear.

Figure 2-1 Cranial bones

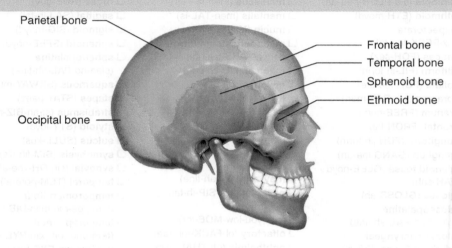

Parietal bone
Frontal bone
Temporal bone
Sphenoid bone
Ethmoid bone
Occipital bone

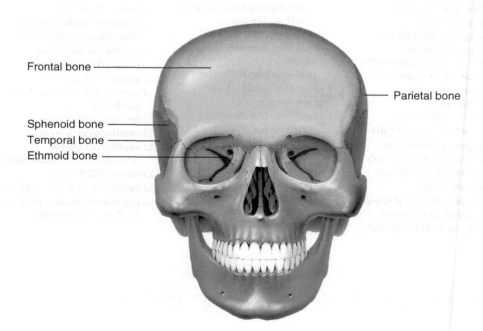

Frontal bone
Parietal bone
Sphenoid bone
Temporal bone
Ethmoid bone

- **parietal** (pah-**RYE**-eh-tal): two bones, one on each side, that make up the roof and side walls covering the brain.
- **frontal** (**FRON**-tal): a single bone in the frontal or anterior region that makes up the forehead.
- **occipital** (ock-**SIP**-ih-tahl): one large, thick bone in the lower back of the head that forms the base of the skull and contains a large opening for the spinal cord passage to the brain.
- **ethmoid** (**ETH**-moyd): a spongy bone located between the eye orbits that helps form the roof and part of the anterior nasal fossa of the skull.
- **sphenoid** (**SFEE**-noyd): a large bat-shaped bone at the base of the skull between the occipital and ethmoid in front, and the parietal and temporal bones at each side.

Facial Bones

Fourteen bones make up the facial division of the cranium (see Figure 2-2). All are paired with one on each side, except there is only one vomer in the nose and one mandible extending from right to left. The facial bones are:

- **zygomatic** (zye-goh-**MAT**-ick): two facial bones, one under each eye, that form the cheekbone and give character to the face. The zygomatic bones are also called the **malar** (**MAY**-lar) bones.
- **maxilla** (**MACK**-sih-lah): two large facial bones, one under each eye, that unite in the center in the *median suture* to form the upper jaw that supports the maxillary teeth in the *alveolar process*. Also present in this bone is the *maxillary sinus* (Atrium of Highmore) and the *infraorbital frenum* under each eye that permits the passage of nerves.
- **palatine** (**PAL**-ah-tine): two bones, one left and one right, that unite at the *median palatine suture* to form the hard palate of the mouth and the nasal floor. Present in this bone are multiple foramina, the largest, the *incisive foramen,* is directly behind the central incisors.

Figure 2-2 Facial bones

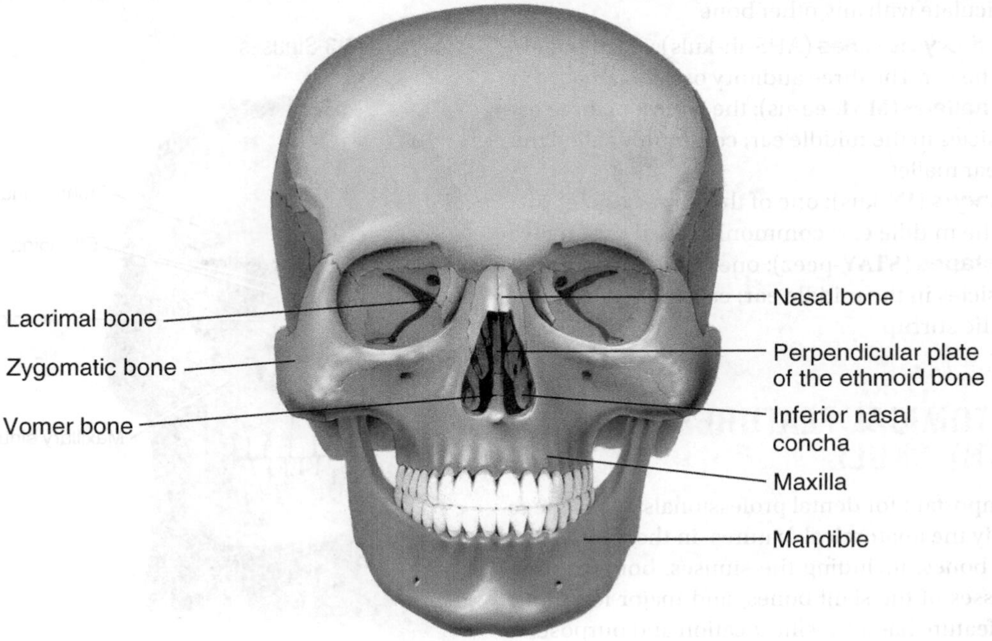

Lacrimal bone

Zygomatic bone

Vomer bone

Nasal bone

Perpendicular plate of the ethmoid bone

Inferior nasal concha

Maxilla

Mandible

- **nasal** (**NAY**-zal): two bones, one left and one right, that join side by side to form the arch or bridge of the nose.
- **lacrimal** (**LACK**-rih-mal): two small bones, one each on the inner side or nose site of the orbital cavity, that make up the corner of the eye where the *tear ducts* are located.
- **inferior concha** (**KONG**-kah in singular use or (conchae) **KONG**-kee in plural use): two thin scroll-like bones that form the lower part of the interior of the nasal cavity.
- **mandible** (**MAN**-dih-bull): the strong, horseshoe-shaped bone that forms the lower jaw (described in further detail later in this chapter).
- **vomer** (**VOH**-mer): a single bone that forms the lower posterior part of the nasal septum and separates the nose into two chambers.

Miscellaneous Bones of the Skull

There are several bones that are not considered bones of the face or cranium, but they are present in the head or skull. These bones include:

- **hyoid** (**HIGH**-oyd): a horseshoe-shaped bone lying at the base of the tongue. It does not articulate with any other bone.
- **auditory ossicles** (AHS-ih-kuls): small bones in the ear. The three auditory ossicles are:
  - **malleus** (**MAL**-ee-us): the largest of three ossicles in the middle ear; commonly called the ear mallet.
  - **incus** (**IN**-kus): one of the three ossicles of the middle ear; commonly called the anvil.
  - **stapes** (**STAY**-peez): one of the three ossicles in the middle ear; commonly called the stirrup.

ANATOMICAL FEATURES OF THE SKULL

It is important for dental professionals to be able to identify the anatomical features in the cranial and facial bones, including the sinuses, bone sutures, processes of the skull bones, and major foramina. Each feature has a specific location and purpose.

Sinus

A **sinus** (**SIGH**-nus) is an air pocket or cavity in a bone that lightens the bone, warms the air intake, and helps form sounds. These sinus cavities are named after the bone they are occupying (Figure 2-3). The **accessory paranasal sinuses** that empty into the nasal cavity are:

- **frontal:** larger accessory sinus, located in the frontal bone or the forehead above each eye.
- **ethmoid:** multiple, smaller sinuses located in the ethmoid bone, at the side of each eye.
- **sphenoid:** multiple, small sinuses located in the sphenoid bone situated behind the eyes.
- **maxillary:** located in the maxilla; the maxillary sinus is the largest and is called the **Atrium** (**A**-tree-um) **of Highmore**; this cavity is easily seen and is used as a landmark for identifying radiographs in the mounting of films.

Sutures of the Skull

A **suture** (**SOO**-chur) is a line where two or more bones unite in an immovable joint. Several main sutures are located in the cranium (Figure 2-4):

Figure 2-3 Sinuses

Frontal sinus

Ethmoidal sinuses

Sphenoidal sinus

Maxillary sinus

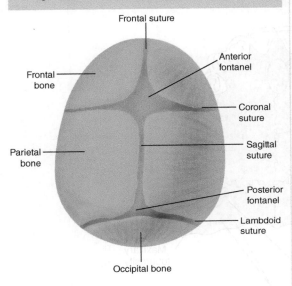

Figure 2-4 Sutures of the skull

Frontal suture

Anterior fontanel

Frontal bone

Coronal suture

Parietal bone

Sagittal suture

Posterior fontanel

Lambdoid suture

Occipital bone

- **coronal** (kor-**OH**-nal): junction of the frontal and the parietal bones; this area is soft at birth and shortly afterward, and it has been called the baby's "soft spot" or **fontanel** (**fon**-tah-**NELL** = *little fountain*), sometimes spelled *fontanelle*.
- **sagittal** (**SAJ**-ih-tahl): the union line between the two parietal bones on the top of the skull.
- **lambdoid** (**LAM**-doyd): located between the parietal bone and the upper border of the occipital bone.
- **temporoparietal** (**tem**-poe-roe-pah-**RYE**-eh-tal): located between the temporal and parietal bones; also known as the **squamous** (**SKWAY**-mus) suture (not visible in Figure 2-4).

Bone Structures of the Hard Palate

Oral cavity sutures indicate an area where bones are joined together. The hard palate is composed of four main processes united by two palatine sutures, the *median* and the *transverse palatine sutures*. The left and right palatine processes and the left and right processes of the maxilla meet at the median palatine suture. All four edges of the processes combine at the transverse palatine suture, completing the hard palate. Five foramina

are present in this hard palate bone. The largest, the *incisive foramen*, is situated behind the incisors; a *greater* and a *lesser palatine foramina* are present on each side in the rear (Figure 2-5).

Processes of the Cranium

A **process** (**PROS**-es) is a projection or outgrowth of bone or tissue. This bone projection is not to be confused with the fusion line where two bones develop into one, such as the mandible. The **symphysis** (**SIM**-fih-sis) is in the center of the mandible, forms the chin, and is called the **mental** or chin **protuberance** (pro-**TOO**-ber-ans = *projection*). The skull has eight main processes or bony growths related to dentistry:

- **alveolar** (al-**VEE**-oh-lar): bone growth or border of the maxilla and the mandible; makes up and forms the tooth sockets.
- **condyloid** (**KON**-dih-loyd): posterior growth on the **ramus** (**RAY**-mus) of the mandible;

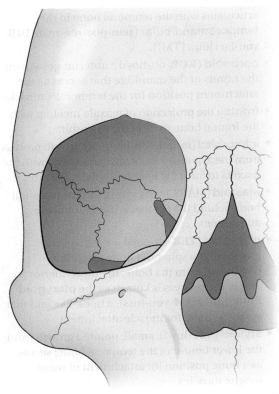

Figure 2-5 Anatomy of the palate

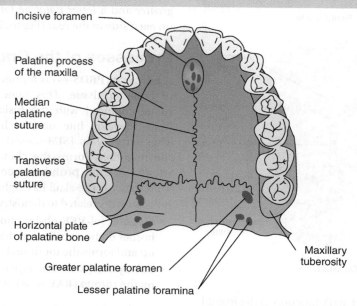

Incisive foramen

Palatine process
of the maxilla

Median
palatine
suture

Transverse
palatine
suture

Horizontal plate
of palatine bone

Greater palatine foramen

Lesser palatine foramina

Maxillary
tuberosity

articulates with the temporal bone in the **temporomandibular** (**tem**-poe-roe-man-**DIB**-you-lar) joint (TMJ).

- **coronoid** (**KOR**-oh-noyd): anterior growth on the ramus of the mandible that serves as the attachment position for the temporalis muscle.
- **frontal:** the projection of maxilla meeting with the frontal bone to form the eye orbit.
- **infraorbital** (**in**-frah-**OR**-bih-tahl): growth process from the zygomatic bone that articulates with the maxilla to form the lower side of the eye orbit.
- **mastoid** (**MASS**-toyd): growth on the temporal bone behind the ear that is used for muscle attachment.
- **pterygoid** (**TER**-eh-goyd = *wing shaped*): growth of the sphenoid bone extending downward from the bone; the most inferior end of the process is known as the **pterygoid hamulus** (**HAM**-you-luss), a hook-like end that serves as a site for muscle attachment.
- **styloid** (**STY**-loyd): small, pointed growth from the lower border of the temporal bone; serves as a bone position for attachment of some tongue muscles.

Foramina of the Cranium

A **foramen** (for-**RAY**-men) is an opening or hole in the bone for nerve and vessel passage. A foramen is not to be confused with the **external auditory meatus** (mee-**AY**-tus), a large opening in the temporal bone used for the passage of auditory nerves and vessels. Knowing the location of the foramina is important because many injections for anesthesia are placed in these areas. There are nine main **foramina** (foh-**RAY**-men-ah = *plural of foramen*) of the head related to dentistry:

- **magnum** (**MAG**-num): opening in the occipital bone for spinal cord passage; largest of all foramina.
- **mandibular:** located on the lingual side of the ramus of the mandible; permits nerve and vessels passage to teeth and mouth tissues.
- **mental** (**MEN**-tal = *Latin for chin*): opening situated on left and the right anterior areas of the mandible; used for passage of nerve and vessels.
- **lingual** (**LIN**-gwal): small opening in the center of the mental spine for nerve passage to the incisor area.
- **incisive** (in-**SIGH**-siv): opening in the maxilla behind the central incisors on the midline.

- **supraorbital** (**soo**-prah-**OR**-bih-tal): an opening in the frontal bone above the eye orbit.
- **infraorbital:** an opening in the maxilla under the eye orbit.
- **palatine:** anterior and posterior openings in the hard palate.
- **zygomaticofacial** (**zye**-go-**MAT**-ee-coe-**fay**-shal): an opening in the zygomatic bone.

All bones are covered by a fibrous membrane called the **periosteum** (pear-ee-**AHS**-tee-um) that forms a lining on all surfaces, except for the areas in the oral cavity. The tissues inside the oral cavity have a mucous surface layer, called the mucoperiosteum (**MYOU**-koh-**pear**-ee-**AHS**-tee-um). The oral cavity has three types of oral **mucosa** (**MU**-ko-sa):

- **lining mucosa:** mucous membrane that lines the inner surfaces of the lips (*labial mucosa*) and the cheeks (*buccal mucosa*).
- **masticatory** (mass-**TIH**-kah-toe-ree) **mucosa:** elastic type of mucous membrane that undergoes stress and pull; located around the alveolar area of the teeth and lines the hard palate.
- **specialized mucosa:** smoother mucous tissue found on the dorsal side of the tongue.

LANDMARKS AND FEATURES OF THE MANDIBLE

The mandible is the only movable bone in the skull. It is the strongest bone in the face and supports many features (see Figure 2-6). The mandible has seven major anatomical parts:

Figure 2-6 Lateral and lingual view of the mandible

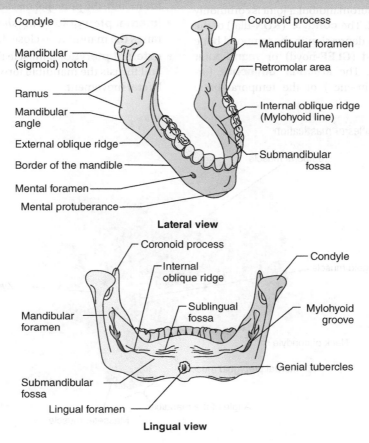

Condyle

Mandibular (sigmoid) notch

Ramus

Mandibular angle

External oblique ridge

Border of the mandible

Mental foramen

Mental protuberance

Coronoid process

Mandibular foramen

Retromolar area

Internal oblique ridge (Mylohyoid line)

Submandibular fossa

Lateral view

Coronoid process

Internal oblique ridge

Sublingual fossa

Condyle

Mylohyoid groove

Mandibular foramen

Submandibular fossa

Lingual foramen

Genial tubercles

Lingual view

- **ramus:** ascending part of the mandible that arises from the curved, lower arch.
- **angle of the mandible:** area along the lower edge of the mandible where the upward curve of the mandible forms.
- **sigmoid notch:** S-shaped curvature between the condyle and coronoid processes; upper border of the mandible; also called the mandibular notch.
- **mylohyoid ridge** (my-loh-**HIGH**-oyd): bony ridge on the lingual surface of the mandible.
- **oblique** (oh-**BLEEK**) **line:** slanted, bony growth ridge on the facial side of the mandible.
- **retromolar** (ret-row-**MOLE**-ar) **area:** space located to the rear of the mandibular molars.
- **symphysis:** center of mandible (chin); also known as *mental protuberance* (projection).

The mandible **articulates** (are-**TICK**-you-lates) or comes together as a joint with the temporal bone of the cranium. This temporomandibular joint is commonly abbreviated as TMJ. The **condyle** (**KON**-dial) of the mandible rests in a depression in the temporal bone called the **glenoid** (**GLEE**-noyd) or **mandibular fossa** (**FAH**-sah). The **articular eminence** (ar-**TICK**-you-lar **EM**-in-ence) of the temporal bone forms the anterior boundary of the fossa and helps maintain the mandible in position. Between the contact area of these two bones is the articular disc, a **meniscus** (men-**IS**-kus) and **synovial** (sin-**OH**-vee-al) **fluid** that cushions and lubricates the joint that works in a hinge-action movement.

MUSCLES OF MASTICATION

Mastication (mass-tih-**KAY**-shun = *chewing*) is controlled by paired (left-right) muscles, named for their placement area. Each performs a specific function. The four major muscles of mastication (Figure 2-7) are:

- **temporal:** a fan-shaped muscle on each side of the skull; elevates and lowers the jaw and can draw the mandible backward.
- **masseter** (mass-**SEE**-ter): the muscle that closes the mouth; the principal mastication muscle.
- **internal pterygoid** (*wing shaped*): muscle that raises the mandible to close the jaw.
- **external pterygoid:** muscle that opens the jaw and thrusts the mandible forward; assists with lateral movement.

Figure 2-7 Muscles of mastication

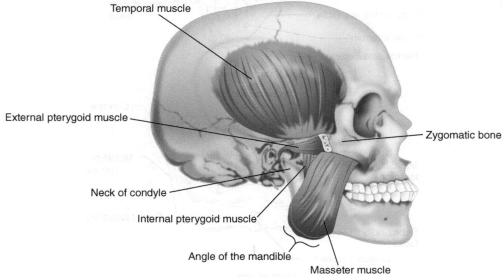

Temporal muscle

External pterygoid muscle

Zygomatic bone

Neck of condyle

Internal pterygoid muscle

Angle of the mandible

Masseter muscle

Figure 2-8 Muscles of facial expression

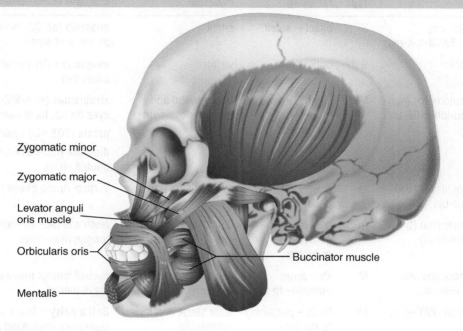

Zygomatic minor

Zygomatic major

Levator anguli
oris muscle

Orbicularis oris

Mentalis

Buccinator muscle

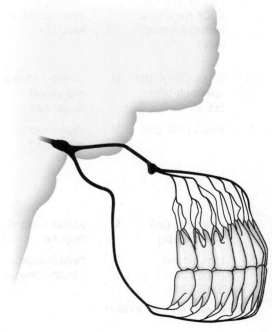

Several other muscles of the head are important to dentistry. These essential muscles relate to or control some of the anatomy concerned with dental care (Figure 2-8):

- **orbicularis oris** (or-bick-you-**LAIR**-iss **OR**-is): Also known as the "kissing muscle," a circular muscle surrounding the mouth that compacts, compresses, and protrudes the lips.
- **buccinator** (**BUCK**-sin-ay-tore): principal cheek muscle; compresses the cheek, expels air through the lips, and aids in food mastication.
- **mentalis** (men-**TAL**-iss): muscle of the chin (mental) that moves the chin tissue and raises or lowers the lower lip.

TRIGEMINAL NERVE LOCATION AND FUNCTIONS

Muscle movement and the registration of sensations are accomplished by nerves, the communication lines to the brain. The head contains 12 pairs of cranial nerves. Each pair is numbered; one of each pair is on the left and one on the right. Table 2-1 lists the cranial

Table 2-1 The Cranial Nerves and Their Function

Nerve		Type	Meaning	Function	Example Malfunction(s)
I	Olfactory (ol-**FACK**-toh-ree)	S	olfact – *smell*	smell	**anosmia** (an-**OZ**-me-ah) loss of sense of smell
II	Optic	S	optic – *eye*	vision	**anopia** (an-**OH**-pee-ah) blindness
III	Oculomotor (auk-you-loh-**MOE**-tor)	M	oculo – *eye*, motor – *movement*	upper-eyelid and eyeball movement	**strabismus** (stra-**BIZ**-mus) eyes do not fix at same point **ptosis** (**TOE**-sis) eyelid droop **diplopia** (dip-**LOW**-pee-ah) double vision
IV	Trochlear (**TRAH**-klee-ur)	M	trochle – *small pulley*	eye movement and sensation	vertical droop of eye
V	Trigeminal (try-**JEM**-in-al)	B	tri – *three*, geminal – *branches*	dental and face nerve	teeth and face sensation, tongue movement
VI	Abducens (**AB**-due-sense)	M	ab – *away*, ducens – *to lead*	lateral eye sense and movement	eyeball cannot move laterally—stays medial
VII	Facial (**FAY**-shal)	M	facial – *pertaining to the face*	taste sense and facial expression	**Bell's palsy** – face contraction, taste loss, decreased saliva
VIII	Vestibulocochlear (ves-**tib**-you-loh-**COCK**-lee-ar) also termed acoustic nerve	M	vestibulo – *small opening or cavity*, cochlear – *snail-like*	equilibrium, hearing, sensation	acoustic loss **vertigo** (**VER**-tee-go) dizziness **tinnitus** (tin-**EYE**-tis) ear ringing **ataxia** (ah-**TACKS**-ee-ah) muscle incoordination
IX	Glossopharyngeal (**gloss**-oh-fair-en-**JEE**-al)	M	glosso – *tongue*, pharyngeal – *throat area*	taste sensation, swallowing, regulation of O_2 and CO_2 breaths	loss of taste sensation, swallowing difficulty, reduced saliva flow of parotid gland
X	Vagus (**VAY**-gus)	M	vaga – *vagrant, wander*	taste sensation of epiglottis, pharynx, blood pressure, smooth muscle of gastrointestinal system, heart rate, digestion	paralyze vocal cords, heart rate increase, sensation interference of swallowing, GI organs
XI	Accessory (ack-**SESS**-ore-ee)	M	access – *assist, help out*	body sensation, muscles of shoulders	difficulty in raising shoulders and moving head
XII	Hypoglossal (**high**-poe-**GLOSS**-al)	M	hypo – *under*, glosso – *tongue*	body sensation, tongue movement in speech and swallowing	difficulty in chewing, speaking, and swallowing

Note: S = sensory; M = motor; B = mixed

nerves, type (S for sensory, M for motor, or B for mixed), meaning, function, and example malfunctions.

The most important nerve connected with dentistry is the fifth cranial nerve, the **trigeminal**. This combination motor and sensory nerve emerges from the brain and branches at the **Gasserian** (**GAS**-er-in) or semilunar, **ganglion** (**GANG**-glee-on = *mass of nerves*). The trigeminal nerves are classified as *ophthalmic, maxillary*, or *mandibular*:

- **ophthalmic** (off-**THAL**-mick): The smallest sensory nerve of the three main divisions, also has three branches:
  - **lacrimal:** carries sensation from the lacrimal gland and eye conjunctiva.
  - **frontal:** carries sensation from the forehead, scalp, upper eyelid, and nasal root.
  - **nasociliary** (**nay**-zoh-**SIL**-ee-air-ee): carries sensation from the nose, eye, and eyebrow.
- **maxillary:** a sensory division of the trigeminal nerve that has several branches:
  - **anterior palatine:** carries sensation from the hard palate, periosteum (pear-ee-**AH**-stee-um), and mucous membrane of the molars and premolar teeth; sometimes considered the greater palatine nerve.
  - **middle palatine:** carries sensation from the soft palate, the **uvula** (**YOU**-view-lah), and upper or soft part of the palate, along with the posterior palatine nerve; may be grouped as lesser palatine nerves.
  - **posterior palatine:** carries sensation from the tonsils and the soft palate.
  - **nasopalatine** (**nay**-zoh-**PAL**-ah-tine): carries sensation from the nose and the anterior area of the palate.
  - **infraorbital:** subdivides into three parts:
    - **anterior superior alveolar branch:** carries sensation from the maxillary centrals, laterals, and canines.

- **middle superior alveolar branch:** carries sensation from the maxillary premolars and the mesiobuccal root of the maxillary first molar.
- **posterior superior alveolar branch:** carries sensation from the maxillary second and third molar, and the remaining roots of the maxillary first molar.
- **zygomatic:** carries sensation from the lacrimal and upper cheek.
- **sphenopalatine** (**sfee**-no-**PAL**-ah-tine): sensory nerve ending for the maxillary anterior mucosal and palatine tissues.
- **mandibular:** *mixed* nerve division that registers sensation and causes movement (see Figure 2-9). It has several branches:
  - **inferior alveolar:** carries sensation from the mandibular teeth and mucosa of the mouth floor and some tongue areas.
  - **mental:** carries sensation from the skin of chin and the lower lip.
  - **incisive:** carries sensation from the anterior teeth and alveoli, chin, and lip areas.
  - **buccal:** carries sensation from the buccal gingiva and mucosa of the molar region.
  - **lingual:** carries some sensation from the tongue and causes some movement of the tongue and mastication muscles; thereby the classification of the trigeminal nerve is mixed.

BLOOD SUPPLY OF THE CRANIUM

Blood is supplied to the head by a vascular (**VAS**-kyou-lar = *small vessels*) system of arteries and veins. An artery (**ARE**-ter-ee) carries blood away from the heart, and a vein (**VAYN**) takes blood to the heart. Knowledge of the vascular system is important for controlling bleeding and also for administering local anesthesia. In dentistry there are three major areas of concern: capillaries, carotid arteries, and jugular veins:

Figure 2-9 Mandibular branch of the trigeminal nerve

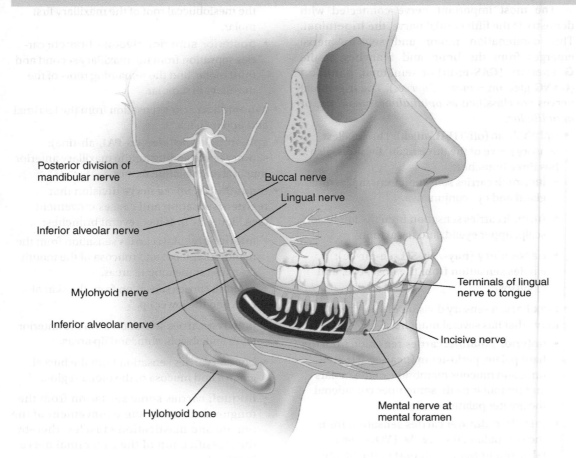

Posterior division of
mandibular nerve

Buccal nerve

Lingual nerve

Inferior alveolar nerve

Terminals of lingual
nerve to tongue

Mylohyoid nerve

Inferior alveolar nerve

Incisive nerve

Hylohyoid bone

Mental nerve at
mental foramen

- **capillaries** (**KAP**-ih-lair-eez): tiny blood vessels that help to transport blood from the veins to the arteries.
- **carotid** (kr-**AA**-tuhd) **artery:** rises from the aorta right and left, and divides in the neck to form two arteries (Figure 2-10):
  - **internal carotid artery:** provides the blood supply to the brain and eyes.
    - **external carotid artery:** provides blood to the throat, face, mouth, tongue, and ears through these branches:

- **infraorbital (under eye orbit):** provides blood to the maxillary anterior teeth and surrounding tissues.
- **inferior alveolar (lower alveolar process):** provides blood to the mandibular teeth, periodontal ligaments, and surrounding tissues.
- **facial (pertaining to face):** provides blood to the face, tonsils, palate, and submandibular gland.

Figure 2-10 Carotid arteries

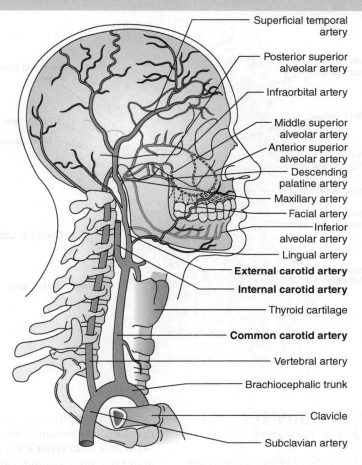

- Superficial temporal artery
- Posterior superior alveolar artery
- Infraorbital artery
- Middle superior alveolar artery
- Anterior superior alveolar artery
- Descending palatine artery
- Maxillary artery
- Facial artery
- Inferior alveolar artery
- Lingual artery
- **External carotid artery**
- **Internal carotid artery**
- Thyroid cartilage
- **Common carotid artery**
- Vertebral artery
- Brachiocephalic trunk
- Clavicle
- Subclavian artery

- **lingual (tongue):** divides into branches to serve the tongue, tonsil, soft palate, throat, and floor of the mouth.
    - **maxillary:** largest of the branches the external carotid; provides blood to the maxillary teeth, periodontal ligaments, muscles, sinus, and palate.
- **jugular (JUG**-you-lar) **vein:** carries blood from the head to the heart through two divisions (Figure 2-11):
    - **internal jugular vein:** collects and drains blood from the brain, cranium, face, and neck.
    - **external jugular vein:** collects and drains blood through assorted branches. The major branches are:
    - **facial division:** carries blood from the face structures and mouth area.
    - **maxillary division:** carries blood from the maxillary region.
    - **pterygoid venus plexus (PLECK**-sus = *network*): collects the blood supply from the head, nasal cavity, palate, teeth, and muscles.

Figure 2-11 Jugular veins

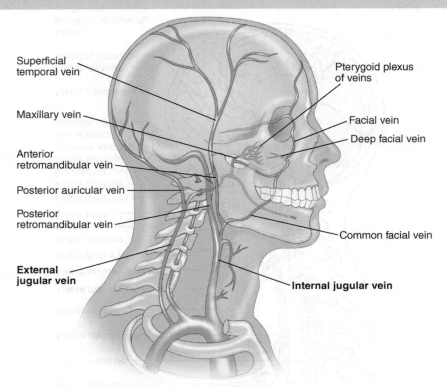

Superficial temporal vein

Maxillary vein

Anterior retromandibular vein

Posterior auricular vein

Posterior retromandibular vein

External jugular vein

Pterygoid plexus of veins

Facial vein

Deep facial vein

Common facial vein

Internal jugular vein

LOCATIONS AND PURPOSES OF THE SALIVARY GLANDS

Salivary glands supply secretions to the oral cavity that protect the lining of the mouth, help moisten food, assist in speech, and make saliva to **expectorate** (ex-**PECK**-toe-rate = *spit*). The major salivary glands produce large amounts of secretions, and the minor salivary glands maintain moist oral tissue.

Secretions may produce **serum** (**SEAR**-um = *watery fluid*) or **mucin** (**MYOU**-sin = *sticky, slime, secretion*) that forms mucus. Some glands produce both with **enzymes** (**EN**-zimes = *body-produced chemicals*) to digest food. In dentistry, the three major pairs of salivary glands are (Figure 2-12):

- **parotid** (pah-**ROT**-id): the largest salivary gland, located near the ear, produces serus saliva that empties into the mouth near the maxillary second molar through the Stenson's **duct** (**DUCKT** = *to lead*). This gland becomes swollen when infected by mumps.
- **submandibular:** a smaller gland located on the lower side of the face that secretes mucin and serus fluids with enzymes; empties through the submandibular duct (Wharton duct) openings in the small fleshy growths, called **caruncles** (**CAR**-un-kuhls). These growths may be seen under the tongue on each side of the lingual frenum.
- **sublingual:** smallest major salivary gland, situated in the floor of the mouth; secretes mucin through multiple ducts; many other small glands are nearby, and they function to keep the mouth tissues moist.

Figure 2-12 Salivary glands, lateral view

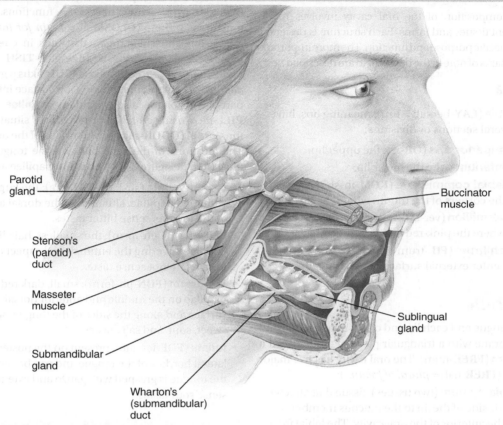

Parotid gland

Stenson's (parotid) duct

Masseter muscle

Submandibular gland

Wharton's (submandibular) duct

Buccinator muscle

Sublingual gland

AGENTS AND FUNCTIONS OF THE LYMPHATIC SYSTEM

The lymphatic system's presence throughout the body helps protect the body from disease and assists with immunity. The lymphatic system is composed of a variety of structures:

- **lymph** (LIMF): vessels that transport lymph fluid of plasma and water and waste products.
- **lymph capillaries:** tiny vessels or tubes that carry lymph fluid.
- **lymph node:** a mass of lymph cells forming a unit of lymphatic tissue that is named after the formation site, for example:
  - **axillary** (**ACK**-sih-lair-ree = *pertaining to the armpit*): lymph nodes located under the armpit.

- **cervical** (**SIR**-vih-kul = *pertaining to the neck*): lymph nodes located in the neck.
- **inguinal** (**IN**-gwee-nal = *pertaining to the groin*): lymph nodes found in the groin area near the abdomen.
- **tonsil** (**TAHN**-sill): lymphatic tissue masses found in the posterior of the throat between the anterior and posterior fauces (*palatine tonsil*) and on the back of the tongue (*lingual tonsil*). Tonsils act as filters, aid in the production of disease-fighting immune responses, and may help immunity.
- **adenoid** (**ADD**-eh-noyd): lymphatic tissue found in the nasopharynx area; sometimes called the *pharyngeal tonsil*.

More specific information on this system is found in Chapter 5, Infection Control.

IMPORTANT STRUCTURES IN THE ORAL CAVITY

The composition of the oral cavity involves many different tissues and forms. Each structure is designed for a specific purpose and function. The more important landmarks of note in the dental field are described next.

Labia

- **Labia** (**LAY**-bee-ah = *lips*), meaning lips, have several sections or divisions:
  - **superior oris** (**OR**-is): the upper lip.
  - **inferium oris:** the lower lip.
  - **labial commissure** (**KOM**-ih-shur): area at the corners of the mouth where the lips meet.
  - **vermillion** (ver-**MILL**-yon) **border:** area where the pink-red lip tissue meets facial skin.
  - **philtrum** (**FIL**-trum): median groove in the center external surface of the upper lip.

FRENUM

The tongue and each lip and cheek attach to the oral membrane with a triangular piece of tissue called a **frenum** (**FREE**-num). The oral cavity has five major **frena** (**FREE**-nah = *plural of frenum*):

- **labial frenum** (two tissues): tissue that attaches the inside of the lip to the mucous membrane in the anterior of the oral cavity. The labial frena occur in both the maxillary and the mandibular arches. The maxillary labial frenum is a common site for a surgical frenectomy to permit closure of the two central incisors' gap caused by a labial frenum that is too large or thick.
- **lingual frenum** (one tissue): attaches the lower side of the tongue to the floor membrane. Openings for the Wharton's duct are found on each side of this frenum in the fleshy tissue elevations called caruncles. If the lingual frenum is too short, **ankyloglossia** (**ang**-key-loh-**GLOSS**-see-ah), a "tongue-tied" condition, can result.
- **buccal frenum** (two tissues): attaches the inside of the cheek to the oral cavity in the maxillary first molar area. This frenum occurs one each on the left and the right sides.

Tongue Structures

The tongue is an important organ in the oral cavity that performs many necessary functions. The tongue, or **glossa** (**GLOSS**-ah = *Latin for tongue*), is a strong muscular organ that aids in chewing, talking, and **deglutition** (**dee**-glue-**TISH**-un = *swallowing*). A **median sulcus** (**SULL**-kus = *groove, depression*) divides the tongue's top surface into two parts. The tongue also has many **papillae** (pah-**PILL**-lie = *tissue growths*) or taste buds situated on the **dorsal** (**DOOR**-sal = *back*) surface of the tongue. The locations of the taste buds on the tongue are illustrated in Figure 2-13. The major papillae are:

- **circumvallate** (sir-kum-**VAL**-ate): the largest, V-shaped papillae, situated on the dorsal aspect of the tongue; sense bitter tastes.
- **filiform** (**FIL**-ih-form): the smallest, hair-like papillae covering the entire dorsal aspect of the tongue; do not sense taste.
- **fungiform** (**FUN**-jih-form): small, dark red papillae on the middle and anterior dorsal surface and along the sides of the tongue; sense sweet, sour, and salty tastes.
- **foliate** (**FOE**-lee-ate): present on the posterior lateral borders of the tongue and can be seen if the tongue is grasped with gauze and extended; sense sour tastes.

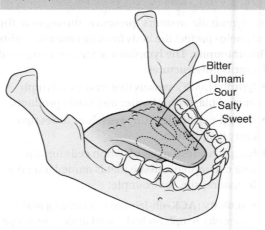

Figure 2-13 View of tongue with taste buds (papillae) noted

Bitter
Umami
Sour
Salty
Sweet

There is a newly discovered fifth taste known as **umami**, which is the taste of monosodium, described as a meaty, savory taste.

Palate Structures

The **palate** (**PAL**-utt) or roof of the mouth is composed of assorted structures. Its two main divisions are the hard palate and soft palate:

- **hard palate:** composed of the palatine processes of the maxillae bones; covered with mucous membrane and has the following features:
  - **rugae** (**RUE**-guy): irregular folds or bumps on the surface.
  - **incisive papilla:** tissue growth that is situated at the anterior portion of the palate behind the maxillary centrals; the site for infiltration injection of local anesthesia.
  - **palatine raphe** (**RAH**-fay = *ridge between the union of two halves*): white streak in the middle of the palate.

- **soft palate:** flexible portion of the palate without bone; area where the gag reflex is present. The soft palate is movable and closes off the nasal passage during swallowing.

Miscellaneous Oral Cavity Structures

Additional oral cavity structures include the following:

- **uvula:** tissue structure hanging from the palate in the posterior of the oral cavity.
- **vestibule** (**VES**-tih-byul): open gum and tissue area between the teeth and the cheek.
- **fauces** (**FOE**-seez): constricted opening or passage leading from the mouth to the oral pharynx, bound by the soft palate, the base of tongue, and the palatine arches. The fauces are considered two pillars of mucous membranes:
  - **glossopalatine arch** (gloss-oh-**PAL**-ah-tine = *glossa* and *palate* area): anterior pillars.
  - **pharyngopalatine** (fare-in-goh-**PAL**-ah-tine = *pharynx* and *palate* area): posterior pillars. The palatine tonsils lay between these pillars.

Review Exercises

Matching

Match the following word elements with their meaning:

1. _____ rugae	**A.** foramen in occipital bone for spinal cord passage	7. _____ buccinator	**G.** upper lip
2. _____ fauces	**B.** tissue structure hanging from the posterior of the palate	8. _____ magna foramen	**H.** border of lip and facial tissue
3. _____ philtrum	**C.** another word for tongue	9. _____ suture	**I.** groove on external middle surface of upper lip
4. _____ superior oris	**D.** irregular folds on palate surface	10. _____ vermillion border	**J.** principal cheek muscle
5. _____ glossa	**E.** mass of lymph cells forming body named for area site	11. _____ mental	**K.** forehead bone
6. _____ parotid	**F.** constricted opening leading from the mouth	12. _____ incus	**L.** bone of middle ear
		13. _____ uvula	**M.** another word for chin
		14. _____ frontal	**N.** immovable junction of two bones
		15. _____ node	**O.** largest salivary gland

Definition

Using the selection given for each sentence, choose the best term to complete the definition.

1. The border area where the pink tissue of the lips meets the facial tissue is called:
   a. circumvallate
   b. vermillion
   c. commissure
   d. frenum

2. Which vessel transports blood from the brain to the heart?
   a. internal jugular
   b. internal carotid
   c. external jugular
   d. external carotid

3. A body-produced chemical helping to break down food for digestion is called:
   a. infragen
   b. enzyme
   c. expectorant
   d. antigen

4. Which artery carries the blood supply to the head and brain?
   a. jugular
   b. carotid
   c. capillary
   d. radial artery

5. The branch of the ophthalmic nerves that provides sensation for the tear gland is the:
   a. lacrimal
   b. nasociliary
   c. maxillary
   d. plexus

6. The principal muscle of mastication that closes the mouth is the:
   a. internal pterygoid
   b. external pterygoid
   c. masseter
   d. common pterygoid

7. Which of the following is not an auditory ossicle?
   a. stapes
   b. malleus
   c. tympanic
   d. anvil

8. The protective mucous layer covering the bone surface is:
   a. periosteum
   b. mucoperiosteum
   c. calcisopenum
   d. osteoplasta

9. The fusion line in the center/middle of the mandible is the:
   a. symphysis
   b. condyle
   c. ramus
   d. orbit

10. The squamous suture between the two bones in the head is called the:
    a. sagittal
    b. coronal
    c. temporoparietal
    d. symphysis

11. The Atrium of Highmore is another name for:
    a. opening in the occipital bone
    b. oral cavity free space between the cheek/lips
    c. maxillary sinus cavity
    d. opening in the frontal bone

12. Which of the following is not considered a facial bone?
    a. lacrimal
    b. maxilla
    c. zygomatic
    d. occipital

13. The bone that lies in suspension between the larynx and the mandible is:
    a. lambdoid
    b. hyoid
    c. sigmoid
    d. frontal

14. The large bone growth behind the ears on the temporal bone is:
    a. coronoid
    b. sublingual
    c. mastoid
    d. occipital

15. An opening or passage through a bone that is used for nerve or vessel passage is called a/an:
    a. foramen
    b. frenum
    c. alveolar crest
    d. sinus

16. An inferior end of a process that has a hooked end is called a/an:
    a. plexus
    b. hamulus
    c. protuberance
    d. forama

17. The S-shaped curvature between the condyle and coronoid process is the:
    a. ramus
    b. angle of mandible
    c. mandibular notch
    d. coronoid

18. The largest V-shaped papillae present on the dorsal side of the tongue are:
    a. fungiform
    b. foliate
    c. circumvallate
    d. filiform

19. The area located to the rear of the mandibular molars is:
    a. retromolar area
    b. suborbital area
    c. supramandibular area
    d. hyoid area

20. The median sulcus divides the tongue into how many sections?
    a. none
    b. one
    c. two
    d. three

Building Skills

Locate and define the prefix, root/combining form, and suffix (if present) in the following words:

1. **infraorbital**
   prefix _____
   root/combining form _____
   suffix _____

2. **periosteum**
   prefix _____
   root/combining form _____
   suffix _____

3. **glossopalatine**
   prefix _____
   root/combining form _____
   suffix _____

4. **submandibular**
   prefix _____
   root/combining form _____
   suffix _____

5. **temporoparietal**
   prefix _____
   root/combining form _____
   suffix _____

Fill-Ins

Write the correct word in the blank space to complete each statement.

1. The skull is composed of two main bone divisions, the _____ and the cranium.

2. The part of the mandible that rises upward and contains the condyle is the _____.

3. The _____ gland is the largest of the major salivary glands.

4. The mandibular _____ foramen is located in the anterior region of the mandible.

5. The fibrous membrane covering of most bones is called the _____.

6. Another name for the sigmoid notch is the _____ _____.

7. The junction of the frontal and parietal bones at birth is soft and sometimes called the baby's "soft spot" or the _____.

8. Another name for the circular "kissing muscle" surrounding the mouth is the _____ _____.

9. The trigeminal nerve emerges from the brain and branches at the semilunar mass of nerves called the _____.

10. The division of the trigeminal nerve that registers sensation to the maxillary second molar is the _____ division.

11. The internal carotid artery supplies blood to the cranium and the _____.

12. Wharton's duct is the drain opening for the _____ salivary gland.

13. The lymphatic system assists with immunity and protects the body from _____.

14. The vascular vessel that carries blood to the heart is called a/an _____.

15. Small fleshy tissue elevations under the tongue are called _____.

16. In the TMJ, the mandibular condyle rests in the _____ fossa of the temporal bone.

17. The small, dark-red papillae on the middle and anterior dorsal surface and along the sides of the tongue are called the _____ papillae.

18. The _____ is the muscular tissue structure that hangs down from the palate in the rear of the oral cavity.

19. The branch of the mandibular division of the trigeminal nerve that causes movement of the tongue is the _____ branch.

20. The tissue body that is situated between the glossopalatine and pharyngopalatine pillars is the _____.

Word Use

Read the following sentences and define the word written in boldface letters.

1. Many people complain of **sinus** problems when the temperature or humidity is high.

   _____

2. Touching the **uvula** or soft palate area will cause a gag-reflex action.

   _____

3. X-ray examination revealed a fracture of the left **coronoid** process and the presence of an unerupted maxillary tooth.

   _____

4. The patient was given a prescription for treatment of enlarged tonsils and an acute infection in the **mastoid** area.

   _____

5. The orthodontist recommended a labial **frenectomy** before the orthodontic treatment would be started.

   _____

CHAPTER 3

TOOTH ORIGIN AND FORMATION

✔ Learning Objectives

On completion of this chapter, you should be able to:

1. Discuss the primary and secondary dentitions and terms related to them.

2. Identify each developmental stage of tooth formation from initiation to attrition; list the eruption dates for the primary and secondary teeth.

3. Identify and determine the makeup of each of the tooth tissues and conditions related to their development.

4. Name and discuss the various tissues and membranes that make up the periodontium.

5. Discuss the attributes and characteristic terms that are common to teeth.

6. Name and identify the tooth surfaces and characteristic landmarks.

CLASSIFICATION OF THE HUMAN DENTITION

Each human receives two sets of teeth. The first set or **deciduous** (deh-**SID**-you-us = *falling off*) teeth are followed by the permanent **dentition** (den-**TISH**-un = *tooth arrangement*). The 20 deciduous teeth erupting first are commonly called "baby teeth" or primary teeth. The 32 permanent teeth that erupt and replace the deciduous teeth are commonly called secondary teeth. The permanent teeth are also termed **succedaneous** (suck-seh-**DAY**-nee-us) because these teeth, with the exception of the molars, replace the deciduous teeth when the latter **exfoliate** (ecks-**FOH**-lee-ate = *scale off*).

Mixed dentition occurs from age 6 to 16, when the dentition contains both deciduous and secondary teeth. Figure 3-1 illustrates mixed dentition. Although human teeth are considered **heterodont**

Vocabulary Related to Tooth Origin and Formation

This list contains selected new and important word parts and terms from this chapter. Take the time to learn these word parts and their meanings. You may use the list to review these terms and practice pronouncing them correctly. When you work with the audio for this chapter, listen to the word, repeat it, and then place a checkmark in the box. Proceed to the next boxed word, and repeat the process.

(hyphen before word means it's a suffix, hyphen after word means prefix, no hyphen means root word.)

Word Parts	Meaning	Word Parts	Meaning
hyper-	over, above	bi-	two
cement/o	cementum	furca	branch
-osis	condition of	-tion	condition or state of
muc/o	mucus	peri-	around
gingiv	gingiva, gums	odont	tooth
-al	relating to	-itis	inflammation
-ology	study of		

Key Terms

- ❏ **acellular** (ay-**SELL**-you-lar)
- ❏ **alveolar** (al-**VEE**-oh-lar)
- ❏ **ameloblast** (ah-**MEAL**-oh-blast)
- ❏ **anodontia** (an-oh-**DON**-she-ah)
- ❏ **antagonist** (an-**TAG**-oh-nist)
- ❏ **apical** (**AY**-pih-kahl)
- ❏ **apposition** (ap-oh-**ZIH**-shun)
- ❏ **attrition** (ah-**TRISH**-un)
- ❏ **bifurcation** (bye-fer-**KAY**-shun)
- ❏ **buccal** (**BUCK**-al)
- ❏ **calcification** (kal-sih-fih-**KAY**-shun)

(Continued)

Key Terms *continued*

- ❑ canaliculi (kan-ah-LICK-you-lie)
- ❑ cementoblasts (see-MEN-toh-blasts)
- ❑ cementoclasts (see-MEN-toh-klasts)
- ❑ cementum (see-MEN-tum)
- ❑ cervix (SIR-vicks)
- ❑ cingulum (SIN-gyou-lum)
- ❑ cuticle (KYOU-tih-kul)
- ❑ deciduous (deh-SID-you-us)
- ❑ dens in dente (DENZ in DEN-tay)
- ❑ denticles (DEN-tih-kuls)
- ❑ dentin (DEN-tin)
- ❑ dentinogenesis imperfecta (den-tin-oh-JEN-eh-sis im-per-FECK-tuh)
- ❑ dentition (den-TISH-un)
- ❑ diastema (dye-ah-STEE-mah)
- ❑ differentiation (dif-er-en-she-AY-shun)
- ❑ distal (DIS-tal)
- ❑ ectoderm (ECK-toh-derm)
- ❑ eminence (EM-in-ence)
- ❑ enamel (eh-NAM-el)
- ❑ epithelium (ep-ith-EE-lee-um)
- ❑ eruption (ee-RUP-shun)
- ❑ exfoliate (ecks-FOH-lee-ate)
- ❑ fibroblasts (FIE-broh-blasts)
- ❑ fissure (FISH-er)
- ❑ fluorosis (floor-OH-sis)
- ❑ fossa (FAH-sah)

- ❑ furcation (fur-KAY-shun)
- ❑ furrow (FER-oh)
- ❑ germination (jerm-ih-NAY-shun)
- ❑ gingiva (JIN-jih-vah)
- ❑ gomphosis (gahm-FOH-sis)
- ❑ granuloma (gran-you-LOH-mah)
- ❑ heterodont (HET-er-oh-dahnt)
- ❑ histodifferentiation (his-toh-dif-er-en-she-AY-shun)
- ❑ hypercementosis (high-per-see-men-TOH-sis)
- ❑ hypocalcification (high-poh-kal-sih-fih-KAY-shun)
- ❑ hypoplasia (high-poh-PLAY-zee-ah)
- ❑ incisal (in-SIGH-zel)
- ❑ keratinized (KARE-ah-tin-ized)
- ❑ labial (LAY-bee-al)
- ❑ lacuna (lah-KYOU-nah)
- ❑ lamellae (lah-MEL-ah)
- ❑ lamina dura (LAM-ih-nah DUR-ah)
- ❑ lingual (LIN-gwal)
- ❑ lobe (LOWB)
- ❑ macrodontia (mack-roh-DAHN-she-ah)
- ❑ mamelon (MAM-eh-lon)
- ❑ mesenchyme (MEZ-en-kime)
- ❑ mesial (ME-zee-al)
- ❑ mesoderm (MESS-oh-derm)
- ❑ microdontia (my-kroh-DAHN-she-ah)

- ❑ morphodifferentiation (more-foh-diff-er-en-she-AY-shun)
- ❑ mucogingival (myou-koh-JIN-jih-vahl)
- ❑ occlusal (oh-KLOO-zahl)
- ❑ odontoblasts (oh-DAHN-toh-blasts)
- ❑ odontoclasts (oh-DAHN-toh-klasts)
- ❑ odontogenesis (oh-dahn-toh-JEN-eh-sis)
- ❑ osteoblasts (AHS-tee-oh-blasts)
- ❑ osteoclasts (AHS-tee-oh-klasts)
- ❑ papilla (pah-PILL-ah)
- ❑ periodontal (pear-ee-oh-DAHN-tahl)
- ❑ periodontium (pear-ee-oh-DANT-ee-um)
- ❑ proliferation (pro-lif-er-AY-shun)
- ❑ pulpitis (pul-PIE-tis)
- ❑ quadrant (KWAH-drant)
- ❑ resorption (ree-SORP-shun)
- ❑ succedaneous (suck-seh-DAY-nee-us)
- ❑ sulcus (SULL-kus)
- ❑ supernumerary (sue-per-NEW-mer-air-ee)
- ❑ tertiary (TERR-shee-air-ee)
- ❑ trifurcation (try-fer-KAY-shun)
- ❑ tubercle (TOO-ber-kul)
- ❑ tubule (TOO-bule)

(**HET**-er-oh-dont = *teeth of various shapes*), all teeth go through the same stages of development.

HISTOLOGICAL STAGES OF TOOTH DEVELOPMENT

The term **odontogenesis** (oh-**don**-toh-**JEN**-eh-sis, odont = *tooth*, genesis = *production*) refers to the formation and the origin of the tooth. During

its evolution and growth, each tooth begins and passes through the developmental stages shown in Figure 3-2.

First Stage of Development

The first, or bud, stage of development is termed the **initiation** (ih-**nish**-ee-**AY**-shun = *beginning*). At the fifth or sixth week **in utero** (in-**YOU**-ter-oh

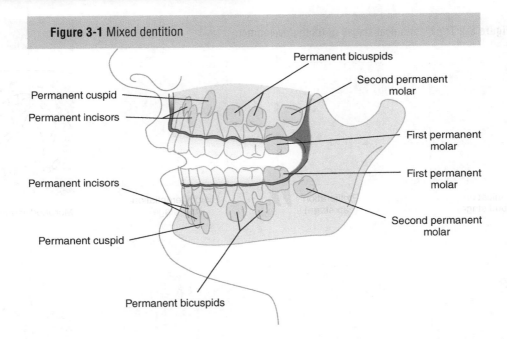

Figure 3-1 Mixed dentition

Permanent cuspid

Permanent incisors

Permanent bicuspids

Second permanent molar

First permanent molar

First permanent molar

Second permanent molar

Permanent incisors

Permanent cuspid

Permanent bicuspids

= *in uterus*), the **dental lamina** (**LAM**-ah-nah = *membrane band containing organs of future teeth*) develops in the primitive oral cavity **epithelium** (**ep**-ith-**EE**-lee-um = *mucous tissue covering and connective tissue layer*). At various points of fetal and age development, these organs present buds or seeds of future teeth.

Second Stage of Development

Proliferation (pro-**lif**-er-**AY**-shun = *reproduction of new parts*), the second stage, includes the bud and early cap stages. Proliferation begins during the fourth or fifth month in utero when small buds appear at different time periods until all deciduous teeth are apparent. Permanent teeth follow the same pattern but begin development in utero and after birth.

The tooth bud consists of three parts:

- **dental organ** (*enamel organ*): derived from the **ectoderm** (**ECK**-toh-derm = *outer layer of development*), gives the tooth bud its covering.

- **dental papilla** (pah-**PILL**-ah = *tissue development giving rise to dentin, pulp*): makes up the inner structures of the tooth, such as the dentin and the pulp, and is derived from the **mesoderm** (**MESS**-oh-derm = *middle layer*), in particular from the **mesenchyme** (**MEZ**-en-kime = *connective tissue cells*).

- **dental sac** (**SACK** = *pocket covering*): derived from the mesoderm; makes up the surrounding covering for the dental organ and papilla. It gives rise to the cementum, or root-covering tissue, the periodontal ligaments that hold the tooth in the alveolar socket, and the alveolar bond; also called *dental follicle*.

Third Stage of Development

Differentiation (**dif**-er-en-she-**AY**-shun = *acquiring different functions from the original*) stage (C and D) causes changes in the tooth bud shape and makeup.

It occurs in two ways:

- **histodifferentiation** (**his**-toh-dif-er-en-she-**AY**-shun = *branch into different tissues*)

Figure 3-2 The histological stages of tooth development

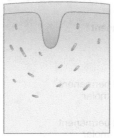

Initiation
(bud stage)

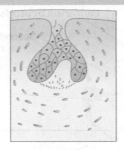

Proliferation
(cap stage)

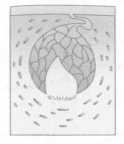

Histodifferentiation
(bell stage)

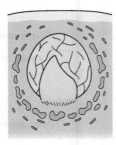

Morphodifferentiation

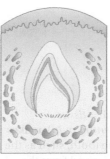

Apposition
(maturation stage)

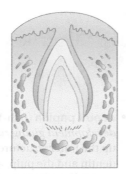

Calcification

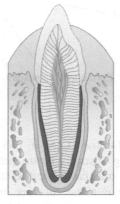

Eruption

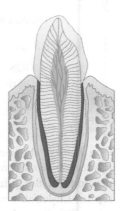

Attrition

- **morphodiffernetiation** (more-**foh**-dif-er-en-she-**AY**-shun = *change into other shape*)

TOOTH DEVELOPMENT

After the makeup and shape change from the tooth cap to the early bell stage, the various tissues of the tooth begin to develop and function. This process occurs because of the appearance of specialized germ cells:

- **odontoblasts** (oh-**DAWN**-toh-blasts = *dentin-forming cells*): encourages cell growth to form the dentin, the bulk of the tooth.
- **ameloblasts** (ah-**MEAL**-oh-blasts = *enamel-forming cells*): encourages cell growth to form the enamel covering tooth tissue.

- **cementoblasts** (see-**MEN**-toh-blasts = *cementum-forming cells*): encourages cell growth to form the root-covering cementum tissue.
- **fibroblasts** (**FIE**-broh-blasts = *fiber-forming germ cells*): encourages cell growth to form the periodontal ligaments.
- **osteoblasts** (**AHS**-tee-oh-blasts = *bone-forming germ cells*): encourages cell growth to form alveolar bone and the alveolar plate.

Fourth Stage of Development

Apposition (**ap**-oh-**ZIH**-shun = *addition of parts*) is the fourth stage when mineral salts and organic matter are set down and in place for tissues and tooth formation.

Fifth Stage of Development

Calcification (**kal**-sih-fih-**KAY**-shun = *deposit of lime salts*) is characterized by the hardening and setting of tooth tissues. It continues after eruption (the sixth stage until total development is accomplished, which takes approximately two years).

Sixth Stage of Development

Eruption (ee-**RUP**-shun = *breaking out*), the sixth phase of tooth development, is commonly called "cutting of the teeth." It occurs when the tooth moves toward the oral cavity and enters through the tissues.

Final Stage of Development

Attrition (ah-**TRISH**-shun = *chafing or abrasion*) is the last stage of development. This wearing away occurs where teeth interact through mastication and speech.

SPECIALIZED CELLS

The stages of tooth development occur at different times according to the tooth involved and its normal developmental schedule, from the first growth stage at the fourth or fifth week in utero to the final calcification of the permanent third molars. In addition to the constructive developing actions, some degenerative periods are necessary to remove the deciduous teeth, making room for the permanent dentitions. Several specialized cells cause root **resorption** (ree-**SORP**-shun = *removal of hard tooth surface*) and degeneration of deciduous teeth:

- **odontoclasts** (oh-**DAWN**-toh-klasts): cells that bring about absorption of primary tooth roots.
- **cementoclasts** (see-**MEN**-toh-klasts): cells that destroy tooth cementum.
- **osteoclasts** (**AHS**-tee-oh-klasts): cells that destroy or cause absorption of bone tissue.

TOOTH ABNORMALITIES

Changes or disturbances during any of the development stages can cause a variety of tooth irregularities or abnormalities that are called **anomalies** (ah-**NOM**-ah-lees = *not normal*):

- **amelogensis** (ah-**meal**-oh-**JEN**-ih-sis = *process of forming tooth enamel*) **imperfecta** (im-per-**FECK**-tuh): a genetic disorder resulting in the formation of defective enamel.
- **anodontia** (an-oh-**DON**-she-ah = *absence of teeth*): partial or total lack of teeth.
- **dens in dente** (**DENZ**-in-**DEN**-tay = *tooth in tooth*): a tooth enfolds on itself to form a small cavity that holds a hard structure or mass, found most commonly on the lingual surface of the maxillary laterals.
- **dentinogenesis imperfecta** (**den**-tin-oh-**JEN**-eh-sis = *occurring in dentin formation,* im-per-**FECK**-tuh = *inadequacy*): a genetic disorder characterized by weakened or gray-colored teeth or shell teeth resulting from poor formation.
- **fluorosis** (floor-**OH**-sis = *reaction to overfluoridation*): also called "mottled enamel."
- **fusion** (**FEW**-shun = *joining together*): union of tooth buds resulting in large crown or root.
- **germination** (**jerm**-ih-**NAY**-shun = *development of germ cell*): single tooth germ separating to form two crowns on a single root.
- **Hutchinsonian incisors:** saw-like incisal edges of maxillary incisors, caused by maternal syphilis during tooth formation (see Figure 3-3).
- **hypocalcification** (**high**-poh-kal-sih-fah-**KAY**-shun = *underbonding or incomplete calcification*): lack of hardening of tooth tissue resulting in weak, susceptible teeth.
- **hypoplasia** (high-poh-**PLAY**-zee-ah = *underdevelopment of tissue*): enamel hypoplasia is a lack of enamel covering.
- **macrodontia** (**mack**-roh-**DAWN**-she-ah): abnormally large teeth.
- **microdontia** (**my**-kroh-**DONT**-she-ah): unusually small teeth.

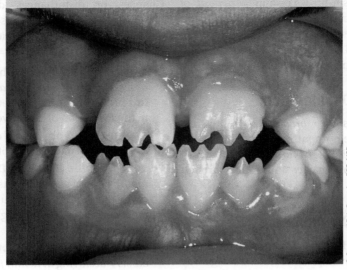

Figure 3-3 Hutchinson's incisors from prenatal syphilis

© Courtesy of Dale Ruemping, DDS, MSD

- **peg-shaped teeth:** a condition of small rounded teeth that usually occurs in the maxillary lateral incisors.
- **supernumerary (sue**-per-**NEW**-mer-air-ee = *extra*): more than the normal amount of teeth.

TOOTH ERUPTION

The eruption (cutting) or appearance of the teeth follows a pattern or schedule. Knowledge of expected eruption can be of value in dental treatment. Delay of tooth appearance or overextended time before exfoliation (shedding) could be responsible for later malocclusion. Also, past diseases (fevers) or reactions from some medications or chemicals (excessive fluoride) could show evidence in newly erupted teeth.

Some variations of tooth eruption may include:

- Lower teeth erupt before their maxillary counterparts (mandibular centrals before maxillary central, etc.).
- Primary teeth shed approximately three months to six months before their replacement teeth.

- Permanent teeth require approximately two or more years after eruption to finish calcification.

A general eruption pattern in orderly sequence is shown in the following table.

Months	Tooth
Primary Dentition	
6–12 months	Mandibular central incisor, 6–10 months
	Maxillary central incisor, 6–10 months
	Mandibular lateral incisor, 7–10 months
	Maxillary lateral incisor, 9–12 months
12–18 months	Mandibular first molar, 12–18 months
	Maxillary first molar, 12–18 months
16–22 months	Mandibular cuspid/canine, 16–22 months
	Maxillary cuspid/canine, 16–22 months
20–32 months	Mandibular second molar, 20–32 months
	Maxillary second molar, 24–32 months

(*Continued*)

Months	Tooth
Permanent Dentition	
6–8 years	Mandibular first molar, 6–7 years
	Maxillary first molar, 6–7 years
	Mandibular central incisor, 6–7 years
	Maxillary central incisor, 7–8 years
9–12 years	Mandibular cuspid/canine, 9–10 years
	Maxillary cuspid/canine, 11–12 years
10–12 years	Mandibular first premolar/bicuspid, 10–11 years
	Maxillary first premolar/bicuspid, 10–11 years
	Mandibular second premolar/bicuspid, 11–12 years
	Maxillary second premolar/bicuspid, 11–12 years
11–13 years	Mandibular second molar, 11–13 years
	Maxillary second molar, 12–13 years
17–21 years	All third molars (if present and erupting)

TISSUE STRUCTURE OF THE TEETH

All teeth possess the same tissue formations, anatomical basics, and structural landmarks. There are four types of teeth:

- incisors
- canines/cuspids
- premolars/bicuspids
- molars

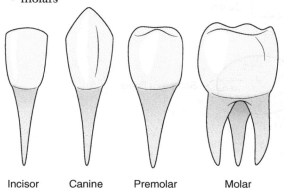

Incisor   Canine   Premolar   Molar

Enamel

Enamel (eh-**NAM**-el) is a hard tooth covering that is 96 percent inorganic. Tooth enamel exhibits a variety of unique structures and characteristics:

- **cuticle** (**KYOU**-tih-cal): also called **Nasmyth** (**NAHS**–myth) **membrane**, a tissue layer covering the tooth surfaces; soon wears away after eruption.
- **lines/stripes of Retzius** (**RET**-zee-us = *Swedish anatomist*): lines in enamel; also called bands or striae of Retzius (see Figure 3-4).
- **lamellae** (lah-**MEL**-ah = *thin plate or scale*): developmental cracks or imperfections in enamel tissue extending toward or into the dentin.
- **tuft** (*abnormal clump of rods*): irregular grouping of undercalcified enamel.
- **spindles** (**SPIN**-duls = *spindle-like processes*): end areas of union for odontoblasts and enamel rod endings.
- **rods:** slightly curved prism-like structures that extend from the dentinoenamel junction to the outer surface; tightly packed with an organic matrix material to give a smooth, hard surface (see Figure 3-4).
- **gnarled enamel** (**NARLD** = *twisted*): enamel rod twisting and curving within the tooth tissue.

Dentin

Dentin (**DEN**-tin), the main tissue of tooth surrounding the pulp, is less inorganic (70 percent) than enamel. It is slightly yellow-brown in color and gives bulk to the tooth. Dentin is present in both the crown and root and may exhibit two unique characteristics:

- **tubules** (**TOO**-bules = *small tubes*): S-shaped tubes or channels extending from the dentinoenamel wall to the pulp chamber. The tubules (see Figure 3-4) transmit pain stimuli and nutrition throughout the tissues.
- **fibers** (**FIGH**-bers = *thread-like films/elements*): also known as **Tomes' dentinal fibril**, fibers lying within the dentin tubule and help the dentin to nourish and register sensation.

Dentin gives shape to the tooth. It is softer than enamel but harder than the pulp tissue. The three different types of dentin tissue are:

- **primary dentin:** dentin in newly formed tooth, the original dentin.
- **regular secondary dentin:** occurs during regular development and maturing of tooth.
- **irregular secondary dentin:** occurs as protection from irritation, decay, trauma, attrition, and the

like. This irregular secondary dentin is also called "reparative dentin" or **tertiary** (**TERR**-shee-air-ee = *third*) **dentin,** the third type of dentin.

Pulp

Pulp (*soft, vascular tooth tissue*) is found in the center of the tooth. It is encased in the pulp chamber that is found in the crown and the pulp canal located in the root section of the tooth. **Pulp**

Figure 3-4 Posterior tooth with enlarged views of (A) enamel, (B) dentin, (C) cementum with periodontal attachment and pulp horns, pulp chamber, and pulp canal

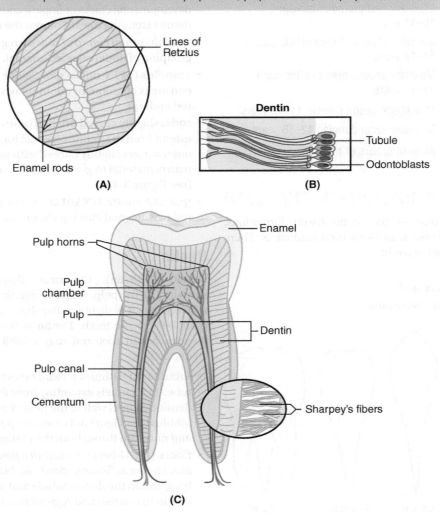

horns are pointed edges or boundaries of the pulp chamber extending toward the chewing surfaces (see Figure 3-4). The most organic tooth tissue, pulp performs four main functions: nourishment, defense, registration of sensation/pain, and dentin protection. The tooth pulp is composed of multiple cells called **fibroblasts** that are capable of developing connective tissue.

Four common diseases of the pulp are:

- **pulpitis** (pul-**PIE**-tis = *pulp inflammation*): also called toothache; occurs for many reasons.
- **pulp stone:** also known as **denticle** (**DEN**-tih-kal), a small growth in a tooth.
- **pulp cyst** (**SIST**): a closed, fluid-filled sac within the pulp tissue.
- **granuloma** (gran-you-**LOH**-mah = *granular tumor or growth*): a growth or tumor usually found in the root area.

Cementum

Cementum (see-**MEN**-tum = *tissue covering of tooth root*) is approximately 55 percent inorganic, rough in texture, and meets the enamel tissue at the **cementoenamel** (cement-enamel union) **junction** that is located at the neck of the tooth. The function of cementum is to protect the root and provide rough surface anchorage for attachment of **Sharpey's fibers**, which are connective tissue fibers of the periodontal ligament. There are two kinds of cementum:

- **Primary cementum:** original cementum that does not contain bone-type cells and is uniform in surface texture; also called **acellular** (ay-**SELL**-you-lar = *without cells*) **cementum**.
- **Secondary cementum:** contains bone-type cells and usually forms on the lower root surface as a result of stimulation, attrition, and wear; also called **cellular cementum**.

In addition to matrix material and cementoblasts, other features may be present in cementum:

- **lacuna** (lah-**KYOU**-nah = *small open space*): tiny cavities that may contain cementocytes (see-**MEN**-toh-sights = *irregular cementum-forming cells*).
- **canaliculi** (**kan**-ah-**LICK**-you-lie): small channels or canals.

- **hypercementosis** (**high**-per-**see**-men-**TOH**-sis = *overgrowth of cementum tissue*): an anomaly resulting in a thickening of cementum; usually occurs as a result of constant stress or occlusal trauma.

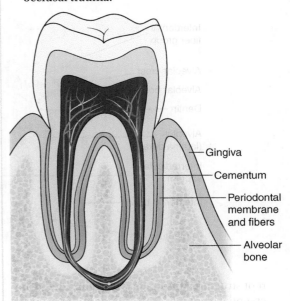

Gingiva
Cementum
Periodontal membrane and fibers
Alveolar bone

TISSUE COMPOSITION OF THE PERIODONTIUM

The anchorage, support, and protection of the teeth is provided by various tissues collectively called the **periodontium** (**pear**-ee-oh-**DANT**-ee-um = *tissues surrounding teeth*). The periodontium is composed mainly of four separate tissues:

- **periodontal** (**pear**-ee-oh-**DAHN**-tahl = *around tooth*): membrane and fibers that anchor the tooth in the alveolar socket.
- **alveolar** (al-**VEE**-oh-lar): bone, bony sockets, or crypts for teeth placement in the maxillae and the mandibular bone; the alveolar bone also gives support to the teeth.
- **gingiva** (**JIN**-jah-vah = *mouth tissue*): mucous tissue surrounding the teeth; also gives protection to the teeth and the underlying tissues.
- **cementum:** although we have discussed cementum as a tissue covering for the tooth

Figure 3-5 Principal fibers of the periodontium

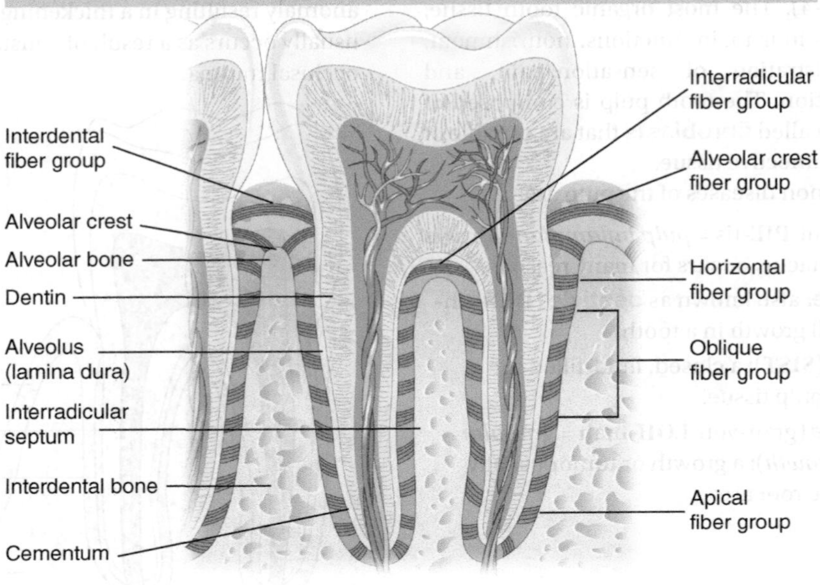

Labels (left side):
- Interdental fiber group
- Alveolar crest
- Alveolar bone
- Dentin
- Alveolus (lamina dura)
- Interradicular septum
- Interdental bone
- Cementum

Labels (right side):
- Interradicular fiber group
- Alveolar crest fiber group
- Horizontal fiber group
- Oblique fiber group
- Apical fiber group

root structure, this tissue is also considered an essential element of the periodontium.

Periodontal Membranes

Periodontal membranes, also called periodontal ligaments, are made up of connective tissues arranged in bundles and dense fibrous tissue groupings. There are five principal types of periodontal membranes or ligaments (Figure 3-5). The functions of each are as follows:

- **alveolar crest fibers:** found at the cementoenamel junction, they help to retain the tooth in its socket and to provide protection for the deeper fibers.
- **horizontal fibers:** connect the alveolar bone to the upper part of the root and assist with the control of the lateral movement.
- **oblique fibers:** attach the alveolar socket to the majority of the root cementum and assist in the resistance of the axial forces.
- **apical fiber bundles:** running from the apex of the tooth to the alveolar bone, these fibers

help prevent tipping and dislocation, as well as protect the nerve and blood supply to the tooth.

- **interradicular fiber bundles:** present in multirooted teeth, extending apically from the tooth furcation, help the tooth resist tipping, turning, and dislocation.

Alveolar Bone

The alveolar bone, also called the alveolar process, is composed of an alveolar socket and a dense covering of compact bone with an inner and outer growth called the **cortical plate**. Lining the alveolar socket is a thin **cribriform** (**KRIB**-rih-form = *sieve-like*) **plate** covering called the **lamina dura** (**LAM**-ah-nah **DUR**-ah = *hard lining*). This outline is easily viewed on radiographs as a thin radiopaque line.

Gingiva

Also known as gum tissue, the gingiva protects the tooth root and underlying tissues. It is composed of various epithelial layers, some of which are attached and some of which are free gingiva. These tissue layers will be discussed more in Chapter 16, Periodontics, but they are listed here as well:

- **attached:** the portion that is firm, dense, stippled, and bound to the underlying periosteum, tooth, and bone.
- **keratinized** (**KARE**-ah-tin-ized = *hard* or *horny*): hard tissue, also called *masticatory mucos,* the area where the gingiva and mucous membrane unite.
- **mucogingival** (myou-koh-**JIN**-jah-vahl), or vermillion border, indicated by the color changes from pink gingiva to red mucosa.
- **marginal:** the portion that is unattached to underlying tissues and helps to form the sides of the gingival crevice, also called the free margin gingiva.
- **sulcus:** a space forming the gingival area between the tooth and attached gingival measuring approximately 1–3 mm in depth.
- **papillary:** the part of the marginal gingiva that occupies the interproximal spaces.
- **interdental papilla:** normally a triangular space that fills the tooth embrasure area.

Cementum

The function of the cementum in the periodontium is to provide surface anchorage for the tooth in the alveolar socket. This is accomplished by the covering of Sharpey's fibers that extend between the rough cementum surface and the alveolar wall.

ODONTOLOGY/MORPHOLOGY

Although teeth differ in size and shape, they have many attributes and characteristics in common. They are composed of the same four tissues arising from the same germ cells and share many common features in form and structure. The study of teeth in general is called **odontology** (oh-dahn-**TAHL**-oh-jee), while the study of tooth form and shape is termed **morphology** (more-**FALL**-oh-gee).

Characteristics

The dentition shares the following mouth division characteristics and terminology, seen in Figure 3-6:

- **maxillary:** upper tooth area; normally the maxilla slightly overlaps the mandible.
- **mandibular:** lower tooth area; moves up and down to meet the maxillary teeth.
- **arch** (*curved-like or bow-like outline*): half of the mouth, either maxillary or mandibular.
- **quadrant** (**KWAH**-drant = *one-fourth*): half of an arch, right or left, and containing eight teeth.
- **anterior** (an-**TEE**-ree-or = *before or in front of*): front area of the mouth, from canine (cuspid) to canine (cuspid).
- **posterior** (pahs-**TEE**-ree-or = *toward the rear*): area back from the corners of the mouth, not including the canine (cuspid) or incisor teeth.

Types of Teeth

The four types of teeth are incisors, cuspids (canines), premolars (bicuspids), and molars. **Incisors** (in-**SIGH**-zors = *cutter*) are single-rooted anterior teeth with a sharp cutting edge. Maxillary incisors are larger than mandibular incisors; their root is approximately 1.5 times longer than the crown area. The central incisor gives character to the face and smile. The lateral incisors resemble the central but are smaller, and the incisal edge turns more distally. The laterals may show irregularities such as a peg shape and are frequently missing as a result of genetic origin. The mandibular laterals are wider than their centrals, while the maxillary centrals are wider than their laterals. The central incisor area is the only place where the mesial edge of one tooth is adjacent to the mesial side of another tooth.

Cuspids (**KUSS**-pids) are single-rooted anterior teeth at the corner of the mouth; they are also called the **canines** (**KAY**-nines). The cuspid is the longest tooth in the mouth and divides the anterior from the posterior. The mandibular cuspid resembles the maxillary cuspid but is not as pointed and is thicker in the distal portion.

Premolars (pree-**MOH**-lers = *before a molar*) are the fourth and fifth teeth posterior from the center of the mouth. The maxillary teeth are sometimes called *bicuspids* because the cusps are large and well defined. The mandibular teeth are called premolars because they resemble a molar in form. Either name

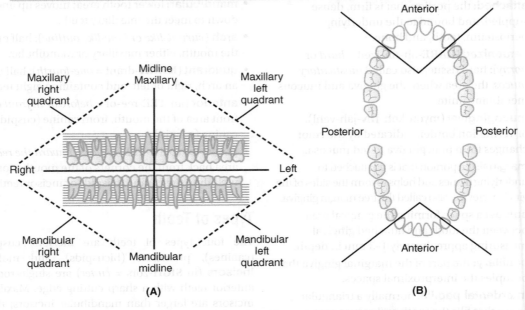

Figure 3-6 Divisions of the human dentition

Midline Maxillary

Maxillary right quadrant

Maxillary left quadrant

Right — Left

Mandibular right quadrant

Mandibular midline

Mandibular left quadrant

(A)

Anterior

Posterior — Posterior

Anterior

(B)

is correct. The maxillary first bicuspid exhibits two root canals even if the root's bifurcation is not apparent to the eye, and it is normally smaller than its second bicuspid. The mandibular premolars are rounder and imitate the molar teeth to follow.

Molars (**MOH**-lars = *grinding tooth*) are the most posterior teeth, excluding the premolars. The maxillary molar teeth have three roots, termed **trifurcation** (**tri**-fur-**KAY**-shun = *branching into three parts*). The mandibular molars have two roots, termed **bifurcation** (**bye**-fer-**KAY**-shun = *branching into two parts*). The maxillary first molar, the largest of the three, can exhibit an extra cusp on the meso-lingual cusp area, which is called the **cusp of Carabelli**. The second molar resembles the first but is smaller. The mandibular second molar is smaller than the first molar but resembles it in shape. The maxillary molars are more diamond or round shaped, while the mandibular molars have more of a box shape. The maxillary and mandibular third molars are often misshapen or distorted due to their placement. These molars are termed "wisdom teeth" because their eruption dates are late, from 17 to 21 years of age (presumably when wisdom is supposed to come!).

Tooth Anatomy/Morphology

The anatomy of the tooth involves a variety of parts, some of which are illustrated in Figure 3-7, and all of which are described here:

- **crown:** the top part of the tooth containing the pulp chamber, dentin, and enamel covering. The crown is classified in one of two ways:
  - **anatomical crown:** covered with enamel and may not be totally visible but will be present the entire life of tooth.
  - **clinical crown:** surface visible in the oral cavity; may not be totally visible for various reasons, such as impaction, hyperplasia, mal-position, immaturity, and the like.
- **root:** bottom part of a tooth; may have a single root, be bifurcated into two roots, or as in the maxillary molar teeth, be trifurcated into three roots.
- **cervical line:** the place where the enamel of the crown meets the cementum of the root. This area is called the cementoenamel junction or the **cervix** (**SIR**-vicks = *neck*) of the tooth.

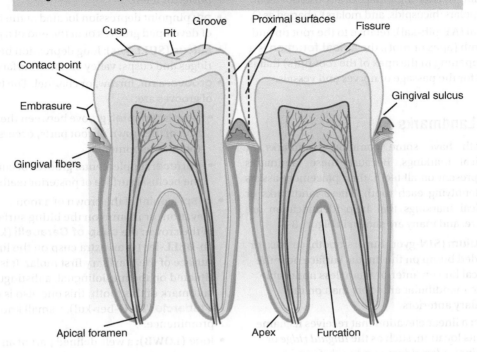

Figure 3-7 Examples of common tooth terms

Cusp · Pit · Groove · Proximal surfaces · Fissure
Contact point
Gingival sulcus
Embrasure
Gingival fibers
Apical foramen · Apex · Furcation

TOOTH SURFACES

A tooth has six major surfaces, of which the apical surface end is actually only a tip. The following terms indicate the various surfaces of teeth:

- **buccal** (**BUCK**-al = *cheek*): posterior tooth surface toward the cheeks; charted as B.
- **facial** (**FAY**-shal): anterior tooth surface toward the lips; charted as F.
- **lingual** (**LIN**-gwal = *tongue*): the surface of all teeth toward the tongue; charted as L.
- **mesial** (**ME**-zee-al = *to the middle*): side surface of a tooth closest to the midline (middle) of the face; charted as M.
- **distal** (**DIS**-tal = *to the distant, away*): side surface of a tooth farthest from the midline of the face; charted as D.
- **incisal** (in-**SIGH**-zel = *to cut*): cutting edge of anterior teeth (centrals, laterals, and cuspids/canines); charted as I.

- **apex** (**AY**-pecks = *the root end*): the tip end of a tooth; one apex is at each end of each root tip.
- **contact area:** surface point or area where two teeth meet side by side (widest part of tooth); if no contact occurs, the open area is referred to as a **diastema** (dye-ah-**STEE**-mah).
- **embrasure:** a V-shaped area located between the contact point of two teeth and the gingival crest.
- **proximal surface:** side wall of a tooth that meets or touches the side wall of another tooth.
- **axial surfaces:** long-length surface of the tooth.
- **line angle:** meeting of two surfaces on a tooth, such as mesial and incisal surfaces.
- **point angle:** the meeting of three surfaces on a tooth, such as mesial, incisal, and labial.
- **midline:** imaginary vertical line bisecting the head at the middle; determines the right and left sides.
- **antagonist** (an-**TAG**-oh-nist = *opposing tooth*): tooth that counteracts, occludes, or contacts with another tooth in the opposing arch.

- **occlusal** (oh-**KLOO**-zal = *to grind, meet*): grinding or chewing surface of all posterior teeth (premolars/bicuspids, and molars); charted as O.
- **apical** (**AY**-pih-kal): relative to the root tip end of tooth (apex or root); the **apical foramen** is a tiny opening in the apex of the root tip(s) that is used for the passage of nerves and vessels.

Tooth Landmarks

The teeth have some common landmarks or anatomical markings. Because these landmarks are not present on all teeth, their placement assists us in identifying each tooth. These landmarks or anatomical markings that help identification are listed here, and many are shown in Figure 3-7:

- **cingulum** (**SIN**-gyou-lum): smooth, convex, or rounded bump on the lingual surface near the cervical line on anterior teeth; less noticeable on the mandibular anteriors than on the maxillary anteriors.
- **ridge:** a linear elevation that receives its name from its location, such as the *lingual ridge* or *marginal ridge*; ridges commonly found on teeth include the following:
  - **marginal ridges:** rounded enamel elevations on the occlusal surface of the posteriors, the linguals of anteriors, and the mesial and distal surfaces of all teeth.
  - **transverse ridge:** occurs on occlusal surface of the posterior teeth at a point where two triangular ridges meet.
  - **triangular ridge:** named after the cusps involved in the triangular ridge, from the cusp tips to the central groove on the occlusal surface of posterior teeth.
  - **oblique ridge:** a slanting ridge found on the maxillary molars, which is present more on the first molar than the second molar.
- **fissure** (**FISH**-er): a groove or natural depression, slit, or break; also may be an incomplete lobe union in enamel surface of a tooth.
- **fossa** (**FAH**-sah): a shallow, rounded, irregular depression or concavity on the lingual surface of anterior teeth and on the occlusal surfaces of posterior teeth.
- **pit:** pinpoint depression located at the junction of developed grooves or at the end of a groove.
- **sulcus** (**SULL**-kus): long depression between ridges and cusps; valley on tooth surface.
- **groove:** a rut, furrow, or channel. The two types of grooves are:
  - **developmental:** groove between the junction of the crown or root parts; occurs during tooth development.
  - **surface:** supplemental grooves occurring on the occlusal surface of posterior teeth.
- **cusp:** a point of the crown of a tooth, elevation, or mound on the biting surface of the crown; the **cusp of Carabelli** (kare-ah-**BELL**-lee) is an extra cusp on the lingual surface of the maxillary first molar. It is situated on the mesiolingual, a distinguishing landmark of this tooth; this one also is called a **tubercle** (**TWO**-ber-kul), a small knob-like prominence.
- **lobe** (**LOWB**): a well-defined part of an organ that develops into a tooth formation; a developing cusp that eventually unites with other lobes to form a complete tooth.
- **furrow** (**FUR**-oh): a shallow concave groove located on either the crown or the root; also called a "developmental depression."
- **eminence** (**EM**-in-ence): a high place, projection, or prominence.
- **furcation** (fur-**KAY**-shun = *fork or branch off*): the place where tooth roots branch apart.
- **mamelon** (**MAM**-el-lon): bumps forming a scallop border of the incisal edge of newly erupted anteriors; because of attrition, mamelons wear away shortly after eruption and become remnants of lobe forms. The presence of mamelons on an older child or adult is usually an indication of malocclusion.

Figure 3-8 A to D illustrates each tooth in the dentition, giving notice to important landmarks on specific teeth and the identification of tooth surfaces.

Figure 3-8 Tooth identification (*Continues*)

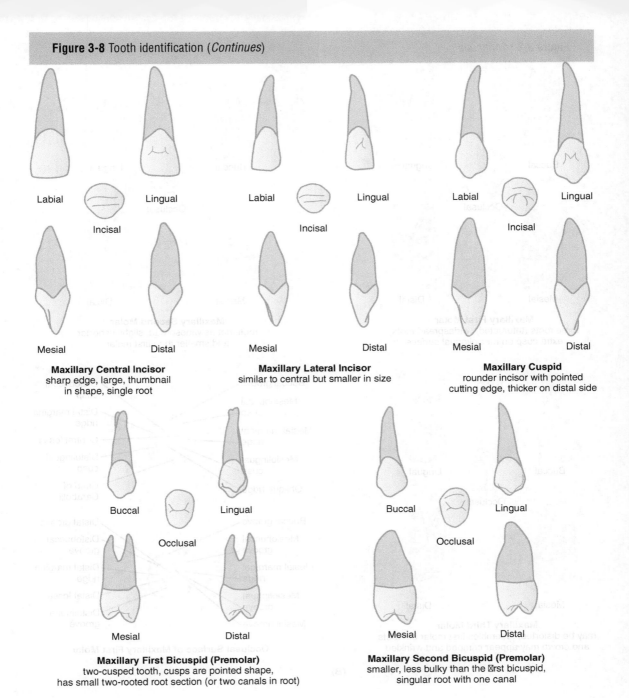

Labial   Lingual
Incisal
Mesial   Distal

Maxillary Central Incisor
sharp edge, large, thumbnail
in shape, single root

Labial   Lingual
Incisal
Mesial   Distal

Maxillary Lateral Incisor
similar to central but smaller in size

Labial   Lingual
Incisal
Mesial   Distal

Maxillary Cuspid
rounder incisor with pointed
cutting edge, thicker on distal side

Buccal   Lingual
Occlusal
Mesial   Distal

Maxillary First Bicuspid (Premolar)
two-cusped tooth, cusps are pointed shape,
has small two-rooted root section (or two canals in root)

Buccal   Lingual
Occlusal
Mesial   Distal

Maxillary Second Bicuspid (Premolar)
smaller, less bulky than the first bicuspid,
singular root with one canal

(A)

53

Figure 3-8 (*Continued*)

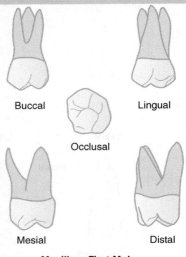

Buccal

Lingual

Occlusal

Mesial

Distal

Maxillary First Molar
three roots (trifurcated), widespread roots,
extra cusp on mesiolingual surface

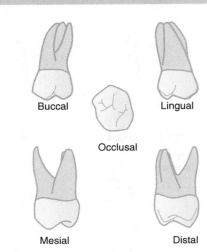

Buccal

Lingual

Occlusal

Mesial

Distal

Maxillary Second Molar
roots not as widespread, slightly shorter
and smaller than first molar

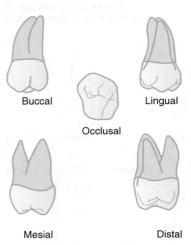

Buccal

Lingual

Occlusal

Mesial

Distal

Maxillary Third Molar
may be distorted, resembles first molar but roots
and crown may appear crimped and wrinkled

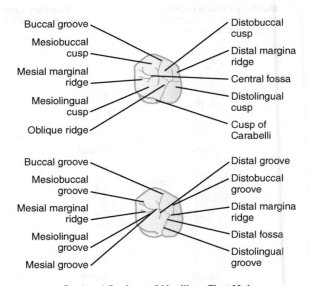

Buccal groove
Mesiobuccal cusp
Mesial marginal ridge
Mesiolingual cusp
Oblique ridge

Distobuccal cusp
Distal marginal ridge
Central fossa
Distolingual cusp
Cusp of Carabelli

Buccal groove
Mesiobuccal groove
Mesial marginal ridge
Mesiolingual groove
Mesial groove

Distal groove
Distobuccal groove
Distal marginal ridge
Distal fossa
Distolingual groove

Occlusal Surface of Maxillary First Molar

(B)

Figure 3-8 (*Continued*)

Labial   Lingual

Incisal

Mesial   Distal

Mandibular Central Incisor
no cingulum, resembles maxillary,
central but smaller, single root

Labial   Lingual

Incisal

Mesial   Distal

Mandibular Lateral Incisor
larger than central incisal edge,
incisal edge curves toward distal

Labial   Lingual

Incisal

Mesial   Distal

Mandibular Cuspid
bulkier, pointed cutting edge,
single root

Buccal   Lingual

Occlusal

Mesial   Distal

Mandibular First Bicuspid (Premolar)
lingual cusps smaller than buccal cusps, single root,
smaller than second premolar,
occlusal view may appear as bell shape

Buccal   Lingual

Occlusal

Mesial   Distal

Mandibular Second Bicuspid (Premolar)
larger than first bicuspid, lingual cuspid may split
or look like two buccal cusps, single root,
sometimes looks like a three-cusped tooth

(C)

Figure 3-8 (*Continued*)

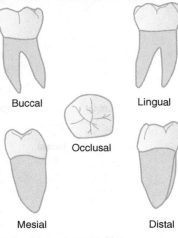

Mandibular First Molar
two roots (bifurcated), widespread,
box shape with five cusps

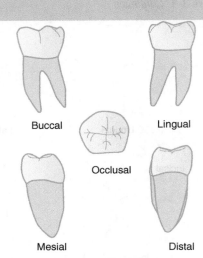

Mandibular Second Molar
two roots, rectangular, box
shape with four regular cusps

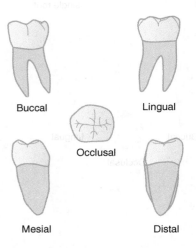

Mandibular Third Molar
two roots and cusps underdeveloped,
usually wrinkled

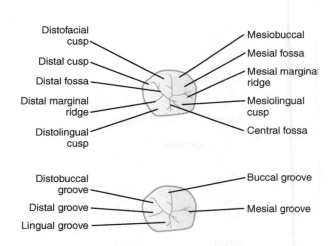

Occlusal Surface of Mandibular First Molar

(D)

Review Exercises

Matching

Match the following word elements with their meanings.

1. _____ microdontia
2. _____ odontology
3. _____ exfoliate
4. _____ heterodont
5. _____ ameloblasts
6. _____ fibroblasts
7. _____ fusion
8. _____ quadrant
9. _____ anomaly
10. _____ diastema
11. _____ occlusal
12. _____ lingual
13. _____ succedaneous
14. _____ deciduous
15. _____ pulp
16. _____ anodontia
17. _____ fluorosis
18. _____ cuticle
19. _____ initiation
20. _____ pulpitis

A. toothache
B. pulp tissue cells
C. not normal
D. chewing surface of posterior teeth
E. Nasmyth membrane
F. mottled enamel
G. one-fourth of oral cavity, one-half of arch
H. surface of tooth touching tongue
I. unusually small teeth
J. without teeth
K. soft, vascular tissue, center of tooth
L. joining together, union
M. open space between adjacent teeth, open contacts
N. enamel forming cell
O. scale off, shed
P. primary teeth
Q. permanent teeth
R. study of teeth and their form
S. teeth of various shapes
T. first stage of tooth development

Definitions

Using the selection given for each sentence, choose the best term to complete the definition.

1. Which bicuspid/premolar exhibits two root canals even if the tooth bifurcation is not apparent to the eye?
   a. maxillary first bicuspid/premolar
   b. mandibular first premolar/bicuspid
   c. mandibular second premolar
   d. maxillary second bicuspid/premolar

2. The stripes or bands of Retzius are found in which tooth tissue?
   a. enamel
   b. cementum
   c. dentin
   d. pulp

3. The building cell that forms the bulk tissue of the tooth is:
   a. ameloblast
   b. fibroclast
   c. odontoblast
   d. cementoclast

4. Newly formed or original dentin is which type of dentin?
   a. primary
   b. secondary
   c. teritary
   d. reparative

5. Morphodifferentiation refers to a change of tooth:
   a. tissues
   b. materials
   c. position
   d. shape

6. Sharpey's fibers are:
   a. connective tissues that make up and compose the pulp tissues
   b. nerve fibers that register sensation
   c. part of the periodontal ligament system

7. Which tooth is the longest tooth of the maxillary arch?
   a. first molar
   b. first bicuspid
   c. canine
   d. incisor

8. Anchoring and support of the teeth is provided by the:
   a. periodontium
   b. periodontosis
   c. cribriform plate
   d. tubules

9. An overgrowth of cementum tissue on the root area is called:
   a. rootoexcession
   b. hypercementosis
   c. hypocementosis
   d. anacementa

10. Bud stages of tooth development for the deciduous anterior teeth begin about what age?
    a. five or six weeks in utero
    b. third month of pregnancy
    c. birth
    d. one year of age

11. Which of the following is not a gingival tissue?
    a. lamina dura
    b. papillary
    c. marginal
    d. keratinized tissue

12. What is the name of the permanent teeth that replace the deciduous teeth?
    a. heterdont
    b. dentition
    c. succedaneous
    d. primary

13. Peg-shaped laterals are most common on which maxillary teeth?
    a. cuspids
    b. incisors
    c. premolars
    d. laterals

14. The cusp of Carabelli may be found on which tooth?
    a. maxillary central incisor
    b. mandibular second molar
    c. mandibular lateral
    d. maxillary first molar

15. During tooth formation, the middle layer of tissue is called:
    a. mesoderm
    b. ectoderm
    c. entoderm
    d. bioderm

16. The surface of the tooth closest to the midline is called:
    a. distal
    b. mesial
    c. occlusal
    d. saggital

17. A groove, natural depression, or slit in the enamel of the tooth is called:
    a. ridge
    b. fissure
    c. mamelon
    d. sulcus

18. A high place or projection of a tissue is called a(n):
    a. eminence
    b. apex
    c. sulcus
    d. occlusion

19. The single-rooted tooth found at the corner of the mouth is called:
    a. bicuspid
    b. incisor
    c. canine
    d. lateral

20. The Nasmyth membrane is another word for the tooth:
    a. surface
    b. periodontal tissues
    c. cuticle
    d. enamel

Building Skills

Locate and define the prefix, root/combining form, and suffix (if present) in the following words.

1. **hypercementosis**
   prefix _____
   root/combining form _____
   suffix _____

2. **mucogingival**
   prefix _____
   root/combining form _____
   suffix _____

3. **bifurcation**
   prefix _____
   root/combining form _____
   suffix _____

4. **periodontitis**
   prefix _____
   root/combining form _____
   suffix _____

5. **odontology**
   prefix _____
   root/combining form _____
   suffix _____

Fill-Ins

Write the correct word in the blank space to complete each statement.

1. Because the human dentition contains teeth of various sizes and shapes, the dentition is considered to be _____.

2. The last stage of tooth development is called _____.

3. Amelogenesis is a genetic disorder resulting in the production of defective _____ _____ tissue.

4. A hard tooth-like mass that develops in a small cavity inside the tooth is called _____ _____.

5. Tomes' tubules are small S-shaped tubes or channels within the _____ _____ tissues of a tooth.

6. Another word for primary teeth is _____ _____.

7. A minute depression located at the junction of a developed groove or at the end of the grooves is called a _____.

8. The reaction of overfluoridation to enamel is called _____.

9. Developmental lobes or bumps on the incisal edge of new maxillary anteriors are called _____ _____.

10. The main tissue of the tooth that surrounds the pulp is _____.

11. The small opening in the apex of the root that permits the passage of the nerve and vessels is called the _____.

12. A V-shaped area between the contact point of two adjacent teeth and the gingival crest is a/an _____ _____.

13. The lining of the alveolar socket is completed by the cribriform plate called the _____ _____.

14. The chewing surface of the posterior teeth is the _____ surface.

15. The presence of both deciduous and permanent teeth in the mouth is termed a/an _____ _____ dentition.

16. The condition of having more than the normal amount of teeth is called _____.

17. A line angle is the union or junction of _____ tooth surfaces.

18. The facial surface of the tooth that touches the lip is also called the _____ surface.

19. A convex, rounded bump on the lingual surface of anterior teeth is called a/an _____ _____.

20. A tooth that comes in contact with or meets in occlusion with the opposing tooth is called a/an

_____.

Word Use

Read the following sentences, and define the meaning of the word written in boldface letters.

1. The process of **calcification** is not complete until two years after eruption of the tooth.

_____

_____

2. An enlarged frenum could be the reason for a **diastema** of the maxillary incisors.

_____

_____

3. During the exam and prophylaxis, the hygienist records the **sulcus** measurements.

_____

_____

4. The assistant prepared the anesthetic syringe for infiltration anesthesia of the lower-left **quadrant**.

_____

_____

5. The dentist explained that deciduous teeth have widespread roots to make room for the **succedaneous** teeth.

_____

_____

CHAPTER 4

PRACTICE AND FACILITY SETUPS

✔ Learning Objectives

On completion of this chapter, you should be able to:

1. Name and discuss the different roles of the professionals who render dental care.

2. Describe the various places and organizational structures in the field of dentistry where qualified and interested parties work.

3. List and explain the use of the major hand instruments used in dental procedures.

4. List and explain the use of the major rotary instruments in dental care procedures.

5. Describe the common operative equipment used in the dental operatory and office environments.

DENTAL PROFESSIONALS

Each profession speaks a language of its own, using terms or words connected with its common procedures, personnel, techniques, and instrumentation. People who are involved with, use the language of, and participate in each of these occupations are said to be *professionals* of that occupation. Others who are not related to or familiar with this profession are called *lay people*. Each of the many different types of personnel associated with the dental profession performs a special function or meets a particular need. Some are directly involved with the practice, and others provide support.

Dentist

The dentist, who is a Doctor of Dental Surgery (DDS) or a Doctor of Medical Dentistry (DMD), diagnoses, performs, and monitors the dental care of patients. Various specialists, who complete extended studies, training, and testing, perform the following specific duties or skills of their particular specialty. The official ADA-recognized special areas are listed here:

- **prosthodontist (prahs**-thoh-**DOHN**-tist): replaces missing teeth with artificial appliances such as dental crowns, full mouth dentures, or partial bridgework.

Vocabulary Related to Practice and Facility Setups

This list contains selected new and important terms from this chapter. Take the time to learn these word parts and their meanings. You may use the list to review these terms and practice pronouncing them correctly. When you work with the audio for this chapter, listen to the word, repeat it, and then place a checkmark in the box. Proceed to the next boxed word and repeat the process.

Key Terms

- ❑ **armamentarium (ar**-mah-men-**TARE**-ee-um)
- ❑ **cleoid (KLEE**-oyd)
- ❑ **curette** (kyou-**RETT**)
- ❑ **cuspidor** (kuss-pih-**DORE**)
- ❑ **dentated (DEN**-tay-ted)
- ❑ **denturist (DEN**-ture-ist)
- ❑ **endodontist** (en-doh-**DAHN**-tist)
- ❑ **excavator (ECKS**-kah-vay-tore)
- ❑ **forensic** (for-**EN**-sick)
- ❑ **mandrel (MAN**-drell)
- ❑ **matrix (MAY**-tricks)
- ❑ **maxillofacial (mack**-sill-oh-**FAY**-shul)
- ❑ **operatory (AH**-purr-ah-tore-ee)
- ❑ **orthodontist** (ore-thoh-**DON**-tist)
- ❑ **pediatric** (pee-dee-**AT**-trick)
- ❑ **periodontist** (pear-ee-oh-**DAHN**-tist)
- ❑ **prosthodontist** (prahs-thoh-**DAHN**-tist)
- ❑ **rheostat (REE**-oh-stat)
- ❑ **scalpel (SKAL**-pell)
- ❑ **truncated (TRUN**-kay-ted)

- **periodontist** (pear-ee-oh-**DOHN**-tist): treats diseases of periodontal (gingiva and supporting) tissues.
- **orthodontist** (**or**-thoh-**DON**-tist): corrects malocclusion and improper jaw alignment.
- **pediatric** (pee-dee-**AT**-trick) **dentist:** performs dental procedures for the child patient, also called **pedodontist** (**PEE**-doh-**don**-tist).
- **endodontist** (en-doh-**DAHN**-tist): treats the diseased pulp and periradicular structures.
- **oral and maxillofacial** (**mack**-sill-oh-**FAY**-shal) **surgeon:** performs surgical treatment of the teeth, jaws, and related areas.
- **public health dentist:** works on causes and prevention of common dental diseases and promotes dental health to the community or general population.
- **oral pathologist:** studies the nature, diagnosis, and control of oral diseases.
- **oral and maxillofacial radiologist:** concerned with the production and interpretation of radiant energy images or data regarding the oral and maxillofacial regions.
- **forensic** (for-**EN**-sick) **dentist:** discovers and uses pathological evidence for legal proceedings; forensic dentistry is not yet established as a recognized specialty but is organized and related to a particular type of dental care.

Each licensed dentist is permitted to perform general dental procedures in any or all of the various areas of dentistry. Some dentists, while not technically specialists, may limit their practice to only one specialty area such as oral surgery, orthodontics, or the like, servicing only those types of patients. Other dentists may advertise and perform procedures in special dental areas of interest, such as amalgam free, cosmetic, diagnostic, implant, sedation, TMJ, holistic dentistry, and so forth.

The official organization of the dentists and dental specialists, the **American Dental Association (ADA),** has branches on the state (constituent) and local (component) levels. As

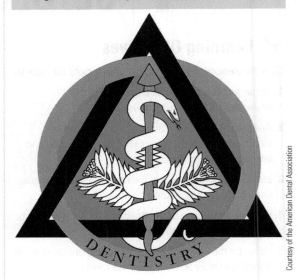

Figure 4-1 ADA logo

Courtesy of the American Dental Association

illustrated in Figure 4-1, the official seal of the ADA is a triangle containing the Greek letter D (triangle) for dentistry and a serpent on the staff indicating a healing art. The branch on one side contains 20 leaves for the deciduous teeth, and the branch with 32 leaves on the other side represents the permanent teeth. All symbols are encircled with the ring of health.

Registered Dental Hygienist

The **registered dental hygienist (RDH)** completes postsecondary education in dental hygiene instruction. An RDH is board-tested in theory and proficiency and state registered. Most states require the presence of the responsible dentist in the clinical setting, but some states permit independent dental hygiene practice in outside areas. The hygienist is concerned with the prevention of dental disease, specializing in the cleaning, polishing, and radiographing of teeth, periodontal treatment, fluoride and sealant application, and patient education. The hygienist, if educated, tested, and certified as state approved, may also perform some operative or supportive procedures such as nitrous oxide and/or anesthetic injection administration, application of microbial agents, patient assessment, and interpretation of X-rays and testing results. The dental hygienist who completes the advanced ADHA educational curriculum may earn **ADHP (advanced dental hygiene practitioner** or **dental therapist)** certification. The official organization of hygienists is the **American Dental Hygienist Association (ADHA)**, with branches at the state (constituent) and local (component) levels.

Dental Assistant

The **dental assistant** aids the dentist in diagnosis, treatment, dental care, and general duties. The dental assistant may be an **RDA** (state registered dental assistant), a **CDA** (nationally certified dental assistant), or an expanded functions dental assistant **(EFDA)**. Each state regulates the permissible duties, functions, and designated titles of expanded function duty personnel. Dentists will delegate restorative and preventative duties to the EFDA.

Specialized certifications are offered by the **Dental Assisting National Board (DANB)**. These certifications include **CDA (Certified Dental Assistant)** and **COA (Certified Orthodontic Assistant)**. Certificates of Competency can be earned in Radiation Health and Safety (RHS) and Infection Control (ICE). The official dental assistant organization is the **American Dental Assistants Association (ADAA)**, with constituent, component, and local level branches.

Dental Laboratory Technician

The **dental laboratory technician** performs dental lab procedures under written orders from a licensed dentist. The technician may receive on-the-job training (OJT) or be educated in a laboratory or school setting. The technician may be a **certified dental technician (CDT)**. The official organization for these professionals is the **National Association of Dental Laboratories (NADL)**, which also has state and local level branches.

Other Dental Professionals

Other related dental professionals include dental supply/detail persons, dental equipment technicians, and dental manufacturers and suppliers. Some dental professionals dedicate their careers to research, education, and the development of oral medicine.

PLACES OF EMPLOYMENT

Qualified and interested parties may work in various places and organizational structures in the field of dentistry, as described in the following list:

- **Solo:** dental practice owned and operated by a single dentist or a practice that is owned by a dentist who contracts with another dentist (an associate) to work in the establishment with the owner.
- **Partnership:** dental practice owned and operated equally by two or more dentists.
- **Group:** dental practice employing a multitude of dentists. It might be incorporated and owned by the working dentists or owned and operated by an outside corporation or dental health plan.
- **Clinics and hospitals:** a clinic setting or hospital care center that offers dentistry services. Many hospitals grant privileges to dentists to bring difficult or compromised patients for dental care using hospital services. Oral surgeons may be staff members and work in the hospital and in their private offices.
- **Specialty practice:** various specialists work in private offices or facilities concerned with their training. Public health specialists may work in outpatient clinics, field establishments, schools, and offices. Forensic specialists may work in the lab, field, and court.
- **Miscellaneous practice sites:** includes research, insurance companies, education, publication, specialty houses, employment and recruiting agencies, charity clinics, and other areas.

DENTAL HAND INSTRUMENTS

Each profession employs its own type and kind of instrumentation. Just as a baseball team requires balls, bats, masks, and gloves, dentistry requires specialized equipment for operation. Some tools are in common use in all aspects of dentistry, and others are constructed for various specialized procedures. Following are the standard instruments, grouped by their related family of use.

Hand Grasp Instruments

Hand instruments may have one working end (single-ended) or a working end at each of the opposite sides (double-ended). Working ends on the same instrument may vary in size, function, or location of operative site locations. Many instruments are named for an inventor or school where they were designed. Instruments are grouped into families according to function and are constructed of various materials from stainless steel to hard resin. All instruments have the following three components, as shown in Figure 4-2:

- **Shaft or handle:** used to grasp the instrument; supplied in various weights, diameters, and surfaces that may be smooth, padded (tactile), grooved or serrated; may be rounded or octagonal-shaped plastic or metal with manufacturer's name and/or formula code etched on one side.
- **Shank:** connects the handle to the working end; sometimes called the *instrument neck*. The shank may be straight, curved, or angled to accommodate specific areas of the mouth.
- **Working end:** also called *blade* or *nib*; rounded end is the *toe*; the pointed end is the *tip*, which may be beveled, curved, scooped, or spoon shaped and present on both ends.

Basic Dental Setup

Dental hand instruments are conveniently grouped into families of use, such as diagnostic, restorative, finishing, surgical, periodontal, and so forth, but this

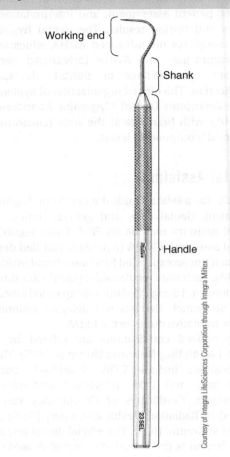

Figure 4-2 Components of hand instruments

Working end
Shank
Handle

does not limit their use. A hand instrument may be used at the operator's choice in any specific duty or function desired. The instruments in this chapter will be grouped and shown in families.

Basic or Diagnostic Grouping

The basic or diagnostic dental setup is an instrument collection composed of a mouth mirror, explorer, periodontal probe, cotton forceps or pickup, and a piece of 2 × 2 gauze and is used in most arrangements, alone or with other instruments (Figure 4-3). A setup is also called an **armamentarium** (**ar**-mah-men-**TARE**-ee-um).

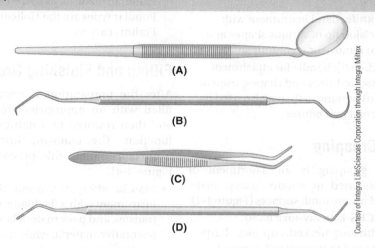

(A)

(B)

(C)

(D)

Courtesy of Integra LifeSciences Corporation through Integra Miltex

- **mouth mirror:** used for reflection, retraction, and visual observation; supplied in various sizes from 1 (16 mm) to 6 (26 mm) and may have one side or double-sided plain faces or faces that magnify the view. Some are solid, one piece; others have cone screw-in handles.

- **explorer:** a sharp, flexible, pointed instrument used to detect caries and calculus; to explore restorations, surfaces, and furcations; to make location marks; and to pick up cotton points or materials. This tool is supplied in multiple shapes as single or double ended with an explorer edge on one side and another type of edge on the opposite side.

- **cotton forceps:** tweezer-like pinchers used to transport materials to or from the mouth; also called *dressing pliers*; available with or without serrated tips.

- **periodontal probe:** a longer pointed instrument with measured marks on the tip; used to assess depths of tissue pockets; available with a round or flat blade and may be color-coded to help determine measurements.

- **expro** (**EX**-pro): double-ended instrument with a diagnosing probe tip at one end and an explorer tip at the other end.

Periodontal Grouping

The periodontal group is a family of instruments used to treat and care for the gingival and periodontal tissues. They will be discussed more in Chapter 16, Periodontology.

- **scaler:** thin-bladed hand instrument with pointed tip and two cutting edges; used to scale or (scrape off) supragingival hard deposits from teeth; designed for quadrant use.

- **sickle scaler:** sharp blade in the shape of a sickle; used to remove calculus from tooth surfaces.

- **scallette:** hygiene instrument combining a scaler on one tip and a curette on the other tip to save time and tray space during treatment.

- **curette** (kyou-**RETT**): rounded-tipped thin blade with a longer neck and two cutting edges; designed for specific tooth area and used to remove subgingival deposits.

- **implant scaler/curette:** nonmetallic, resin-tipped instrument, designed to remove deposits around titanium implant abutments. Some thin bladed, titanium scalers/curettes have been developed to use safely and not mar the metal implant abutments.

- **periodontal file:** hand instrument with rough edge or teeth working surface; used to smooth in root planning.
- **periodontal knife:** hand instrument with flat-bladed incision tip of various shapes and angles; used to remove or recontour soft tissue.
- **scalpel** (**SKAL**-pell): handle for attachment of blades of assorted sizes and shapes; used to incise (cut into) or remove tissue; also used in specialized dental procedures.

Restorative Grouping

The restorative grouping is an assortment of hand instruments used to remove decay, make preparations, and restore tooth surfaces (Figure 4-4):

- **excavator** (**ECKS**-kah-vay-tor): hand instrument with long-necked, cup-like, sharp-edged blades; used to remove soft decayed tissue from preparations; also may be called *spoon excavators*.
- **gingival margin trimmer:** hand instrument with long, slender, curved, flat blade; used to break away enamel margins during tooth preparations and smooth or refine the cavity preparation.
- **hoe:** smaller bladed instrument with a tip resembling a farm hoe; used to break or pull away enamel tissue during preparations.
- **hatchet:** hand instrument with a sharp-edged hatchet-like tip; used to remove hard tissue.
- **chisel:** hand instrument with cutting edge that is used to cut and plane away enamel and dentin. Chisels have straight shanks, or a curved shank, such as the Wedelstaedt chisel, or may have an extra angled shank, such as the bin-angle chisels.
- **cleoid** (**KLEE**-oyd)/**discoid** (**DISK**-oyd) **carver:** double-ended, long-necked, carving instrument with a pointed tip on one end (cleoid) and a disc-shaped blade on the other end (discoid); used to carve anatomy features in newly placed restorations or can be used to remove decay and tooth tissue during cavity preparations.

- **carver:** thin-bladed hand instrument used to remove decay or carve newly placed restorative material; blade faces come in various shapes. Popular types are the Hollenback, Wards, and Frahms carvers.

Filling and Finishing Grouping

After the preparation is complete, it must be filled with an appropriate restorative material and then restored to a natural appearance and function. The following instruments may be used to complete this process (also shown in Figure 4-4).

- **plastic filling instrument (PFI):** hand instrument with a flat blade; used to carry, transfer, and pack materials, or to carve restorative material while it is still in a movable or plastic stage.
- **condenser:** hand instrument with a thick, rounded, or oval-shaped flat head that is sometimes serrated. It is used to pack or condense restorative material into the cavity preparation. Double-ended ones vary in sizes and/or surfaces.
- **burnisher:** hand instrument with a smooth, rounded head that comes in various shapes; used to smooth out restorative material or other metal surfaces, such as a matrix strip.
- **amalgam carrier:** hand instrument with holding cylinder for the transfer of amalgam material while in a plastic form; it has a spring lever pusher to expel the material into the preparation. The instrument is supplied in assorted sizes from 1.5 to 3.2 mm with various cylinder materials on the end tips. They are color-coded for size (red = jumbo, yellow = large, and white = medium). Another type of amalgam carrier is the amalgam gun with a thumb spring push to expel the material. Both amalgam carriers may be loaded by pressing the plastic load of restorative material into the **amalgam well**.
- **matrix** (**MAY**-tricks) **holder, matrix strip,** and **wedge:** holder device used to maintain

(A) Excavator

(B) Spoon Excavator

(C) Cleoid/Discoid

(D) Gingival Margin Trimmer

(E) Hoe

(F) Hatchet

(G) Chisel/ bin-angle

(H) Chisel/Wedelstaedt

(I) Chisel/straight

(J) Carver/Hollenback

(K) Carver/Frahm

(L) Plastic Filling Instrument

Courtesy of Integra LifeSciences Corporation through Integra Miltex

Figure 4-4 (*Continued*)

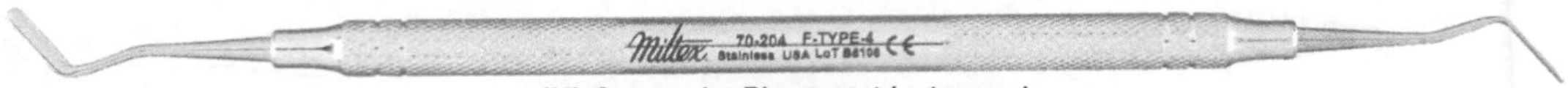

(M) Composite Placement Instrument

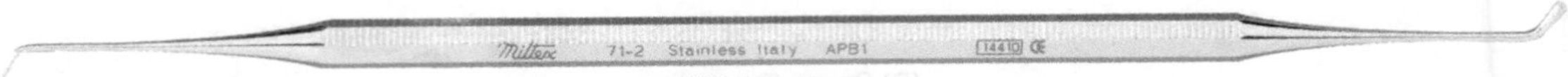

(N) Condenser

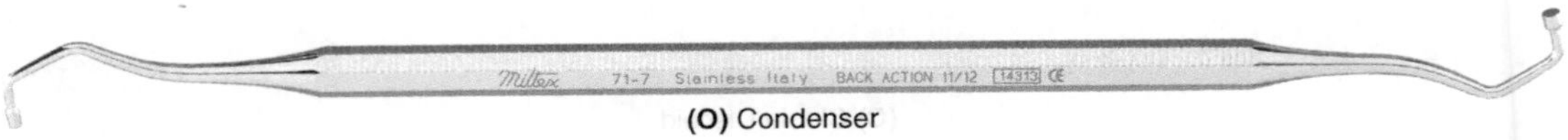

(O) Condenser

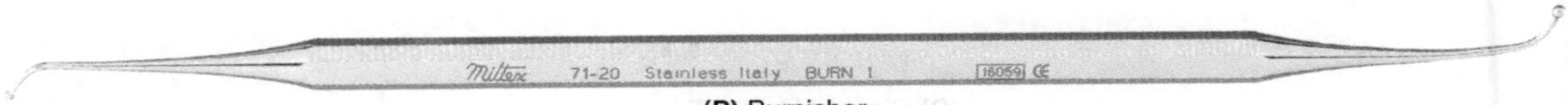

(P) Burnisher

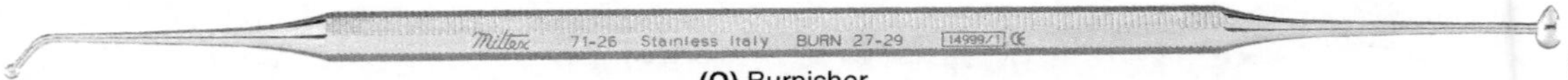

(Q) Burnisher

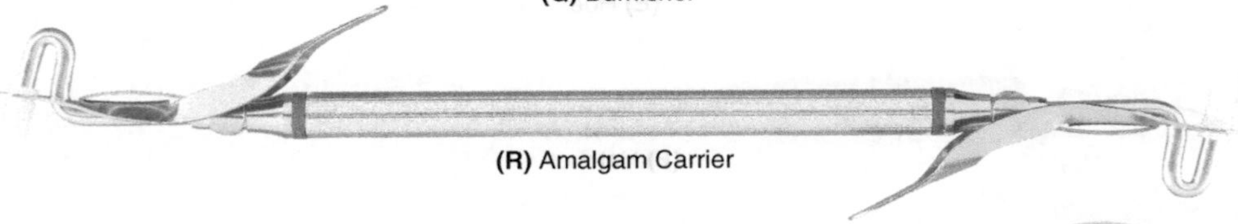

(R) Amalgam Carrier

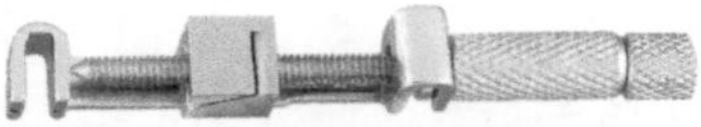

(S) Matrix

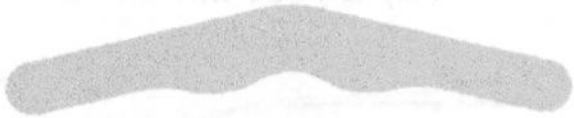

(T) Band

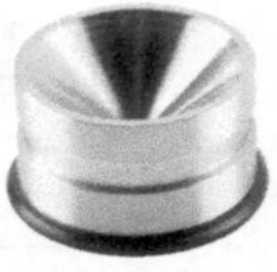

(U) Well

Courtesy of Integra LifeSciences Corporation through Integra Miltex

artificial wall (matrix strip) around the tooth preparation. A wooden or resin triangular wedge is used to hold the strip in place and prevent the material from leaking. Matrix retention will be discussed further in Chapter 10, Tooth Restorations.

- **loupes:** though not considered an instrument, eye loupes are glasses used for magnification, precision, and identification purposes, and are required in many procedures. Magnification power is from 2× to 8× and may have light sources and a splash side for sanitary purposes.

Evacuation

Evacuation of the mouth is accomplished by using tips that are inserted into suction tubing. These tips are placed in the mouth and used to remove moisture, debris, and other matter. The two types of handheld evacuator tips commonly used in saliva evacuation are:

- **high volume evacuator (HVE):** curved, metal or resin, beveled tip with a large hole, inserted into a high evacuation tube system handle with off/on and intensity controls; used for gross removal of fluids and debris from the mouth.

- **saliva ejector tip:** smaller suction tip that is inserted into the evacuation tubing from the dental unit; used for a steady, constant fluid removal from the oral cavity.

Various mechanical devices are used to isolate and maintain a dry field such as the disposable *Isolite* illuminator (see Figure 4-5), a device placed into the mouth that will serve as a tongue retainer, and a luminated evacuation unit that is maintained by the patient in a bite block position. Insertion of gauze pads or commercial absorbent pads near the saliva duct in the cheek and rubber dam placement can help to maintain some fluid control. Some units have a **cuspidor** (**KUSS**-pih-dore = *basin*) nearby for patients to empty their mouths.

Assorted Instruments

Other instruments, such as scissors, spatulas, knives, and pliers, are used interchangeably in any family or instrument group. Each dental procedure will need specific variations of the basic instruments mentioned previously and call for specialized instruments and materials as required. Instruments may be color-coded by placing a colored band on the shaft to indicate the type of instrument, the operatory/treatment room of use, the operator, the type of setup, or any other way of grouping. They may be sterilized in colored trays arranged in a pre-setup to match this coding. Use of sterilizing

Figure 4-5 Isolite—one unit delivers isolation, illumination, retraction, and aspiration.

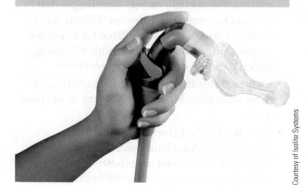

Courtesy of Isolite Systems

cassettes or trays will be discussed in Chapter 5, Infection Control.

ROTARY DENTAL INSTRUMENTS

Rotary instruments are power-driven tools that operate in a circular motion at various speeds. The rate of speed or rpm (rotations per minute) determines the classification of the instrument. The handpiece holds and operates the inserted instrument. It is classified as slow, high, or ultra-high speed, depending on its rpm (10,000 to 400,000). Rotation is achieved by a belt-driven electric turbine or a compressed air system. High-speed handpieces have an attached angled head that holds a friction grip (FG) bur, diamond, or point that is inserted into the head and tightened into place. Slower handpieces may be used independently or may accommodate the following smaller handpieces (Figure 4-6):

- **contra-angle handpiece (CAHP):** handpiece with an obtuse angled head (more than 90 degrees). A CAHP is inserted into the power unit's straight handpiece and is used to gain access to posterior teeth and difficult areas.
- **right-angle handpiece (RAHP):** handpiece with the head at a 90-degree angle; is inserted and connects into the power unit's handpiece; employed in general use throughout the oral cavity.
- **prophy** (**PRO**-fee) **angle handpiece (PHP):** small prophylaxis handpiece rotary angle with a 90-degree angle head; has a limited opening in the working end for polishing cups or brush placement. The PHP is inserted into a slow-speed handpiece and used to polish teeth. Many PHPs are disposable, and some may be battery powered with swivel heads and optical light sources.
- **fiber-optic handpiece:** specific slow or high-speed handpiece that supplies a light source to the operative site for improved vision.
- **rheostat** (**REE**-oh-stat): a foot pedal or lever that is used to regulate the speed of the handpiece.

Figure 4-6 Low-speed handpiece with attachments: (A) handpiece, (B) contra-angle, (C) right-angle or prophy angle, with rubber cup, (D) round bur with long shank

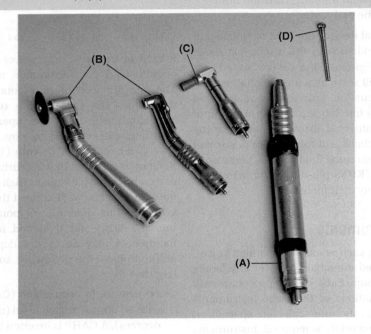

Although not considered standard operative handpieces used for restorative and tissue-removing procedures, other dental instruments that are handheld can be attached to the specialized mobile stand or movable over-the-patient tray called a **delivery system**. Each practice chooses which types of handpieces to have available for that practice (see Figure 4-7). Along with the basic air/water syringe, the selective combination can be chosen from:

- **air abrasion:** air-powered handpiece delivering abrasive aluminum oxide powder or sodium bicarbonate under force to clean or prepare tooth surfaces or remove some carious tissue (Figure 4-8).
- **ultrasonic handpiece:** high-speed vibration-scaling tips used for scaling and curettage purposes; sometimes called *ultrasonic scaler*.
- **curing light handpiece:** handheld device that focuses a light beam to cure or "set" specified materials.

- **intraoral camera:** handpiece with a small camera situated in the head; used to transmit various views of the oral setting.
- **electrosurgery handpiece:** combination of assorted metal tips that fit into a probe handle; these tips pass electrical currents that incise and coagulate the blood in a surgical procedure.
- **laser handpiece:** photon handpiece that emits a precise light energy wavelength that is concentrated to perform specialized tasks; various wavelengths are utilized for a specific target or procedure, such as tooth whitening, caries removal, or surgical gingivectomy.
- **caries detection scanner:** a noninvasive laser scan that detects early decay in occlusal areas.
- **implant drilling unit:** lighted, digitally controlled drilling handpiece with sterile irrigation that is used to smooth alveolar bone, drill operative sites, and install implants.

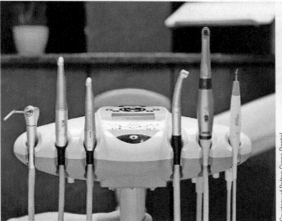

Courtesy of Pelton Crane Dental

Figure 4-8 Air abrasion unit

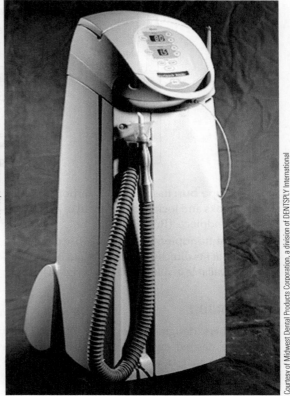

Courtesy of Midwest Dental Products Corporation, a division of DENTSPLY International

All dental handpieces are expensive items and must be maintained, sterilized, and cared for in the manner specified by the manufacturer of the instrument.

Handpieces may be used to hold the burs, mandrels, mounted stones, and discs that are used in restorations and chairside dental procedures. The dental bur is the most commonly used rotary item and is employed in cavity preparation and restorations. A bur has three parts (see Figure 4-9):

- **Shank:** the end of the bur that is inserted into the handpiece. The type of end is determined by the requirements of the power handpiece. The assortment of burs includes the friction grip (FG), right angle (RA), or handpiece (HP) that is placed directly into a straight handpiece. The length of the shank—long, short, or pedodontic—varies according to the type of bur or area involved.

- **Neck:** connecting area between the shank and the working end or head of the bur.

- **Working end or head:** end that cuts tissue or works on the tooth or material involved. Each shape or type is designed for a specific purpose or position.

Bur Types

Rotary burs may be typed according to style or handpiece placement. Burs are supplied in graduated sizes and are numbered according to the shape of the head, and some are color-coded according to the amount of cutting edges. Burs that have extra teeth in a crosscut pattern are called **dentated** (**DEN**-tay-ted = *dented, depressed*), and shortened burs are called **truncated** (**TRUN**-kay-ted = *cut part off, lop off*). Three types of burs are:

- **friction grip bur:** smooth-ended bur, held in the handpiece by the friction grip chuck inside the handpiece head. (FG)

71

Figure 4-9 Parts of bur

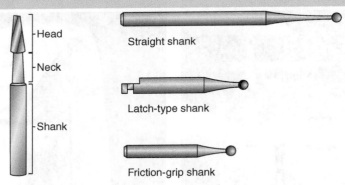

- Head
- Neck
- Shank
- Straight shank
- Latch-type shank
- Friction-grip shank

- **latch-type bur:** has grooved insertion bur end that hooks and locks into the head of a latch type handpiece. (RA)
- **straight handpiece:** has a smooth, extended shaft that fits directly into the straight handpiece (HP); available in mini, regular, or surgical lengths.

Bur Numbers

Bur numbers designate the shape of the rotary head. The desired cut for the tooth dictates the bur number that is used in the procedure. The more popular shapes are the round, inverted cone, and plain or tapered fissured burs. While the bur number determines a specific shape, the handpiece determines which type: straight (HP), latch type (RA), or friction grip (FG).

Specialized burs also include surgical burs with longer shafts, lab burs called vulcanite or acrylic, and finishing burs with a wide variety of cutting edges or blades in their working head (see Figure 4-10 for examples of burs).

Miscellaneous Rotary Instruments

Several other instruments may be used in a rotary handpiece:

- **mandrel** (**MAN**-drell): a slim, metal holding device that fits into slow handpieces and is used to smooth and cut. They may have RA or HP end fittings and come in various lengths. Mandrels hold abrasive and rubber discs by a screw-on or snap-on method (see Figure 4-11). The **Joe Dandy**, a thick, carborundum disc, is very popular.
- **stone, wheel, and discs:** abrasive or chemically treated discs, wheels, cups, and points with various shapes that can be permanently mounted or glued on a shaft or placed on discs for mandrels. They are supplied in assorted sizes and **grit** (abrasiveness) and are used for smoothing at chairside or in the lab (see Figure 4-12).
- **diamond rotary instruments:** pulverized industrial diamonds glued on a shaft or disc and commonly called *burs* or *points*. They are used to cut, smooth, and rapidly reduce tissues; they follow the same numbering pattern and color-coding as steel burs.
- **bur block:** a tray device used to hold the small rotary instruments during use at the chair and while being sterilized; may be metallic or resin and may or may not have a cover.

DENTAL FACILITY OPERATIVE EQUIPMENT

Each dental facility or clinic contains specialized dental equipment that is used to perform necessary treatments. Although many items are available, some for general dentistry and some for specialty use, all facilities need the basic items shown in Figure 4-13 and described here:

Figure 4-10 Examples of burs

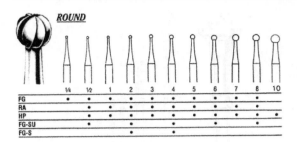

ROUND

	¼	½	1	2	3	4	5	6	7	8	10
FG	•	•	•	•	•	•	•	•	•	•	•
RA		•	•	•	•	•	•	•	•		
HP		•	•	•	•	•	•	•	•	•	
FG-SU	•			•			•		•		
FG-S				•		•					

INVERTED CONE

	33½	34	35	36	37	38	39	36L	37L	
FG	•	•	•	•	•	•	•	•	•	○
RA	•	•	•	•	•	•	•			
HP	•	•	•	•	•	•	•			
FG-SU							•			
FG-S			•							

PLAIN FISSURE STRAIGHT

	56	57	58	59	60	57L	58L
FG	•	•	•	•	•	•	•

CROSSCUT FISSURE STRAIGHT

	556	557	558	559	560	557L	558L
FG	•	•	•	•	•	•	•
RA	•	•	•	•	•		
HP	•	•	•	•			
FG-SU		•	•	•			
FG-S			•				

PLAIN TAPER FISSURE

	169	170	171	172	169L	170L	171L
FG	•	•	•	•	•	•	•
RA							•
HP							
FG-SU		•		•			
FG-S					•		

CROSSCUT FISSURE TAPER

	699	700	701	702	703	699L	700L	701L
FG	•	•	•	•	•	•	•	•
RA	•	•	•	•	•			
HP		•	•	•	•			
FG-SU		•	•	•	•			
FG-S		•						

END CUTTING

	957	958
FG	•	•

WHEEL

	14
FG	•

PEAR

	329	330	331	332	331L
FG	•	•	•	•	•
RA					
HP					
FG-SU					
FG-S			•		

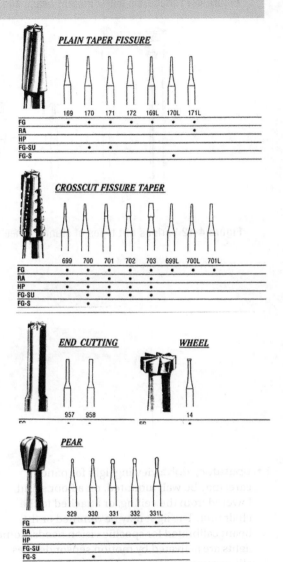

- **operatory** (**OPERA**-tory): small treatment room equipped with dental appliances. Some practices, such as orthodontic, and some clinics have a single large operatory area containing several chairs and necessary equipment separated with half walls or room dividers.

- **dental chair:** chair appliance, usually electrically powered, that raises, lowers, and tilts to provide easy access and proper vision; may be a lounge or upright chair style. Most chairs are operated by remote foot controls to eliminate hand use and contamination.

Figure 4-11 Mandrels with different heads and shanks

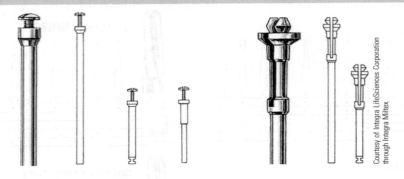

Courtesy of Integra LifeSciences Corporation through Integra Miltex

Figure 4-12 Various grit types of stones, wheels, and points

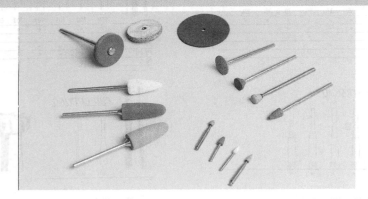

- **operatory light:** viewing light for patient care; may be wall mounted, on a floor stand, lowered from the ceiling, or attached to the chair unit. The light may be dimmed or the beam calibrated for specific vision needs. Some lights are activated by motion sensor devices, eliminating touching and contamination.
- **stools:** movable seats for the dental personnel. Stools have height adjustment and back rests. Some stools have torso rests extending in front for forward-leaning support.
- **dental unit:** upright, stationary, or movable table-style working appliance that provides handpiece power, aspiration, water, and air. Some units also provide electrosurgical power,

a natural gas outlet, fiber optic power, and custom appliances such as intraoral cameras, laser handpieces, perio-pocket depth sensors, air abrasion units, curing lights, pulp depth indicators, and crown shape fabricators.

- **cabinets:** mobile, floor-, or wall-mounted storage cabinets with drawer space for supplies and equipment.
- **radiographic units:** various configurations; a dental practice may have a radiographic control unit in a central area with the X-ray head or power source in each operatory area; other facilities have head and control units in the operatory room or may use a separate radiographic area for panoramic,

Figure 4-13 Dental operatory or treatment room

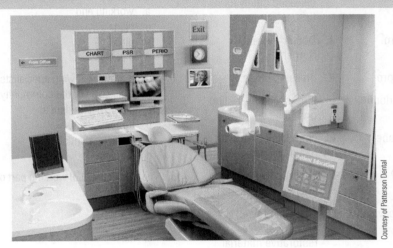

Courtesy of Patterson Dental

cephalometric, or 3D exposures; some have filmless, digitalized radiographic units using sensors, computer-assisted viewing and imaging, or portable X-ray exposure heads.

- **diagnostic or auxiliary units:** include perio-pocket detectors, newly developed electronic diagnostic devices used to assist with a patient

survey; endodontic units detect the depth of instrument probing to avoid accidental penetration of the apex. Laser dental surgery, electronic target anesthesia, computer interaction, charting recording, ultrasonic cleaning methods, and other new units to aid the dental profession are being introduced continually as well.

Review Exercises

Matching

Match the following word elements with their meanings.

1. _____ pedodontist

2. _____ PFI

3. _____ shank

4. _____ cotton forceps

5. _____ endodontist

6. _____ DDS

7. _____ hoe

8. _____ FG

A. bur type used to fit in straight handpiece

B. combination instrument = explorer and periodontal probe

C. fine-pointed instruments with depth-measuring marks

D. rotations per minute, speed of handpiece

E. specialist who performs children's dentistry

F. high-volume evacuation system

G. hand instrument used to remove and dig out decay

H. hand instrument used to break away or pull off enamel

9. _____ HVE   **I.** specialist who treats diseased gingival tissues

10. _____ rpm   **J.** Doctor of Dental Surgery

11. _____ expro   **K.** dressing pliers

12. _____ periodontist   **L.** high-speed or friction grip bur

13. _____ probe   **M.** connects instrument handle to working end

14. _____ HP   **N.** specialist who treats internal pulp tissues

15. _____ excavator   **O.** instrument used to carve pliable restorative material

Definitions

Using the selection given for each sentence, choose the best term to complete the definition.

1. A hand instrument with a thick head, used to push or pack down material is a/an:
   a. condenser
   b. hatchet
   c. curette
   d. discloid-cleoid

2. People who are trained in a specific field and considered knowledgeable in that area are:
   a. lay people
   b. professionals
   c. expertizers
   d. apprentices

3. A person who independently specializes in denture construction is a:
   a. dental detail person
   b. forensic dentist
   c. dental practice consultant
   d. lab technician

4. Which part of an instrument is used to grasp or control the instrument?
   a. working end
   b. blade
   c. nib
   d. handle

5. Which of the following specialists works on common dental diseases of the community?
   a. public health dentist
   b. forensic dentist
   c. pediatric dentist
   d. surgeon

6. The rounded end of working part of a hand instrument is called a:
   a. toe
   b. tip
   c. nib
   d. blade

7. Which of the following specialists replaces missing teeth with artificial appliances?
   a. prosthodontist
   b. periodontist
   c. pedodontist
   d. endodontist

8. A two-edged, rounded toe, cutting instrument used to remove subgingival calculus is a:
   a. scalpel
   b. universal curette
   c. gingival margin trimmer
   d. sickle scaler

9. A nonmetallic, resin-tipped hand instrument used to clean and remove deposits around pegs and abutments is a/an:
   a. periodontal knife
   b. plastic filling instrument
   c. implant scaler/curette
   d. hatchet

10. Another word for the handle of a hand instrument is:
    a. shank
    b. neck
    c. working end
    d. shaft

11. A handpiece with the head set at a 90-degree angle is which type of handpiece?
    a. straight
    b. contra angle
    c. right angle
    d. prophy

12. The end of the bur that is inserted into the handpiece is called the:
    a. shank
    b. neck
    c. head
    d. tip

13. Which of the following would not be inserted into the handpiece to become functional?
    a. mandrel
    b. matrix
    c. mounted stone
    d. bur

14. Which of the following auxiliary units is used to incise and coagulate tissue?
    a. air abrasion
    b. light curing
    c. ultrasonic
    d. electrosurgery

15. Which of the following are group members of the basic instrument setup?
    a. mirror, explorer, cotton pliers, probe
    b. mirror, excavator, matrix, probe
    c. periodontal probe, chart, mirror, hoe
    d. explorer, mirror, handpiece, matrix

16. A hand instrument used to smooth off or contour restorative material or metals is a/an:
    a. matrix
    b. condenser
    c. burnisher
    d. explorer

17. A retaining or holding device used to make an artificial wall in a restoration is a:
    a. retainer
    b. mandrel
    c. matrix
    d. dental dam

18. A hand instrument used to incise (cut into) or remove tissue is a:
    a. carver
    b. scalpel
    c. beaver-tail burnisher
    d. hatchet

19. The national organization for dental assistants is the:
    a. DANB
    b. ADA
    c. ADAA
    d. CDAA

20. A gingival margin trimmer is used to:
    a. break away the enamel side of a tooth during preparation
    b. remove supragingival and subgingival deposits from tooth margins
    c. maintain margin walls during the insertion and condensing of materials

Building Skills

Locate and define the prefix, root/combining form, and suffix (if present) in the following words.

1. **prosthodontist**
   prefix _____
   root/combining form _____
   suffix _____

2. **gingival**
   prefix _____
   root/combining form _____
   suffix _____

3. **evacuator**
   prefix _____
   root/combining form _____
   suffix _____

4. **periodontal**
   prefix _____
   root/combining form _____
   suffix _____

5. **denturist**
   prefix _____
   root/combining form _____
   suffix _____

Fill-Ins

Write the correct word in the blank space to complete each statement.

1. The high-speed vibrating instrument used for scaling and curettage of teeth is called a/an _____ scaler.

2. The portable mobile seats used by dental personnel in the operatory area are called _____.

3. Persons who have not been trained or experienced in a particular trade or study are called _____.

4. When incision and immediate coagulation of the site is desired, the dentist will select the _____ handpiece.

5. A hand instrument used to transfer amalgam while in a plastic stage is a/an _____.

6. Hand instruments may have working heads on each end; this type of instrument is called a/an _____ instrument.

7. The three components of a hand instrument are _____, _____, and _____.

8. A rounded blade end on a hand instrument is called a/an _____.

9. A pointed blade end on a hand instrument is called a/an _____.

10. Name three instruments used in the basic exam setup: _____, _____, and _____.

11. Three purposes for the use of a mouth mirror are _____, _____, and _____.

12. Cotton forceps or pickups are used to _____.

13. Three interworking items used to maintain artificial walls around a cavity prep are _____, _____, and _____.

14. Two initialed titles that indicate a person is trained as a dentist are _____ and _____ _____.

15. A _____ is a device used to hold rotary burs during procedures and through sterilization.

16. Three parts of a rotary instrument called a bur are _____, _____, and _____.

17. Shortened burs are called _____.

18. A latch-type handpiece will require the _____ type of rotary bur.

19. Crosscut or extra teethed burs are called _____.

20. Another name for the foot pedal that controls the speed of the handpiece is a/an _____ _____.

Word Use

Read the following sentences and define the boldfaced words.

1. Many assistants enjoy the diversity of working in a **group practice**.

   _____

2. When faced with the gross removal of tooth structure, the dentist may choose a **dentated** type of rotary bur.

   _____

3. The chemical bleaching treatment of the pulp canal may be performed by the **endodontist.**

   _____

4. It is difficult for a new assistant to learn each specific **armamentarium** for each different procedure.

   _____

5. The patient commented that the **operatory** was bright and colorful.

   _____

✓ Learning Objectives

On completion of this chapter, you should be able to:

1. Discuss the meaning of disease with related signs and symptoms and the various classifications of disease conditions.

2. List and identify sources of disease and the pathogens that may be involved.

3. Identify and explain the action of infectious agents and their method of causing disease.

4. Explain immunity and the methods by which to acquire the various types of immunity.

5. Discuss the importance of preventing disease, and list the common methods used to combat disease and infection potentials.

6. List the principal agencies or government bodies concerned with the control of disease.

DISEASE CONDITIONS

Disease (*pathological condition of the body, abnormal condition*) manifests its presence through **symptoms** (**SIM**-tums = *perceptible change in the body or body function*), which may

Vocabulary Related to Infection Control

This list contains selected new and important word parts and terms from this chapter. Take the time to learn these word parts and their meanings. You may use the list to review these terms and practice pronouncing them correctly. When you work with the audio for this chapter, listen to the word, repeat it, and then place a checkmark in the box. Proceed to the next boxed word, and repeat the process.

(hyphen before word means it's a suffix, hyphen after word means prefix, no hyphen means root word.)

Word Parts	Meaning	Word Parts	Meaning
dis-	away from	gen	birth, coming to be, producing
infec	invade	germ	microorganism
ultra-	above, beyond	-cide	to kill
son	sound	endo-	within
-ic	pertaining to	-ous	pertaining to
-al	relating to	-tion	condition or state of
path/o	disease		

Key Terms

- ❑ **aerobe** (**AIR**-ohb)
- ❑ **aerobic** (air-**OH**-bick)
- ❑ **anaerobic** (an-ah-**ROH**-bick)
- ❑ **antibody** (**ANN**-tih-bod-ee)
- ❑ **antigen** (**ANN**-tih-jen)
- ❑ **antiseptic** (an-tih-**SEP**-tick)
- ❑ **asepsis** (ay-**SEP**-sis)
- ❑ **attenuated** (at-**TEN**-youated)

- ❑ **autoclave** (**AWE**-toh-klave)
- ❑ **autogenous** (awe-toh-**JEE**-nus)
- ❑ **bacteriostatic** (back-tee-ree-oh-**STAT**-ick)
- ❑ **biodegradable** (bye-oh-dee-**GRADE**-ah-bull)
- ❑ **commensal** (koh-**MEN**-sal)

- ❑ **congenital** (kahn-**JEN**-ih-tuhl)
- ❑ **degenerative** (dee-**JEN**-er-ah-tiv)
- ❑ **diagnosis** (die-agg-**NO**-sis)
- ❑ **disinfectant** (dis-in-**FECK**-tant)
- ❑ **disinfection** (dis-inn-**FECK**-shun)
- ❑ **endemic** (en-**DEM**-ick)

(Continued)

Key Terms *continued*

- **endogenous** (en-**DOH**-je-nus)
- **endospore** (**EN**-dough-spore)
- **etiology** (ee-tee-**ALL**-oh-jee)
- **exogenous** (ecks-**AH**-je-nus)
- **flagella** (fla-**JEL**-ah)
- **fungus** (**FUNG**-us)
- **immunocompromised** (im-you-no-**KOM**-proh-mized)
- **inoculation** (inn-ock-you-**LAY**-shun)
- **nematodes** (**NEM**-ah-toads)
- **nosocomial** (noh-soh-**KOH**-me-al)
- **odontalgia** (oh-don-**TAL**-jee-ah)
- **opportunistic** (ah-per-too-**NIS**-tick)
- **pandemic** (pan-**DEM**-ick)
- **parenteral** (pare-**EN**-ter-ahl)
- **pathogenic** (path-oh-**JEN**-ick)
- **pathology** (path-**AHL**-oh-jee)
- **prognosis** (prahg-**NO**-sis)
- **protozoa** (proh-toh-**ZOH**-ah)
- **rickettsia** (rih-**KET**-see-ah)
- **sanitation** (san-ih-**TAY**-shun)
- **saprophyte** (**SAP**-roh-fight)
- **sterilization** (stare-ill-ih-**ZAY**-shun)
- **symptom** (**SIM**-tum)
- **syndrome** (**SIN**-drome)
- **vaccination** (vack-sih-**NAY**-shun)
- **virulence** (**VIR**-you-linz)
- **virus** (**VYE**-rus)

be objective or subjective. **Objective symptoms**, also called **signs**, are evidence observed by someone other than the patient, for example, **edema** (ee-**DEE**-mah = *swelling*). **Subjective symptoms** are evidence of a disease as reported by the patient, for example, **odontalgia** (oh-dahn-**TAHL**-gee-ah = *toothache*). An assortment of signs and **symptoms** grouped together that characterize a disease is called a **syndrome** (**SIN**-drome = *running together*).

The study of disease is called **pathology** (path-**AHL**-oh-jee). Pathologists search for disease **etiology** (ee-tee-**AHL**-oh-jee = *cause of the disease*). Symptoms and signs are used to form a **diagnosis** (die-agg-**NO**-sis = *denoting name of disease*), and a **prognosis** (prahg-**NO**-sis) is a prediction about the course of the disease.

Disease Terms

The condition of a disease or its intensity may be seen in various stages. Some terms used to describe the status of a current disease are:

- **acute** (ah-**CUTE** = *sharp, severe*): describes immediate symptoms such as high fever and pain or distress.

- **chronic** (**KRON**-ick = *not acute, drawn out*): describes a condition present over a long time, often without an endpoint, such as a chronic fatigue and anemia.

- **remission** (ree-**MISH**-un = *lessening or abating*): temporary or permanent cessation of a severe condition, such as a case of sinusitis or some stage of cancer.

Terms associated with the geographical area of a disease are:

- **epidemic** (ep-ih-**DEH**-mick = *among people or widespread*): is a disease that affects a large number of people within a community, population, or region.

- **pandemic** (pan-**DEM**-ick = *all people involved*): is an epidemic that's spread over multiple countries or continents.

- **endemic** (en-**DEM**-ick = *in people*): is a problem that belongs to a particular people or country, and is ongoing.

- **outbreak:** is a greater-than-anticipated increase in the number of endemic cases. It can be a single case in a new area. If it's not quickly controlled, an outbreak can become an epidemic.

Classification of Diseases

Diseases may be further classified according to their actions. Some terms used to denote the origin or manifestations are:

- **exogenous** (ecks-**AH**-jeh-nuss = *produced outside*): refers to causes outside the body, such as illnesses arising from trauma, radiation, or hypothermia.
- **endogenous** (en-**DOH**-jeh-nuss = *arising from within the cell or organism*): refers to causes from within the body, such as infections, tumors, and congenital or metabolic abnormalities.
- **congenital** (kahn-**JEN**-ih-tuhl = *present from birth*): refers to condition inherited from parents, such as cystic fibrosis.
- **degenerative** (dee-**JEN**-er-ah-tiv = *breaking down*): refers to conditions resulting from natural aging of the body, such as arthritis.
- **opportunistic** (ah-pore-too-**NISS**-tick = *taking advantage of*): refers to disease or infection occurring when body resistance is lowered, such as with fungal, bacterial, and viral infections.
- **nosocomial** (**noh**-soh-**KOH**-mee-ahl = *disease in caregiving*): refers to diseases passed on from patient to patient in a health care setting, such as staphylococcal bacterial infections, MRSA, and others. The term nosocomial has been replaced by the terminology *hospital-acquired infections* in recent years.

CAUSES OF DISEASE AND INFECTION

Diseases may be caused by a number of **pathogenic** (**path**-oh-**JEN**-ick = *disease producing*) microorganisms, including bacteria, viruses, and other pathogens.

Bacteria

Bacteria (back-**TEER**-ee-ah) (singular, **bacterium**) are one-celled, plant-like microorganisms lacking chlorophyll. These microorganisms have three principal forms: oval/rounded, rod-shaped, and spiral or curved.

Other terms pertaining to specific characteristics of bacteria are:

- **aerobic** (air-**OH**-bick): designates bacteria that require oxygen to live.
- **facultative aerobes** (**AIR**-ohbs): bacteria that can live in the presence of oxygen but do not require it.
- **obligate or strict aerobes:** bacteria that cannot survive without oxygen, such as **diphtheria**.
- **anaerobic** (an-ah-**ROH**-bick): bacteria that do not need oxygen for survival.
- **facultative anaerobes:** bacteria that grow best without oxygen but can survive in its presence, for example, bacterium fusiform (trench mouth).
- **obligate or strict anaerobes:** bacteria that cannot live in the presence of oxygen.
- **flagella** (flah-**JELL**-ah = *whips*): small, whip-like hairs that provide movement for some bacteria.

A **spore** is a thick-walled reproductive cell. Some bacteria, such as anthrax and tetanus, possess a capsule layer of slime, and a few rod-shaped bacteria develop an **endospore** (**EN**-dough-spore) for a resting stage when unfavorable conditions exist. This covering is difficult to destroy. Examples of these bacteria include anthrax and tetanus.

Viruses

Viruses (**VYE**-russes) are tiny parasitic organisms that cause diseases such as polio, hepatitis, smallpox, colds, coronavirus, HIV, herpes, and influenza, among many others. Viruses require living matter to reproduce and grow.

Other Pathogens

While bacteria and viruses are commonly known germs, there is another variety of pathogens that

Forms of Bacteria

Rod-shaped	Curved forms	Circular	Other shapes
Coccobacilli (oval)	Vibrio (curved rod)	Diplo- (in pairs)	Corynebacter (club)
Streptobacilli	Spirochete (spiral)	Strepto- (in chains)	Streptomyces
Mycobacteria	Spirilla (coil)	Staphylo- (clusters)	Helicobacter (helical)

cause disease and body maladies. These pathogens include the following:

- **rickettsia** (rih-**KET**-see-ah): microbes smaller than bacteria but larger than viruses; usually transmitted by **vectors** (**VEK**-tors = *carriers that transmit disease*), such as fleas, lice, and ticks. Rickettsia cause diseases such as Lyme or Rocky Mountain spotted fever.
- **fungi** (**FUN**-guy = *a division of plants that include mold, yeasts, and slimes*); (singular, **fungus** = **FUNG**-us): Some fungi are beneficial, and others are pathogenic, the latter of which cause thrush, athlete's foot, or ringworm, for example. Fungi grow in two forms: **filamentous** (molds) and **unicellular** (yeasts).
- **protozoa** (proh-toh-**ZOH**-ah = *small animal parasites or organisms*): must live upon another organism called the *host*. Protozoan organisms

cause malaria, dysentery, and encephalitis, for example.

- **saprophytes** (**SAP**-roh-fights): organisms living on decaying or dead organic matter, such as tetanus bacillus (lockjaw).
- **nematodes** (**NEM**-ah-toads): small parasitic worms such as threadworms and roundworms.
- **commensal** (koh-**MEN**-sal = *living together*): microbes that live together on a host without harming it, such as mouth flora.
- **blood-borne pathogens:** disease-producing microbes that are present in human blood.

PORT OF ENTRY FOR DISEASE

Disease or infection is contracted through various methods and ports of entry, as follows:

- **droplet infection:** airborne infection in which pathogens discharged from the mouth or nose by coughing or sneezing are carried through the air and settle on objects.
- **indirect infection:** infection resulting from improper handling of contaminated inanimate substances that absorb and transmit infection, such as doorknobs or bedding. Poor sterilization methods permit passage of microbes from one person to another.
- **direct contact infection:** infection that is passed directly from person to person through contact with saliva, blood, or mucous membranes.
- **parenteral** (pare-**EN**-ter-al = *injection*) **entry:** refers to piercing of the skin or mucous membrane; also called "needle stick."
- **carrier infection:** exchange of disease by direct or indirect contact with an infected human or animal that does not have symptoms of a disease.
- **vector-borne infection:** an infection that is transmitted by an organism such as a fly or mosquito.
- **food, soil, or water infection:** infection passed along by microbes present in food, soil, or water. In the dental office, water lines may harbor a **biofilm** containing bacterial cells that adhere to moist surfaces and form a protective slime that can carry pathogens or nematodes. Dust on surfaces also can transport pathogens.

For disease to occur and prosper, a **"chain of infection"** must be present. Any break or elimination of a link or factor in the chain will stop the disease or infection, as shown in Figure 5-1.

IMMUNITY FACTORS

Immunity (im-**YOU**-nih-tee = *resistance to organisms due to previous exposure*) may be affected by the **virulence** (**VEER**-you-lense = *power*) of a disease, which is the strength or concentration of pathological organisms. Immunity can be classified according to either natural or artificial conditions, actively or passively. Various types of immunity are:

Figure 5-1 Chain of infection

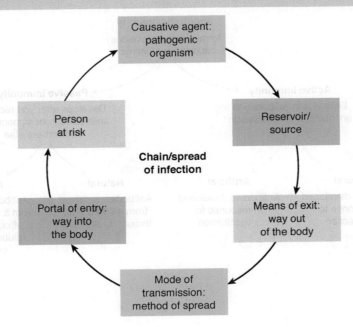

- **natural immunity:** inherited and permanent.
- **natural acquired immunity:** obtained when a person is infected by a disease, produces antibodies, and then recovers from that disease.
- **artificial acquired immunity:** obtained from inoculation or vaccination against a disease.
- **passive acquired immunity:** results from receiving antibodies from another source, such as breast milk, or from injections of gamma globulin, antitoxins, or immune serums.
- **passive natural immunity:** passes from mother to fetus, congenitally or through antibodies in breast milk.
- **immunocompromised** (**im**-you-no-**KAHM**-proh-mized): having a weakened immune system, resulting from drugs, irradiation, disease such as AIDS, or malnutrition.

Immunity may be acquired by an inoculation or vaccination of an antigen that enables the body to produce an antibody to the disease. The vaccine used may contain killed pathogenic microbes or attenuated antigens. Terms related to acquired immunity are:

- **inoculation** (in-**ock**-you-**LAY**-shun): injection of microorganisms, serum, or toxin into the body.
- **vaccination** (**vack**-sih-**NAY**-shun): inoculation with weakened or dead microbes.
- **antigen** (**ANN**-tih-jen): substance that induces the body to form antibodies.
- **antibody** (**ANN**-tih-bod-ee): protein substance produced by the body in response to an antigen.
- **vaccine** (**VAK**-seen): solution of killed or weakened infectious agents injected to produce immunity.
- **autogenous** (**awe**-toe-**JEE**-nus) **vaccine:** vaccine produced from a culture of bacteria

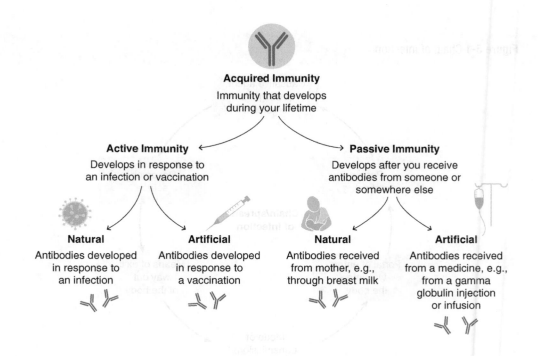

taken from the patient who will receive the vaccine.

- **attenuated** (ah-**TEN**-you-**ate**-ed): diluted or reduced virulence of pathogenic microbes.

DISEASE PREVENTION

Prevention is the best protection method to combat disease and infection in the dental facility. Proper sanitation habits, effective sterilization, and careful handling are primary ways to obtain sanitary conditions. Relevant terminology includes the following:

- **asepsis** (ay-**SEP**-sis): free from germs.
- **sanitation** (san-ih-**TAY**-shun): application of methods to promote a favorable germ-free state.
- **disinfection** (**dis**-inn-**FECK**-shun): application of chemicals to kill, reduce, or eliminate germs.
- **sterilization** (stare-ill-ih-**ZAY**-shun): the process of destroying all micro-organisms.
- **universal precautions:** assuming *all* patients are infectious and applying every method of combating disease and infection.

Procedures and Methods Used to Prevent Disease

Various methods and procedures are employed in the destruction of pathogens. The Centers for Disease Control and Prevention (CDC) has divided instruments and equipment used in the dental office into infection-risk categories and has recommended the type of sterilization for each:

- **Critical:** instruments used to penetrate soft tissue or bone, or enter into the bloodstream. These include forceps, scalpels, scalers, chisels, and surgical burs. Steam under pressure (autoclave), dry heat, or heat/chemical vapor sterilization are suggested.
- **Semi-critical:** instruments that do not penetrate soft tissues or bone but contact

the mucous membrane or non-intact skin. High-level disinfection is appropriate if heat/pressure/chemical is not feasible.

- **Noncritical:** instruments that come into contact with intact skin, such as blood pressure cuffs and X-ray heads. EPA-registered "hospital disinfectant" such as phenols, iodophors, and chlorine-containing compounds and some quaternary ammonium compounds are acceptable.

Sterilization and Disinfection of Dental Instruments and Materials

All instruments and dental equipment should be sterilized after each use. *Sterilization* is the total killing of all microbes; *disinfection* is obtaining a germ-free area as much as possible. After use (or exposure), instruments should be cleaned of debris with enzymatic solutions and then rinsed, dried, packed, and wrapped in cassettes/trays, or prepared as recommended by their manufacturer. Methods used to sterilize or disinfect are the following:

- **autoclave** (**AWE**-toh-klave): apparatus for sterilization by steam pressure. Temperature (121°C, 250°F), pressure (15 psi), and time (20 minutes) are regulated. Liquids with lids ajar and linen-wrapped packs require longer exposure. Liquids need cooling down and depressurizing periods before removal from units (see Figure 5-2).
- **"flash" autoclave:** smaller autoclave with higher temperature setting (132°C, 270°F) will lessen exposure time (3–5 minutes) required to obtain sterilization.
- **dry heat sterilization:** oven apparatus used for a hot-air bake at high temperature (170°C, 340°F) for a longer period of time (2 hours). This method is not useful for plastic materials or some paper objects.
- **molten metal** or **glass bead heat:** devices holding superheated (234°C, 450°F) molten metal or small glass beads; used mainly in

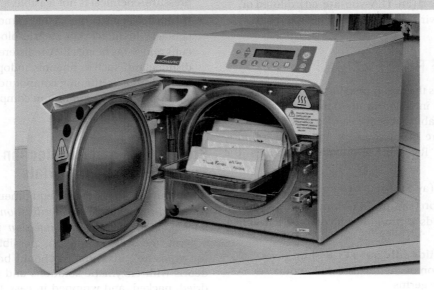

Figure 5-2 The autoclave is the most popular method for sterilization in the dental office. Packages and items are loosely packed to permit circulation of the steam

endodontic practice. (The CDC no longer recommends this method of sterilization.)

- **chemical vapor sterilization:** use of chemicals and heat of 132°C or 270°F unit for 20 minutes. Noncorrosive method that is used on loose or unwrapped articles, particularly metals. Proper ventilation and manufacturer's directions must be followed.

- **ethylene oxide:** sterilizing unit used at room temperature and requires prolonged exposure and devaporization time (10–12 hours). Heated units (49°C or 120°F) require less time (2–3 hours). Useful for plastics and materials that do not tolerate heat. Not a popular method used in dental office because of size, cost, and toxic devaporing requirements.

- **VPH (vaporized hydrogen peroxide):** gas plasma sterilization using hydrogen peroxide that is ionized to release vaporized gas molecules capable of killing microorganisms and endospores in a short period (less than 1 hour) with no vapor clear-off time concerns; compatible with most materials, except liquids, powders, and absorbents. *Plasma* is

the fourth stage of matter—liquid, solid, gas, and plasma. Because of the size and expense of these machines, they are found in hospitals, institutions, and larger dental clinics.

- **chemical agents:** liquids containing chemicals that kill microbes and spores and require longer immersion time. Some chemicals may be disinfectants and/or sterilizers. Chemicals classified as sterilants require long (6–10 hours) soaking to kill spores.

- **indicator strips or commercial spore vials:** placed in or on wrapped items during the sterilization cycle to indicate the effectiveness of the sterilizing process. Two types of indication are:

  ○ **biological:** monitoring of sterilization cycle by office spore strips, culture tubes, and vials with encased germs spore indicators that are routinely sent out for laboratory testing to assure that the sterilization process has been achieved.

  ○ **process:** tapes or marked autoclave sleeves indicate that heat conditions have been obtained but do not guarantee that pressure and time have completed the sterilization. The markings on the autoclave bag or sleeve tape change color when exposed to the proper sterilizing conditions. The wrapping or sleeving of the articles provides protection from contamination in handling after sterilization.

- **cassette trays:** used to contain instrument setups that travel from operatory use to the ultrasonic cleaning, rinsing, and wrapping for sterilizing and storage until the next use. These cassettes are marked and dated; they may be color-coded to signify which operatory, procedure, operator, or any designation desired for organization (see Figure 5-3).

Handpieces and other special items such as camera wands, probes, optic light ends, and so forth are expensive equipment that should be lubricated and sterilized according to the manufacturer's directions. Figure 5-4 is an example of a handpiece maintenance system.

Disinfection is the application of chemicals to kill, reduce, or eliminate germs through soaking, spraying, foams, sponges, or wipes. Newer, faster-acting chemicals are manufactured each with

its own efficiency or directive, such as Surfacine, Cidex OPA, Endoclens, and others. Choice of a disinfectant depends on the item to be processed, timing (from 3–15 minutes), safety to items and operator (skin irritation, vapors, corrosion), shelf and efficiency life, and cost. Because of this diversity, use of each disinfectant must follow the manufacturer's recommendation for that product. Terms related to the disinfection process are:

- **disinfectant** (**dis**-inn-**FECK**-tant): chemical or agent that kills many microbes. Choice of type, concentration, and use is necessary for each item.
- **antiseptic** (an-tih-**SEP**-tick): usually a diluted disinfectant that prevents the growth or inhibits the development of microbes.
- **bacteriostatic** (back-tee-ree-oh-**STAT**-ick): inhibiting or retarding bacterial growth.
- **germicide** (**JER**-miss-eyed): substance that destroys some germs.
- **holding solution:** disinfectant solution with **biodegradable** (**bye**-oh-dee-**GRADE**-ah-bull = *chemical or metabolic material that breaks down protein material*) ingredient that is used to soak instruments until they are properly cleaned and sterilized.

Figure 5-3 Examples of cassette trays

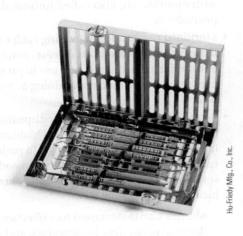

Hu-Friedy Mfg. Co., Inc.

Integra Life Sciences Corporation (through Integra Miltex)

(A)   (B)

Figure 5-4 Handpiece maintenance system

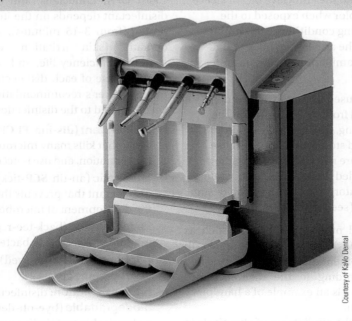

Courtesy of KaVo Dental

- **ultrasonic cleaner:** mechanical apparatus with a reservoir to contain a solution that cavitates (**implodes** = *bursts inwardly*) or bubbles off debris; this machine cleanses items prior to sterilization.

Miscellaneous Methods for Sanitation

Many items, procedures, and techniques are employed to obtain a sanitized, clean area with protection for the patient and operator as well. To maintain sanitation and safety in a dental facility, the following are relevant:

- **PPE:** *personal protective equipment*, such as gloves, eyeglasses, clinical attire, face shields, and masks to help protect the area and the wearer from disease microbes. Also included in PPE are hepatitis vaccinations (an OSHA requirement for health workers).
- **barrier techniques:** drapes, covers, plastic instrument sleeves, X-ray film covers, and the like, which are used to prevent contamination and help to protect the patients.

- **SOP:** *standard operating procedures* for sanitation of operators and patients, including the training and use of proper handling and storage of dental equipment and supplies, hand washing and transfer methods, use of evacuation methods, rubber dams, and preoperative rinse of oral cavity with mouthwash; also called universal procedures.
- **standard precautions:** treating each case as if the patient has a serious disease, handling and sterilizing with each new use to prevent contamination; called maintaining a *sterile field*.
- **proper disposal techniques:** disposing of all contaminated items in a marked biohazard bag; laundry and other materials used in patient care should be considered contaminated by splatter or aerosol matter. Disposal containers include the following:
  - **sharps container:** used for collection and disposal of needles, broken glass, and sharp items.

- ○ **biohazard container:** labeled container for items contaminated with body fluids or life-threatening contaminates.
- ○ **hazardous waste container:** receptacle for used, unsanitary items.

- **MSDS papers:** manufacturer's *material safety data sheet*, covers chemical content, labeling, storage, and safety advice; labels are marked with four colors to specify each danger potential:
  - ○ **Red (fire):** examples are flash point and relative fire hazards.
  - ○ **Yellow (reactivity):** examples are instability, such as harsh chemical, unreliable if heated; chemical reactions when mixed with others.
  - ○ **White (personal protection):** examples are corrosive, acid, radiation.
  - ○ **Blue (health):** examples are hazardous material, inhalation of irritants, toxic fumes.

- **saturate-wipe-saturate disinfection cleaning of operative area:** Many dental facilities fear that on a spray-wipe-spray method of disinfection and use of aerosol spreads and spatters germs from the contaminated sites. Instead, the personnel use disposable cloths saturated with a disinfecting solution to wipe up contaminated surfaces and then use another clean disposable, saturated

cloth to leave behind a wet surface that is wiped dry after a 10-minute soak (see Figure 5-5).

AGENCIES CONCERNED WITH DISEASE CONTROL

Boards of health at the state and local levels apply restrictions and monitoring services to ensure proper health practices for service to the general public. Each state licenses and restricts the practice of dentistry within its borders. In addition, several government agencies and controlling bodies are involved with licensing, infection control, and hazard management in the dental facility. The following are federal agencies involved with disease control and a national professional organization:

- **OSHA (Occupational Safety and Health Administration):** issues and enforces restrictions and guidelines for infection control; sets standards and regulates conditions for employers to provide safety to their employees at work.
- **CDC (Centers for Disease Control and Prevention):** sets regulations and issues suggestions for infection control, which are enforced by OSHA.
- **EPA (Environmental Protection Agency):** regulates and approves materials, equipment, medical devices, and chemicals used in dental

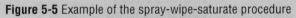

Figure 5-5 Example of the spray-wipe-saturate procedure

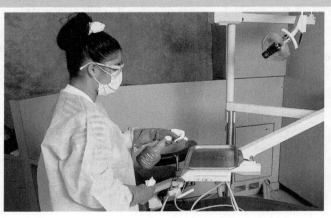

practices. Local EPA agencies regulate dental waste disposals.

- **FDA (Food and Drug Administration):** regulates and approves marketing products and solutions used in infection control.

- **OSAP (Organization for Safety and Asepsis Procedures):** national organization of health professionals that studies and makes suggestions for regulations and guidelines for infection control.

Review Exercises

Matching

Match the following word elements with their meanings.

1. _____ etiology
2. _____ fungus
3. _____ droplet infection
4. _____ pathology
5. _____ antigen
6. _____ immunity
7. _____ germicide
8. _____ sterile
9. _____ endospores
10. _____ protozoa
11. _____ edema
12. _____ implode

13. _____ staphylococcus
14. _____ vector
15. _____ disease

A. burst inward

B. capsulated rod-shaped bacillus

C. cluster-form bacteria

D. condition free from microbes

E. division of plants; includes molds and slimes

F. substance that induces body to form antibody

G. swelling

H. study of disease

I. small animal parasite

J. pathological body state, abnormal condition

K. carries or transmits disease

L. study of the cause of a disease

M. substance that destroys germs

N. resistance to microbes due to previous exposure

O. method of airborne carriage of germs

Definitions

Using the selection given for each sentence, choose the best term to complete the definition.

1. Using sanitation procedures that assume each patient is infectious is called:
   a. standard operating procedures
   b. exposure procedure
   c. universal precautions
   d. chain of infection

2. Symptoms of a disease that are reported by the patient are considered to be:
   a. subjective
   b. objective
   c. cumulative
   d. chronic

3. Diseases such as athlete's foot, thrush, and ringworm are caused by:
   a. viruses
   b. bacteria
   c. fungus
   d. cocci

4. A solution of weakened attenuated or weakened infectious agents used to produce immunity is a/an:
   a. vaccine
   b. disinfectant
   c. antibiotic
   d. toxin

5. Immunity that is inherited and permanent is called:
   a. passive
   b. active
   c. natural
   d. neutral

6. A protein substance that induces the body to form antibodies is called a/an:
   a. biodegradable
   b. immunity
   c. T bar
   d. antigen

7. When disease conditions are present over a long time, it is considered:
   a. acute
   b. endemic
   c. remission
   d. chronic

8. The process of destroying all microorganisms is called:
   a. disinfection
   b. sterilization
   c. sanitation
   d. soaking

9. An oven apparatus used to bake or heat microorganisms to attain sterilization is a/an:
   a. radiation bin
   b. dry heat sterilizer
   c. chemclave
   d. ultrasonic cleaner

10. The use of drapes, wraps, and foil coverings is considered to be what kind of technique?
    a. wrap
    b. ultrasonic
    c. barrier
    d. sepsis

11. A disease that occurs continuously in the same population or location is termed:
    a. pandemic
    b. epidemic
    c. chronic
    d. endemic

12. Which of the following items is not considered part of the PPE for the assistant?
    a. shoe covers
    b. face mask
    c. glasses
    d. gloves

13. The agency concerned with a healthy work environment for employees is:
    a. CDC
    b. OSHA
    c. OSAP
    d. EPA

14. Instruments are precleaned before sterilization in a/an:
    a. ultrasonic cleaner
    b. autoclave unit
    c. chemclave machine
    d. hot oil

15. Microbes that live together on a host without harming the host are called:
    a. saprophytes
    b. nematodes
    c. fungi
    d. commensal

16. Instruments used to penetrate soft tissue and bone are classified as which type of risk?
    a. blood-borne
    b. semi-critical
    c. noncritical
    d. critical

17. Bacteria that do not require oxygen to survive are:
    a. aerobic
    b. obligate
    c. anaerobic
    d. flagella

18. Improper handling of equipment in the dental facility would be an example of:
    a. airborne infection
    b. droplet infection
    c. indirect infection
    d. cross infection

19. A microorganism smaller than a bacterium but larger than a virus is a:
    a. flagella
    b. rickettsia
    c. fungus

20. The prediction of the course of a disease is known as a/an:
    a. assessment
    b. diagnosis
    c. estimate
    d. prognosis

Building Skills

Locate and define the prefix, root/combining form, and suffix (if present) in the following words.

1. **disinfection**
   prefix _____
   root/combining form _____
   suffix _____

2. **ultrasonic**
   prefix _____
   root/combining form _____
   suffix _____

3. **pathogenic**
   prefix _____
   root/combining form _____
   suffix _____

4. **germicidal**
   prefix _____
   root/combining form _____
   suffix _____

5. **endogenous**
   prefix _____
   root/combining form _____
   suffix _____

Fill-Ins

Write the correct word in the blank space to complete each statement.

1. Data sheets covering safety features of a product supplied by the manufacturer are called _____ _____ sheets.

2. A container for items contaminated with body fluids or life-threatening contaminants is labeled _____.

3. A machine used to bubble or cavitate dirty instruments before sterilization is called a/an _____ _____.

4. A pathological condition of the body or a body function is called a/an _____ _____.

5. The resistance to organisms due to previous exposure is called _____ _____.

6. Direct germ passage through intimate relationship is called _____ _____ infection.

7. Indicator strips are used to test the conditions of the _____ process.

8. Used needles and syringes are placed in the _____ _____.

9. Disease-producing microbes that are present in human blood are called _____ _____.

10. Another word for airborne infection is _____ _____ infection.

11. The study of diseases in general is called pathology, while the study of the cause of the disease is called _____.

12. A prediction of the course of a disease is a/an _____.

13. A carrier that transmits a disease is called a/an _____.

14. A/an _____ is a solution of killed or weakened infectious agents.

15. Instruments that do not penetrate the bloodstream but contact mucous membranes are in the _____ _____ classification of infection risk.

16. Pathogenic microbes that have been weakened or reduced in virulence are said to be _____ _____.

17. The term or act of naming a disease affecting a patient is called a/an _____.

18. Encapsulated rod-shaped bacteria encased in a resting stage are called _____.

19. A/an _____ is a group of common symptoms, signs of a disease.

20. A/an _____ is an injection of microorganisms, serum, or toxin into the body to produce immunity.

Word Use

Read the following sentences and define the boldfaced words.

1. The dentist questioned Mrs. Bailer regarding all the **symptoms** that have occurred with her tooth condition.

_____

2. Careless handling of instruments can cause a **parenteral** injury that must be reported and recorded.

_____

3. The dental assistant read that this particular disinfectant was not effective when dealing with TB **endospores**.

_____

4. The dental hygienist reviews the patient's **immunizations** when completing the health records.

_____

5. When placing an order for a new material, the office manager will request an **MSDS** sheet that applies to the item.

_____

CHAPTER **6** | **EMERGENCY CARE**

✓ Learning Objectives

On completion of this chapter, you should be able to:

1. Discuss the importance of prevention, the procedures taken to prepare for emergencies, and procedures for taking vital signs.

2. List and identify the major equipment and materials needed in emergency prevention and treatment.

3. Discuss the methods to clear the airway, and define the terms related to resuscitation.

4. List and discuss the various types of shock.

5. List and describe the most frequent medical emergencies and conditions affecting dental care.

6. Describe the most common emergencies occurring in the dental facility.

EMERGENCY-PREVENTION TECHNIQUES

The best treatment for emergencies is to prevent them from happening. With careful training, observation, and preparation, many medical and dental emergencies can be averted. Two of

---

Vocabulary Related to Emergency Care

This list contains selected new and important word parts and terms from this chapter. Take the time to learn these word parts and their meanings. You may use the list to review these terms and practice pronouncing them correctly. When you work with the audio for this chapter, listen to the word, repeat it, and then place a checkmark in the box. Proceed to the next boxed word and repeat the process.

(hyphen before word means it's a suffix, hyphen after word means prefix, no hyphen means root word.)

Word Parts	Meaning	Word Parts	Meaning
arteri/o	artery	trache	windpipe, trachea
sclero	hardening	otomy	cutting into
-sis	state of	hyper	above, beyond
psych/o	mind	ventila	air vent
fibrilla	irregular rhythm		

Key Terms

- ❏ **anaphylactic** (an-ah-fih-**LACK**-tick)
- ❏ **aneroid** (**AN**-er-oyd)
- ❏ **aneurysm** (**AN**-you-rizm)
- ❏ **antecubital fossa** (an-tee-**CUE**-bee-tal **FAH**-sah)
- ❏ **aorta** (ay-**ORE**-tah)
- ❏ **apnea** (**AP**-nee-ah)
- ❏ **arrhythmia** (ah-**RITH**-mee-ah)
- ❏ **arteriosclerosis** (ar-**teer**-ee-oh-skleh-**ROH**-siss)

- ❏ **asphyxiation** (ass-**fick**-see-**AY**-shun)
- ❏ **atherosclerosis** (**ath**-er-oh-skleh-**ROH**-sis)
- ❏ **atrioventricular** (ay-tree-oh-ven-**TRICK**-you-lar)
- ❏ **atrium** (**AY**-tree-um)
- ❏ **aural** (**ORE**-ahl)
- ❏ **axillary** (**ACK**-sih-lair-ee)
- ❏ **bradycardia** (bray-dee-**KAR**-dee-ah)

- ❏ **cardiogenic** (kar-dee-oh-**JEN**-ick)
- ❏ **cerebrovascular** (**sare**-ee-broh-**VAS**-kyou-lar)
- ❏ **clonic** (**KLAHN**-ick)
- ❏ **cricothyrotomy** (**kry**-koh-thigh-**ROT**-oh-mee)
- ❏ **cyanosis** (sigh-ah-**NO**-sis)
- ❏ **defibrillation** (dee-fib-rih-**LAY**-shun)
- ❏ **deficit** (**DEF**-ih-sit)
- ❏ **diaphragm** (**DYE**-ah-fram)

Vocabulary Related to Emergency Care *continued*

Key Terms *continued*

- ❏ **diastolic** (dye-ah-**STAHL**-ick)
- ❏ **dyspnea** (**DISP**-nee-ah)
- ❏ **embolism** (**EM**-boh-lizm)
- ❏ **endocardium** (en-doh-**KAR**-dee-um)
- ❏ **epicardium** (epp-ih-**KAR**-dee-um)
- ❏ **epilepsy** (**EP**-ih-lep-see)
- ❏ **epistaxis** (ep-ih-**STACK**-sis)
- ❏ **erythema** (air-ith-**EE**-mah)
- ❏ **expiration** (ecks-purr-**AY**-shun)
- ❏ **febrile** (**FEEB**-ril)
- ❏ **hemiplegia** (hem-ih-**PLEE**-jee-ah)
- ❏ **hyperthermia** (high-per-**THER**-mee-ah)
- ❏ **hyperventilation** (**high**-per-ven-tih-**LAY**-shun)
- ❏ **hypoglycemia** (high-poh-gly-**SEE**-me-ah)
- ❏ **hypothermia** (high-poh-**THER**-mee-ah)

- ❏ **hypoxia** (high-**POCK**-see-ah)
- ❏ **incontinence** (in-**KAHN**-tin-ense)
- ❏ **inspiration** (in-spur-**AY**-shun)
- ❏ **ischemia** (iss-**KEE**-me-ah)
- ❏ **metabolic** (met-ah-**BAHL**-ick)
- ❏ **myocardial infarction** (my-oh-**KAR**-dee-ahl in-**FARK**-shun)
- ❏ **myocardium** (my-oh-**KAR**-dee-um)
- ❏ **neurogenic** (new-roh-**JEN**-ick)
- ❏ **pericardium** (pair-ih-**KAR**-dee-um)
- ❏ **postural** (**PAHS**-tour-al)
- ❏ **psychogenic** (sigh-koh-**JEN**-ick)
- ❏ **respiratory** (**RESS**-purr-ah-tore-ee)
- ❏ **resuscitation** (ree-**SUSS**-ih-tay-shun)
- ❏ **septic** (**SEP**-tick)

- ❏ **sequestra** (see-**KWESS**-trah)
- ❏ **sphygmomanometer** (sfig-moh-man-**AHM**-eh-ter)
- ❏ **sternum** (**STIR**-num)
- ❏ **stethoscope** (**STETH**-oh-scope)
- ❏ **stertorous** (**STARE**-toe-rus)
- ❏ **stoma** (**STOW**-mah)
- ❏ **systolic** (sis-**TAH**-lick)
- ❏ **tachycardia** (tack-ee-**KAR**-dee-ah)
- ❏ **tracheotomy** (tray-kee-**AH**-toh-mee)
- ❏ **trismus** (**TRIZ**-mus)
- ❏ **tympanic** (tim-**PAN**-ick)
- ❏ **urticaria** (yur-tih-**CARE**-ee-ah)
- ❏ **ventricle** (**VEN**-trih-kul)
- ❏ **vesicle** (**VES**-ih-kuhl)
- ❏ **xiphoid** (**ZIF**-oyd)

the fundamental methods employed in facility readiness are:

- **Patient health history:** written and oral communication regarding the patient's present and past health status, including medication, treatment, allergies, and health concerns.
- **Vital signs:** body indications of the patient's present health status, including blood pressure, pulse, respiration, temperature, and the patient's concept of pain.

Blood Pressure

Blood pressure (BP) is an indication of the pulsating force of blood circulating through the blood vessels at rest **diastolic** (dye-ah-**STAHL**-ick) and while under the highest pressure of the circulating blood, the **systolic** (sis-**TAHL**-ick) pressure. BP is recorded in even numbers, with systolic pressure numbers placed before diastolic pressure numbers, for example, 120/80 (systolic/diastolic). Relevant terms are:

- **stethoscope** (**STETH**-oh-scope): device employed to intensify body sounds. It has a set of earpieces inserted into rubber tubing that combines the two ear tubes into one and extends to a metal bell-shaped or flat disc diaphragm. Stethoscopes used in training may have two earpieces combined to one diaphragm for instructional purposes.
- **diaphragm** (**DYE**-ah-fram = *thin covering*): a thin layer over the disc end of the stethoscope that helps to enlarge or amplify pulse and body sounds.

- **sphygmomanometer** (**sfig**-moh-man-**AHM**-eh-ter): an instrument employed to measure the arterial blood pressure. This instrument is available in portable, wall mounted, or mobile floor units and consists of a squeeze bulb on rubber tubing, an arm cuff, and a pressure or **aneroid** (**AN**-er-oyd = *air pressure*) dial or a graduated marked mercury column. Digital sphygmomanometers use only a wraparound cuff with machine read-out gauges; no stethoscope is required. The mercury column unit is considered the most reliable recorder and may be used to calibrate the aneroid system.
- **antecubital fossa** (an-tee-**CUE**-bee-tal **FAH**-sah): interior depression or bend of the elbow; the approximate area for the placement of the stethoscope diaphragm to determine blood-pressure sound.
- **brachial artery:** situated at the inside, upper arm area; selected site of blood-pressure cuff placement.

Pulse

Pulse is the beating force for blood circulating through arteries, which is classified according to rate, rhythm, and condition. Pulse counts may be taken at various body areas. Figure 6-1 shows the sites for pulse and blood-pressure readings. Abnormal pulse rates can be:

- **accelerated:** faster pulse rate than normal or expected, also called "rapid."
- **alternating:** changing back and forth of weak and strong pulsations.

Other terms related to pulse are:
- **arrhythmia** (ah-**RITH**-mee-ah): irregular heartbeat or pulsations.
- **bradycardia** (**bray**-dee-**KAR**-dee-ah): pulse rate under 60 beats per minute (bpm).
- **tachycardia** (**tack**-ee-**KAR**-dee-ah): an abnormal condition of pulse rates over 100 bpm (except in children).
- **deficit** (**DEF**-ah-sit = *lacking*): lower pulse rate at the wrist than at the heart site; "heart flutter."

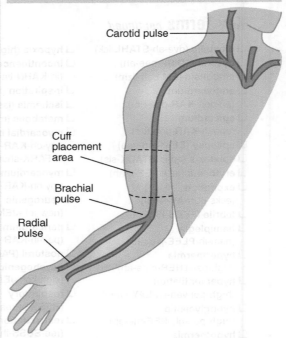

Figure 6-1 Pulse sites used in blood-pressure readings and pulse counts

Carotid pulse

Cuff placement area

Brachial pulse

Radial pulse

Note: The pulse point at the wrist is the radial pulse; in the elbow, the brachial pulse; and in the neck, the carotid pulse.

- **febrile** (**FEEB**-ril): normal pulse rate becoming weak and feeble with prostration or illness.
- **frequency:** pulse count; number of pulsations, which differs with age, sex, body position, health of patient. Frequency can be:
  - **intermittent:** occasional skipping of heartbeats.
  - **irregular:** variation of force or frequency in pulse rate.
  - **regular:** uniform pulse force, frequency, and duration.
  - **thready:** a fine, hard-to-locate, barely perceivable pulse.

Respiration

Respiration is the inhaling or breathing in of oxygen and the exhaling or expelling of carbon dioxide. One

Table 6-1 Vital Signs Ranges

Ages	Blood Pressure	Pulse	Respiration	Temperature
Infants	70–100/50–70	80–160 bpm	30–70 bpm	99.2–99.8
2–5 years	82–110/50–75	80–120 bpm	22–35 bpm	98.5–99
6–12 years	84–120/54–80	75–110 bpm	18–25 bpm	98–98.5
13–18 years	90–140/62–88	60–90 bpm	16–20 bpm	97–99
Adults	90–140/60–90	60–100 bpm	15–20 bpm	97–99
Geriatric +70	90–140/60–90	60–100 bpm	15–20 bpm	96–99

respiration count requires an **inspiration** (**in**-spur-**AY**-shun = *breathing in*) and an **expiration** (ecks-pur-**AY**-shun = *breathing out*). Respirations are described according to rate, character, and rhythm as:

- **absent:** suppresses respiratory sounds.
- **apnea** (**AP**-nee-ah): cessation of breathing, usually temporary.
- **Cheyne-Stokes:** respirations gradually increasing in volume until climax, and then subsiding and ceasing for a short period of time before starting again; may be noted in dying.
- **deep:** strong inhalation of air with exhalation.
- **dyspnea** (**DISP**-nee-ah): out of breath; difficult or labored breathing.
- **frequent:** rapid breathing that may be noted in children, those with disease, those in hysteria, or those in a drug-induced condition.
- **rale** (**RAHL**): noisy, bubbling sounds from lung mucous, heard on inhalation.
- **shallow:** short inhalation with small rise in chest.
- **slow:** fewer than 12 respirations per minute.
- **stertorous** (**STARE**-toe-rus): rattling, bubbling, or snoring sounds that obscure normal breaths.

Temperature

Temperature is the balance of heat loss and production in a body and may be taken at various sites, such as oral, rectal, **axillary** (**ACK**-sih-lair-ee = *armpit*), and aural (**ORE**-ahl = *pertaining to the ear*). Terms relating to temperature are:

- **fever:** elevated body temperature, usually considered over 38.3°C (100–103°F).
- **hyperthermia** (high-per-**THER**-mee-ah): body temperature exceeding 40°C (104°F).
- **hypothermia** (high-poh-**THER**-mee-ah): body temperature, below 35°C (95°F).
- **tympanic** (tim-**PAN**-ick = *pertaining to eardrum*): measurement of body heat registered by an ear thermometer.

The normal ranges of four vital signs are listed in Table 6-1.

Patient's Concept of Pain

A sixth vital sign, the patient's concept of pain, is added to the patient's assessment. Recording the patient's concept of pain endured can be used as a measurement in the determination of the patient's condition. The patient rates the level of pain on a scale of 1–10 in intensity. Any increase or decrease in this pain concept may indicate the course of the disease. This vital sign is subjective because it is received from the patient while the other five listed are objective and can be seen by others and recorded.

EMERGENCY-PREVENTION EQUIPMENT AND MATERIALS

All facilities should maintain the basic equipment and materials necessary to deal with emergencies. Knowledge of the location and use of the following emergency items is essential:

- **emergency call list:** important phone numbers necessary in an emergency, which are located in a prominent position near every available phone.
- **oxygen source:** container with oxygen gas tank, colored green; obtained in various sizes and may be centrally supplied to each work station (see Figure 6-2).
- **oxygen regulator:** device used to control the flow of oxygen.
- **oxygen flowmeter:** gauge used to adjust the flow amount of oxygen.
- **oxygen mask:** device placed over a patient's nose and mouth to administer gas; may be clear or tinted plastic or rubber material.

- **demand-valve resuscitator:** device attached to an oxygen mask to apply pressure to the oxygen flow and thereby inflate the lungs.
- **AMBU-bag:** handheld squeeze device with a mask that is placed over the patient's nose and mouth and used to force atmospheric air into the patient's lungs; may also be attached to the oxygen supply to force oxygen to lungs.
- **emergency tray:** a tray assembled with materials and items necessary for emergencies; often supplied in kit form with medicines, administration items, and chemicals to be used for various emergency events. Emergency trays must be updated frequently and close at hand. All dental personnel should know how to use each item (see Figure 6-3).

Figure 6-2 Oxygen supply unit. All practice personnel should know how to operate the oxygen unit in preparation for an emergency

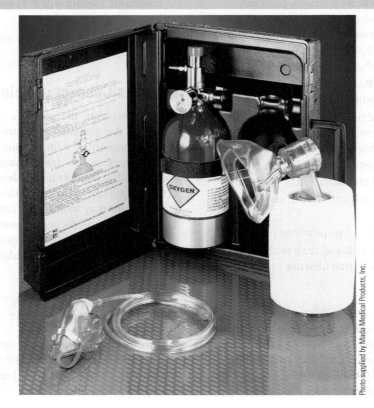

Photo supplied by Mada Medical Products, Inc.

Figure 6-3 An emergency tray is an essential need for most dental-practice emergencies

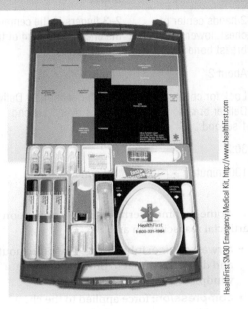

Healthfirst SM30 Emergency Medical Kit, http://www.healthfirst.com

AIRWAY OBSTRUCTION AND RESUSCITATION PROTOCOL

One of the most-feared emergency situations is an airway obstruction, which occurs when a blockage prevents the patient from receiving air into the lungs. Symptoms include an inability to speak or make a noise, fearfulness, opened eyes, clutching of the throat, and **cyanosis** (**sigh**-ah-**NO**-sis = *blue condition*), which is a bluish discoloration of the skin caused by a lack of oxygen. The following are terms related to airway obstruction and resuscitation:

- **abdominal thrust:** quick, jabbing pressure and force at belt line to force air up the windpipe.
- **asphyxiation** (ass-**fick**-see-**AY**-shun): not breathing; a result of oxygen imbalance.
- **chest thrusts:** applying quick pressure on the chest to force air upward in the windpipe to dislodge the obstruction; may be used on pregnant women as a substitute for abdominal thrusts.
- **cricothyrotomy** (**kry**-koh-thigh-**ROT**-oh-mee; crico = *ring*, thyreo = *shield*, tomy = *cut*):

an insert or cut into the thyroid and cricoid cartilage to introduce an emergency air supply.

- **gastric distension:** a condition resulting from air having been forced into the abdomen instead of the lungs.
- **Heimlich maneuver:** procedure in which abdominal thrusts are applied to a choking patient, which forces air from the diaphragm upward to expel a blockage in the airway.
- **hypoxia** (high-**POCK**-see-ah = *lack of oxygen*): a lack of inspired oxygen.
- **stoma** (**STOH**-mah = *mouth*): an artificial opening into the windpipe that is placed between the mouth and lung; the opening is at the frontal base of neck into the windpipe for air intake.
- **tracheotomy** (**tray**-kee-**AH**-toh-mee = *cutting into the trachea*): a cut and an insertion of a tube into the trachea for an emergency air supply.

Cardiopulmonary Resuscitation

Occasionally, an emergency requires **cardiopulmonary resuscitation**, commonly known as CPR, a life-saving measure that combines artificial respiration with external cardiac massage. The American Heart Association (AHA) and American Red Cross believe that air intake is less important than external compression. The following steps, also presented in Table 6-2, are now preferred for anyone who is unresponsive and not breathing normally:

1. **Call 911** for assistance or ask a bystander to call 911, then send someone to get an AED. Stay with the victim if no one else is around.

2. **Open the airway.** With the person lying on his or her back, tilt the head back slightly to lift the chin.

3. **Check for breathing.** Listen carefully, for no more than 10 seconds, for sounds of breathing. If there is no breathing, begin CPR.

4. **Push hard, push fast.** Place your hands, one on top of the other, in the middle of the chest.

Table 6-2 Guidelines for Administering CPR

	Adult	Child	Infant
Hand Position	2 hands center of chest, lower half of breast bone	2 hands center of chest, lower half of breast bone	2–3 fingers in the center of the chest, lower half of the breast bone
Compression Depth	At least 2″	About 2″	About 1½″
Breathing	Look for chest rise; Deliver breaths over 1 second	Look for chest rise; Deliver breaths over 1 second	Look for chest rise; Deliver breaths over 1 second
Compressions:Breaths	30:2	30:2	30:2
Compression Rate	100/minute	100/minute	100/minute

Use your body weight to help you administer compressions that are at least 2 inches deep and delivered at a rate of at least 100 compressions per minute.

5. **Deliver rescue breaths.** With the person's head tilted back slightly and the chin lifted, pinch the nose shut and place your mouth over the person's mouth to make a complete seal. Blow into the person's mouth to make the chest rise. Deliver two rescue breaths, then continue compressions.

6. **Continue CPR steps.** Keep performing cycles of chest compressions and breathing until the person exhibits signs of life such as breathing, an AED (**automated external defibrillator**) becomes available, or EMS or a trained medical responder arrives on scene. An AED is a mechanical/electrical device used to revive and stimulate the heart of a patient in cardiac arrest. Dated electrode pads are placed on the patient's chest to determine if pulseless ventricular tachycardia or a ventricular fibrillation is occurring. After diagnosis, the unit will signal the need for a shock and administer it, analyze the patient, and indicate the need for CPR or administer another shock. Figure 6-4 shows the AED machine and pad placement.

Some common terms used in connection with artificial resuscitation are:

- **airway device:** tube inserted into the mouth and down the throat to provide air to the windpipe.
- **compression:** force applied to the chest, providing pressure on the heart to imitate a heartbeat or pulsation.
- **finger sweep:** using a finger in the mouth of an unconscious person to locate and wipe out any airway obstruction.
- **sternum (STIR**-num): "breastbone," which is the flat bone between the ribs.
- **xiphoid (ZIF**-oyd) process: lowest portion of the sternum (breastbone) with no ribs attached.

CLASSIFICATION OF SHOCK

When a patient incurs a condition that alters the intake of oxygen and its passage and use, the body may react by shutting down any or all of its systems. The most common symptom of shock is **syncope** (**SIN**-koh-pee = *fainting*). The pulse may become weak, fast, or irregular, and blood pressure may drop. Breathing may increase, accompanied by pale skin, sweating, and possibly vomiting. Treatment includes finding the source of shock, providing

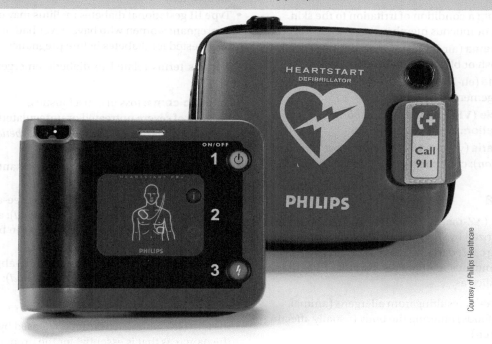

suitable treatment, maintaining body functions, and obtaining assistance. There are nine basic types of shock:

- **anaphylactic** (an-ah-fih-**LACK**-tick): shock arising from a reaction to a body allergen.
- **cardiogenic** (**kar**-dee-oh-**JEN**-ick): shock arising from improper heart action.
- **hemorrhage:** shock arising from excessive blood loss.
- **metabolic** (met-ah-**BAHL**-ick): shock arising from endocrine diseases and disorders, such as diabetes.
- **neurogenic** (**new**-row-**JEN**-ick): shock arising from nervous impulses.
- **postural** (**PAHS**-tour-al): shock arising from a sudden change in body positions.
- **psychogenic** (sigh-koh-**JEN**-ick): shock arising from mental origins.
- **respiratory** (res-per-uh-**TORE**-ee): shock arising from insufficient breathing.

- **septic** (**SEP**-tick): shock arising from a microbial infection.

COMMON MEDICAL EMERGENCIES

During the course of treatment in the dental facility, an occasional medical emergency will arise that complicates the handling and care of the patient. These include allergies, asthma, reactions related to diabetes, epilepsy, hyperventilation, and heart conditions.

Allergies

An **allergic reaction** is caused by a person's sensitivity to a specific antigen that can result in a variety of symptoms. Some are as mild as a slight rash, and others are quite involved, including death from severe anaphylactic shock.

- **anaphylaxis** (an-ah-fill-**ACK**-sis): an allergic reaction of the body resulting in lowered blood pressure, swelling of the throat, shock, and even death.

- **itching:** a condition of irritation to the skin, scalp, or mucous membranes.
- **erythema** (air-ih-**THEE**-mah = *skin redness*): a red rash or blotching of the skin.
- **edema** (eh-**DEE**-mah): a tissue swelling, enlargement of a body area.
- **vesicle** (**VES**-ih-kuhl = *small blister*) **formation:** small, watery blisters.
- **urticaria** (yur-tih-**CARE**-ee-ah = *vascular skin reaction*): commonly called hives or wheals.

Asthma

Asthma (**AZ**-mah = *panting*) is a chronic disorder characterized by shortness of breath, wheezing, and coughing caused by spasms of the bronchial tubes or swollen mucous membranes. Asthmatic conditions are classified as:

- **extrinsic:** resulting from allergens (animal, dust, foods) entering the body (usually affecting children).
- **intrinsic:** resulting from bronchial infection allergens (usually affecting older patients).
- **status asthmaticus** (**AS**-matic-us): severe asthma attack that may be fatal.

Allergies, asthma, diabetes, and other emergencies occurring in the dental practice need immediate attention and sometimes medication that is found in a prepared emergency tray, as shown earlier in Figure 6-3.

Diabetes Mellitus

Diabetes mellitus (dye-ah-**BEE**-tus = *passing through*, mel-**EYE**-tus = *sugar in the urine*) is a disorder of the metabolism of carbohydrates. This disease has been divided into three types:

- Type I, insulin-dependent diabetes (once termed juvenile diabetes), has an early onset and is more severe in course. Treatment consists of insulin intake.
- Type II, noninsulin-dependent diabetes, usually develops later in life and may be

regulated by diet control and/or taking oral medication.

- Type III gestational diabetes mellitus may occur in pregnant women who have never had or been tested for diabetes before pregnancy.

Various terms related to diabetic emergencies are:

- **diabetic coma:** loss of consciousness because of severe untreated or unregulated hyperglycemia, a condition termed *diabetic acidosis.*
- **glucose** (**GLUE**-kose): sugar, an important carbohydrate in body metabolism.
- **hyperglycemia** (**high**-purr-gly-**SEE**-mee-ah; hyper = *over*, glyco = *sweet*, emia = *blood*): a condition characterized by an increase in blood sugar.
- **hypoglycemia** (**high**-poh-gly-**SEE**-me-ah; hypo = *under,* glyco = *sweet*, emia = *blood*): a condition in which the blood sugar is abnormally low.
- **insulin** (**IN**-sahlin): a hormone released by the pancreas that is essential for the proper metabolism of sugar (glucose).
- **insulin shock:** a condition produced by an overdose of insulin resulting in a lowered blood sugar level (hypoglycemia).
- **juvenile diabetes:** onset of diabetes in a person under 15 years of age.
- **ketone** (**KEY**-tone): acidic substance resulting from metabolism; sometimes produces an acetone mouth odor similar to the odor of nail polish remover.

Epilepsy

Epilepsy (**EP**-ih-**lep**-see = *a seizure*) is a disease characterized by recurrent seizures resulting from disturbed brain functioning. Symptoms can range from mild twitching to periods of unconsciousness accompanied with body movements and actions. Caregivers maintain safety by assuring that the patient has an open airway and does not harm himself or herself during this period. Terms related to epilepsy are:

- **petit mal** (**PEH**-teet-mahl) **seizure:** small seizures consisting of momentary unconsciousness with mild body movements or actions of staring off into space; sometimes called *absence seizures* (ab-SAH-ence; French pronunciation).
- **grand mal seizure:** significant epileptic attack that may include an aura, unconsciousness, spasms, mouth frothing, incontinence, and coma.
- **status epilepticus:** a rapid succession of epileptic attacks without the person's regaining consciousness between the occurrences.
- **aura** (**AW**-rah = *breeze*): a subtle sensation of oncoming physical or mental disorder.
- **clonic** (**KLON**-ick = *turmoil*): seizure marked by alternating contraction and relaxation of muscles, producing jerking movements.
- **partial epilepsy:** form of epilepsy consisting of convulsions, without loss of consciousness, that are restricted to certain areas, such as one side of the body.

- **tonic** (**TAHN**-ick) **seizure:** seizure marked by continuous muscular tension, producing rigidity or violent spasms.
- **incontinence** (in-**KAHN**-tin-ense): loss of bladder control, which may occur during a seizure.

Hyperventilation

Hyperventilation (**high**-per-ven-tih-**LAY**-shun) is a condition of increased inspiration resulting in a carbon dioxide decrease (*acapnia*) in the body. This may cause tingling of fingers and/or toes, a drop in blood pressure, dizziness, and possible syncope. Treatment consists of calming the patient's fears, remaining reassuring, and asking the patient to breathe into a paper bag, or to cup the hands over the mouth and take deep breaths. This helps the body regain a carbon dioxide/oxygen balance (see Figure 6-5).

Figure 6-5 Hyperventilation—patient breathing into a paper bag

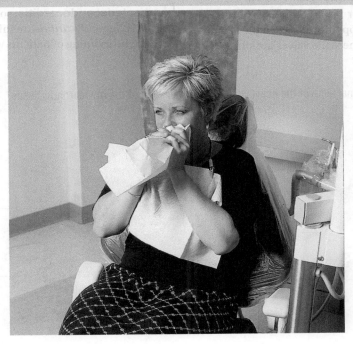

Heart Conditions

Heart problems are cardiac diseases and conditions that are related to the heart, the muscular organ that powers the circulatory system. The heart, as seen in Figure 6-6, is encased in a sac called the **pericardium** (pear-ih-**KAR**-dee-um = *sac around the heart*), which has three layers:

- **epicardium** (epp-ih-**KAR**-dee-um): outer serous layer.
- **myocardium** (my-oh-**KAR**-dee-um): middle cardiac muscular layer.
- **endocardium** (en-doh-**KAR**-dee-um): inner layer lining the four heart chambers.

Various terms are used to describe heart structure, conditions, and diseases:

- **atrium** (**AY**-tree-um = *corridor*; plural is **atria**): two upper chambers of the heart, right and left.
- **ventricle** (**VEN**-trih-kul = *little belly*): two lower chambers of the heart, one on each side, beneath the atrium.
- **valve** (*tiny fold*): a structure for temporary closing of the blood vessels; valves also control the flow of blood through the heart.
- **atrioventricular** (**ay**-tree-oh-ven-**TRICK**-you-lar) **orifice**: an opening between the atrium and ventricle where the valves are situated.

- **semilunar valves:** heart valves. The aortic valve is found at the entrance of the aorta to the heart, and the pulmonary valve or tricuspid valve is situated between the right atrium and the right ventricle of the heart. The mitral, or bicuspid valve, is on the left side between the atrium and the ventricle.
- **aorta** (ay-**ORE**-tah): main artery that exits from the heart.
- **murmur:** abnormal sound heard over the heart or blood vessels, an indication of improper blood flow or valve action.
- **arteriosclerosis** (ar-**teer**-ee-oh-skleh-**ROH**-siss): thickening and hardening of small arteries.
- **atherosclerosis** (**ath**-er-oh-skleh-**ROH**-sis): blocking of larger artery, often from plaque buildup.
- **angina pectoris** (an-**JINE**-ah **PECK** tor-is): a pain in the chest caused by a heart malfunction.
- **myocardial infarction** (my-oh-**KAR**-dee-ahl in-**FARK**-shun): necrosis or death of the myocardium muscle tissue, a heart attack (MI).
- **bacterial endocarditis:** sometimes termed *infective endocarditis*, an inflammation of the heart lining of patients who have had

Figure 6-6 Internal view of the heart with an enlarged view of the myocardium tissue

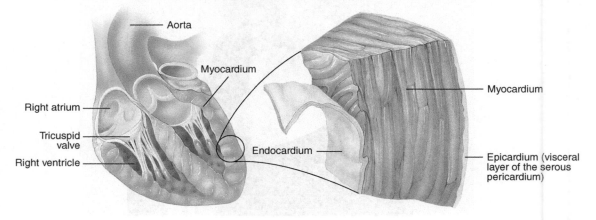

Aorta

Myocardium

Myocardium

Right atrium

Tricuspid valve

Endocardium

Right ventricle

Epicardium (visceral layer of the serous pericardium)

rheumatic fever, open-heart surgery, body part replacements, or implants. Although this is not an immediate emergency chairside threat, these patients require pretreatment with antibiotic therapy to ward off future infections.

- **nitroglycerin:** medication for the immediate relief of heart pains, particularly angina pectoris.

Stroke

A common illness related to the blood supply and circulation is stroke. A stroke is technically termed a **cerebrovascular** (**sare**-ee-broh-**VASS**-kyou-lar = *pertaining to the blood vessels of the brain*) **accident** (abbreviated as CVA). A stroke is the result of insufficient blood supply to the brain because of a rupture or blockage. Recognition of symptoms and immediate care is important because medical attention given within three hours can be of great benefit. There are two types of strokes:

- **hemorrhagic stroke:** occurs when a blood vessel in some part of the brain weakens and bursts open, causing damage to the brain cells; occurs in 15% of strokes.
- **ischemic** (is-**KEY**-mick) **stroke:** caused when the blood supply to the brain is blocked by either a blood clot traveling to the brain (*embolic shock*) or a blood clot forming in an artery (*thrombotic stroke*); occurs in 85% of strokes.

Other terms related to stroke are:

- **transient ischemic attack (TIA):** localized, temporary anemia resulting from an obstruction of the blood circulation; also called a *mini-stroke*. **Ischemia** (iss-**KEE**-me-ah) means a holding back of blood. TIA attacks resolve in less than 24 hours and may be precursors of a stroke (CVA).
- **embolism** (**EM**-boh-lizm): a floating clot or air bubble that may lodge in a blood vessel; if lodged in the brain, it is called *cerebral embolism.*
- **hemorrhage** (**HEM**-or-rij = *blood burst*): a rupture in a brain artery.

- **infarction** (in-**FARK**-shun): a decreased blood supply causing necrosis or tissue death.
- **thrombosis** (throm-**BOE**-siss): a clot forming in a blood vessel; atherosclerosis.
- **hemiplegia** (hem-ih-**PLEE**-jee-ah = *a paralysis on one side of the body*): may result from a brain lesion, thrombosis, hemorrhage, or tumor of the cerebrum.
- **aneurysm** (**AN**-you-rizm = *dilation or bulging of a blood vessel because of wall weakness*): a balloon-like enlargement of a cerebral artery or another vessel.

Signs or symptoms of a possible stroke vary but can be detectable by observers: walking and balance off, speech slurred, face droopy, coordination not working, confusion, and so on.

If you see these symptoms, act FAST:

- **F**ace: Ask the person to smile. Does one side of the face droop?
- **A**rms: Ask the person to raise both arms. Does one arm drift down?
- **S**peech: Ask the person to repeat a simple sentence. Are the words slurred? Was it repeated correctly?
- **T**ime: If the person shows any of these symptoms, call 911. Time is important. Wait for the ambulance or go to the hospital if instructed.

COMMON DENTAL EMERGENCIES

Some emergencies are specifically dental related, occurring as a result of recent dental treatment or the need for dental treatment:

- **alveolitis** (al-**vee**-oh-**LIE**-tis): inflammation of the alveolar area, commonly called "dry socket."
- **avulsed** (uh-**VULST**): a tooth or body part that has been knocked out, forced, or torn away.
- **epistaxis** (ep-ih-**STACK**-sis): nosebleed.
- **hemorrhage:** excessive bleeding. Treatments for hemorrhage are:
  - **astringent** (ah-strin-**JENT**): agent that has a binding effect; constricts.

Figure 6-7 Trendelenburg position; emergency position to restore blood to the brain

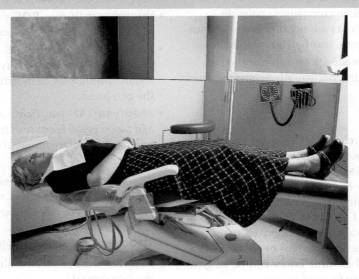

- ○ **coagulant** (koh-**AG**-you-lant): an agent that causes blood to coagulate or congeal.
- ○ **hemostatic** (**hee**-moe-**STAT**-ick): agent that stops bleeding, such as vitamin K.
- **trismus** (**TRIZ**-mus): tonic contraction of muscle, perhaps muscles of mastication (jaw).
- **postural hypotension:** a decrease in blood pressure resulting from quickly raising the body after having been in a lowered position for a period of time; rapid sit-up resulting in dizziness.

- **sequestra** (see-**KWESS**-trah): small bone pieces or spicules working to the surface after surgery, causing bleeding and soreness.
- **syncope** (fainting): the most common emergency in a dental facility. The **Trendelenburg position** refers to the patient being placed in a subsupine position with the feet higher than the head; used in office syncope emergencies (see Figure 6-7).

Review Exercises

Matching

Match the following word elements with their meanings.

1. _____ vesicle

2. _____ apnea

3. _____ dyspnea

4. _____ ketone

5. _____ axillary

6. _____ tonic

7. _____ insulin

A. pulse rate under 60 bpm

B. artificial neck opening for inspiration of air

C. breastbone

D. continuous muscular tension

E. cessation of breathing

F. nosebleed

G. small, watery blister

8.	_____ sternum	**H.**	pulse rate over 100 bpm
9.	_____ thrombosis	**I.**	loss of bladder control
10.	_____ bradycardia	**J.**	clot formed in a blood vessel
11.	_____ epistaxis	**K.**	acid substance resulting from body metabolism
12.	_____ atrium	**L.**	difficult, labored breathing
13.	_____ stoma	**M.**	upper chamber half of heart
14.	_____ tachycardia	**N.**	pertaining to the armpit
15.	_____ incontinence	**O.**	hormone released from pancreas for metabolism

Definitions

Using the selection given in each sentence, choose the best term to complete the definition.

1. The machine that is exclusively used to determine arterial blood pressure is the:
   a. sphygmomanometer
   b. arteriogram
   c. diaphragm
   d. thermometer

2. Which type of shock is caused by a rupture of blood vessel in the head?
   a. atherosclerosis
   b. cardiac
   c. hemorrhagic
   d. ischemic

3. A small epileptic seizure of momentary unconsciousness and mild body involvement is a/an:
   a. grand mal seizure
   b. clonic seizure
   c. aura seizure
   d. petit mal seizure

4. Thickening and hardening of the wall of an artery is termed:
   a. angina pectoris
   b. arterosclerosis
   c. atherosclerosis
   d. arythrocardia

5. What color designates that the gas content is oxygen?
   a. green
   b. blue
   c. red
   d. yellow

6. A body temperature below 35°C (95°F) is termed:
   a. hypothermia
   b. hyperthermia
   c. aurathermia
   d. diathermia

7. Chest thrusts given in cardiac resuscitation on an adult should be how deep?
   a. 2 inches
   b. 1 inch
   c. 3 inches
   d. undetermined

8. The automatic external defibrillator (AED) is used for which type of emergency?
   a. pregnancy
   b. trauma
   c. cardiac
   d. bleeding

9. Which condition exists when air is forced into the abdomen instead of the lungs during CPR?
   a. hypoxia
   b. gastric distension
   c. tracheotomy
   d. stoma

10. What type of shock arises from the body's reaction to an allergen?
    a. anaphylactic
    b. cardiogenic
    c. metabolic
    d. psychogenic

11. The sac covering that encases the heart is the:
    a. pericardium
    b. endocardium

c. myocardium
d. epicardium

12. A bluish cast to the skin due to a lack of oxygen is called:
    a. cyanamide
    b. cyanosis
    c. aura
    d. cryptitis

13. An astringent would be prescribed for which of the following?
    a. diabetes mellitus
    b. epilepsy
    c. asthma
    d. hemorrhage

14. Which type of asthmatic attacks results from an allergen and is usually seen in children?
    a. intrinsic
    b. extrinsic
    c. spastic
    d. status asthmaticus

15. The normal rate of respirations per minute for an adult is:
    a. 8–10
    b. 10–15
    c. 15–20
    d. 20–25

16. The outer serous layer of the heart muscle is the:
    a. epicardium
    b. myocardium
    c. endocardium
    d. mitral

17. The condition caused by increased inhalation resulting in lower body carbon dioxide is:
    a. erythema
    b. gastric distension
    c. hyperventilation
    d. fever

18. The inner layer of the heart, lining the four chambers, is the:
    a. epicardium
    b. myocardium
    c. endocardium
    d. mitral

19. Another term for the common nosebleed is:
    a. apnea
    b. xiphoid
    c. trismus
    d. epistaxis

20. A balloon-like enlargement of a cerebral artery or another blood vessel is a/an
    a. infarction
    b. aneurysm
    c. embolism
    d. hemorrhage

Building Skills

Locate and define the prefix, root/combining form, and suffix (if present) in the following words.

1. **arteriosclerosis**
   prefix _____
   root/combining form _____
   suffix _____

2. **defibrillation**
   prefix _____
   root/combining form _____
   suffix _____

3. **psychogenic**
   prefix _____
   root/combining form _____
   suffix _____

4. **tracheotomy**
   prefix _____
   root/combining form _____
   suffix _____

5. **hyperventilation**
   prefix _____
   root/combining form _____
   suffix _____

Fill-Ins

Write the correct word in the blank space to complete each statement.

1. An artificial opening into the windpipe is called a/an _____.

2. The tympanic temperature reading is obtained by using a/an _____ thermometer.

3. A pulse indicating an occasional skipped beat is termed _____.

4. A/an _____ is an instrument used to intensify body sounds.

5. In a blood-pressure reading, the force of the blow flow at rest is called the _____ reading.

6. One method of removing airway obstructions is to use the _____ maneuver.

7. Another word for the breastbone used in giving CPR is _____.

8. Sensitivity to an allergen present in the body is a/an _____.

9. The _____ bone is situated at the tip of the breastbone.

10. A severe microbial infection may cause _____ shock.

11. The metabolic hormone released by the pancreas is _____.

12. An awareness of an oncoming physical or mental disorder is a/an _____.

13. A quick application of pressure to simulate a heartbeat in CPR is called a/an _____.

14. The _____ are the upper halves of the heart, left and right.

15. The _____ is the main trunk artery exiting the heart.

16. In a health history, body temp, blood pressure, pulse, and respiration are considered the patient's _____ signs.

17. A/an _____ is a tonic concentration of the mastication muscles.

18. _____ or fainting is the most common emergency in the dental facility.

19. Another term for redness or blotching of the skin is _____.

20. The _____ fossa used in BP readings is situated at the inner elbow space.

Word Use

Read the following sentences and define the boldfaced words.

1. The fearful or excited patient can present an elevated **systolic count** in the blood pressure reading.

   _____

2. Since her **cerebrovascular accident (CVA)**, Mrs. Brown's speech and motor skills have been limited.

   _____

3. A patient's complaint of throat swelling and breathing difficulty indicate an oncoming **anaphylactic reaction**.

   _____

4. The receptionist noted that Mr. Harris included **hyperglycemia** as a medical condition on his health history.

   _____

5. The stethoscope's diaphragm is placed on the **antecubital fossa** during the blood pressure procedure.

   _____

7 | EXAMINATION AND PREVENTION

✓ Learning Objectives

On completion of this chapter, you should be able to:

1. Identify and list the various procedures necessary to complete an initial examination.

2. Identify the methods used to examine the oral tissues, cancer screen, and locate diseases associated with oral tissues.

3. Discuss the methods used to examine the teeth and diseases associated with decay and mouth structure.

4. List and explain the various types of teeth-numbering systems and popular mouth-charting symbols.

5. Explain alginate impression and the words related to the procedure and finished product.

6. Define preventive education, and identify the assorted methods of home dental care.

7. Explain the various professional methods used in the dental office to prevent tooth decay.

PROCEDURES INVOLVED WITH THE INITIAL EXAMINATION

This first visit to the dental office is often the most important dental experience for the patient. During this appointment, the dentist assesses the patient's general and dental health. To complete a thorough evaluation, several procedures must be performed. These include taking a health history, checking vital

Vocabulary Related to Examination and Prevention

This list contains selected new and important word parts and terms from this chapter. Take the time to learn these word parts and their meanings. You may use the list to review these terms and practice pronouncing them correctly. When you work with the audio for this chapter, listen to the word, repeat it, and then place a checkmark in the box. Proceed to the next boxed word and repeat the process.

(hyphen before word means it's a suffix, hyphen after word means prefix, no hyphen means root word.)

Word Parts	Meaning	Word Parts	Meaning
a-	without	mal-	disorder, bad
apic	apex	occuls	occlusion, biting together
enam/o	enamel	peri-	around
gloss	tongue	-plasty	surgical repair
-ic	pertaining to	symmetr	same, similar
-itis	inflammation		

Key Terms

- ❏ abfraction (ab-**FRACK**-shun)
- ❏ abrasion (ah-**BRAY**-zhun)
- ❏ alginate (**AL**-jih-nate)
- ❏ ankyloglossia (ang-key-loh-**GLOSS**-ee-ah)
- ❏ ankylosis (ang-kill-**OH**-sis)
- ❏ aphthous (**AF**-thuss)
- ❏ articulation (are-**tick**-you-**LAY**-shun)
- ❏ asculate (awe-**SKUL**-ate)
- ❏ asymmetric (ay-sim-**ET**-rick)
- ❏ attrition (ah-**TRISH**-un)
- ❏ avulsion (ah-**VULL**-shun)
- ❏ bruxism (**BRUCK**-sizm)
- ❏ calculus (**KAL**-kyou-luss)
- ❏ carcinoma (kar-sih-**NO**-mah)
- ❏ caries (**CARE**-eez)
- ❏ cariogenic (care-ee-oh-**JEN**-ick)
- ❏ cellulitis (sell-you-**LIE**-tiss)
- ❏ cheilosis (kee-**LOH**-sis)

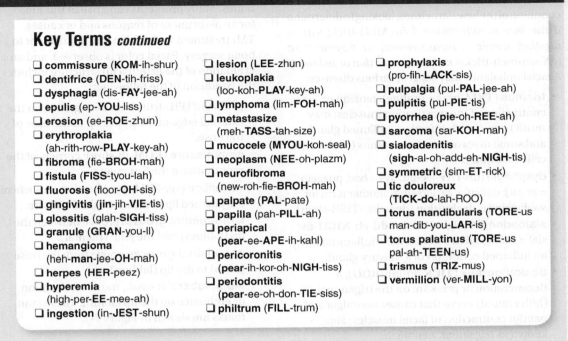

Key Terms *continued*

- **commissure (KOM**-ih-shur)
- **dentifrice (DEN**-tih-friss)
- **dysphagia** (dis-**FAY**-jee-ah)
- **epulis** (ep-**YOU**-liss)
- **erosion** (ee-**ROE**-zhun)
- **erythroplakia**
  (ah-rith-row-**PLAY**-key-ah)
- **fibroma** (fie-**BROH**-mah)
- **fistula (FISS**-tyou-lah)
- **fluorosis** (floor-**OH**-sis)
- **gingivitis (jin**-jih-**VIE**-tis)
- **glossitis** (glah-**SIGH**-tiss)
- **granule (GRAN**-you-ll)
- **hemangioma**
  (heh-**man**-jee-**OH**-mah)
- **herpes (HER**-peez)
- **hyperemia**
  (high-per-**EE**-mee-ah)
- **ingestion** (in-**JEST**-shun)

- **lesion** (**LEE**-zhun)
- **leukoplakia**
  (loo-koh-**PLAY**-key-ah)
- **lymphoma** (lim-**FOH**-mah)
- **metastasize**
  (meh-**TASS**-tah-size)
- **mucocele (MYOU**-koh-seal)
- **neoplasm (NEE**-oh-plazm)
- **neurofibroma**
  (new-roh-fie-**BROH**-mah)
- **palpate (PAL**-pate)
- **papilla** (pah-**PILL**-ah)
- **periapical**
  (pear-ee-**APE**-ih-kahl)
- **pericoronitis**
  (pear-ih-kor-oh-**NIGH**-tiss)
- **periodontitis**
  (pear-ee-oh-don-**TIE**-siss)
- **philtrum (FILL**-trum)

- **prophylaxis**
  (pro-fih-**LACK**-sis)
- **pulpalgia** (pul-**PAL**-jee-ah)
- **pulpitis** (pul-**PIE**-tis)
- **pyorrhea** (pie-oh-**REE**-ah)
- **sarcoma** (sar-**KOH**-mah)
- **sialoadenitis**
  (sigh-al-oh-add-eh-**NIGH**-tis)
- **symmetric** (sim-**ET**-rick)
- **tic douloreux**
  (**TICK**-do-lah-**ROO**)
- **torus mandibularis (TORE**-us
  man-dib-you-**LAR**-is)
- **torus palatinus (TORE**-us
  pal-ah-**TEEN**-us)
- **trismus (TRIZ**-mus)
- **vermillion** (ver-**MILL**-yon)

signs, making a visual assessment, palpating the head structures and mouth conditions, and examining the oral cavity. The initial exam may require additional procedures, including radiographs, alginate impressions, photography by intraoral and extraoral cameras and oral cancer screening, saliva testing, and any other diagnostic test deemed necessary.

Health History

The health history, as reported by the patient and reviewed by the dentist, includes the following:

- The chief complaint that will indicate the patient's symptoms
- General medical condition that will assess the ability to perform treatment
- Allergies that will prevent reactions to materials and injections to be used
- Medication schedule to help plan appointment timing

- Past history of surgeries and illnesses may indicate special treatment conditions or care
- Lifestyle and habit concerns over smoking, exercise, sugar intake, and so forth
- Medical doctor's name for backup information or consultation
- Emergency contact numbers and HIPAA selections for family member involvement

Vital Signs

As discussed in Chapter 6, Emergency Care, vital signs include blood pressure, respiration, temperature, pulse, and pain. These signs might not be taken and recorded at each visit, but during the first, or initial, examination it is important to obtain these measurements. The initial findings, recorded as the *baseline vital signs,* may be used to determine the present condition and also as a comparison or standard for future visits by the patient.

Visual Assessment

During the initial visit, the dentist assesses the condition of the head structures, looking to determine if the face is **symmetric** (sim-**MEH**-trick; sym = *together*, metric = *measurement*) or **asymmetric** (**AY**-sih-meh-trick = *without proportion or balance*). A facial imbalance may suggest various diseases:

- **trismus** (**TRIZ**-mus = *grating*): tension or contraction of the mastication muscles; may result from mouth infection, inflamed glands, and some diseases, such as tetanus (commonly called *lockjaw*).
- **dysphagia** (dis-**FAY**-jee-ah; dys = *bad*, phagein = *to eat*): difficulty swallowing; another term for swallowing is **deglutition** (**dee**-glue-**TISH**-shun).
- **sialoadenitis** (**sigh**-ah-loh-**add**-eh-**NIGH**-tis; sial = *saliva*, aden = *gland*, itis = *inflammation*): an inflamed condition of a salivary gland.
- **tic douloureux** (**TICK** do-luh-**ROO**): a degeneration or pressure on the trigeminal (fifth cranial) nerve that causes neuralgia and painful contraction of facial muscles; also known as *trigeminal neuralgia*.
- **Bell's palsy:** a sudden but temporary unilateral facial paralysis from an unknown cause but may involve swelling of the facial nerve from an immune or viral infection.

- **temporomandibular joint (TMJ):** union of the joints of the temporal and the mandibular bones. Many problems can arise in this area for an assortment of reasons and or causes. TMJ treatment varies from bite adjustment to bone surgery. Facial color is observed, and an evaluation of the external lip structure includes the condition of the following:

  - **philtrum** (**FIL**-trum): median groove on the external edge of the upper lip to the base of the nose.
  - **commissure** (**KOM**-ih-sure): corners of the mouth where the lips meet.
  - **vermillion** (ver-**MILL**-yon) **border:** area where the pink-red lip tissue meets the facial skin.
  - **labio-mental groove:** groove between the lip (labium) and the chin (mental).
  - **naso-labial groove:** groove from the nose (naso) to the lip (labium).
  - **labial tubercle:** small, rounded elevation or eminence on the lip labium. These landmarks are shown in Figure 7-1.

Palpation

One method of determining the condition of a tissue is to **palpate** (**PAL**-pate = *touch or feel*) an area.

Figure 7-1 Landmarks of the lower face area

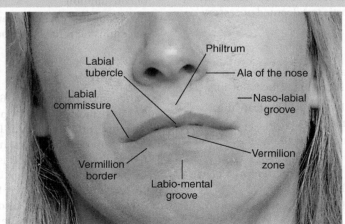

Philtrum

Labial tubercle

Ala of the nose

Labial commissure

Naso-labial groove

Vermillion border

Vermilion zone

Labio-mental groove

The dentist uses finger pressure to sense swellings, softness, irregularities, or movement in skin and mouth tissues. Lymph nodes and neck muscles are tested for lumps or swellings, and lip, cheek, tongue, and mouth tissues are also examined for irregularities. The temporomandibular joint (TMJ) area is palpated for movement and tenderness. The dentist may also use a stethoscope to **ausculate** (awes-**SKUL**-ate = *listen to movement*) the joint area and the blood flow in the carotid arteries in the neck.

EXAMINATION OF THE ORAL TISSUES

Before the dentist examines the teeth, an inspection of the oral tissues is done to determine the condition of the mouth. This usually is performed by visual observation by using regular, dental, and halogen lighting with or without special dyes. The tongue is grasped by a gauze pad and extended to full length, and the gingiva and cheek (*buccal mucosa*) areas are palpated. A variety of diseases may be found in the oral cavity:

- **oral lesion** (**LEE**-zhun = *injury, wound*): altered inflammatory tissue or infected patch in the skin. Causes could be infection, hemorrhage, ulcerations, extra melanoma, fat deposits, amalgam tattoos, dilated veins, or other causes. Associated symptoms might be pain, swelling, or pus. Lesions that affect tooth tissues are called caries.
- **gingivitis** (**jin**-jih-**VIE**-tis = *inflammation of gingiva*): redness and swelling of the gingival tissues that may be caused by irritants, disease, habits, improper hygiene, and poor general or nutritional health.
- **periodontitis** (**pear**-ee-oh-don-**TIE**-tis; peri = *around,* don = *tooth,* itis = *inflammation*): inflammation of the gingiva with involvement of deeper periosteal tissues indicated by formation of pockets and bone loss. A common name for this diseased condition is called **pyorrhea** (**pie**-oh-**REE**-ah = *pus collection*).
- **periodontal** (pear-ih-oh-**DON**-tal) **abscess** (*abscess in periodontal tissues*): abscess originating in and progressing from inflammation of periodontal tissues; differs from periapical abscess, which originates in the pulp and progresses to the apical tip.
- **pericoronitis** (**pear**-ih-kor-oh-**NIGH**-tiss; peri = *around,* corono = *tooth crown,* itis = *inflammation*): inflammation around the crown of a tooth. Pericoronitis happens quite often with erupting third molar teeth.
- **ANUG** (*acute necrotic ulcerative gingivitis*): highly inflamed and dying gingival tissues. ANUG is also called **trench mouth** or **Vincent's infection** (see Figure 7-2A).
- **cellulitis** (sell-you-**LIE**-tiss = *inflammation of cellular or connective tissue*): infection and inflammation extending into adjacent connective tissues.
- **fistula** (**FISS**-tyou-la = *pathway for pus escape, pipe*): tissue opening for pus drainage, providing some pain relief from buildup of pulpal pressure.
- **epulis** (ep-**YOU**-liss = *gumboil*): fibrous tumor of oral tissue.
- **aphthous ulcer** (**AF**-thuss **UHL**-cer; alpha = *little ulcer*): small, painful ulcer within the mouth; also called *canker sore.*
- **Fordyce granules:** small, yellow spots on the mucous membrane, usually the soft palate and buccal mucosa; considered a developmental condition.
- **thrush:** fungus infection of mouth and/or throat; appears as white patches or ulcers on tissues and is caused by *Candidiasis* infection of the oral mucosa (see Figure 7-2B).
- **candida albicans:** sore, white plaque areas resulting from long-term antibiotic therapy permitting fungus buildup.
- **herpes** (**HER**-peez) **simplex virus (HSV):** vesicles or watery pimples that burst and crust; caused by a virus; also called fever blisters or cold sores when on the lips, and gingivostomatitis when present on the oral mucosa. Types of herpes simplex are:
  - **primary herpes:** occurs in young children in the mouth or on the lips.

Figure 7-2 (A) ANUG (acute necrotic ulcerative gingivitis), (B) thrush of the tongue and mouth, (C) herpes (cold sore)

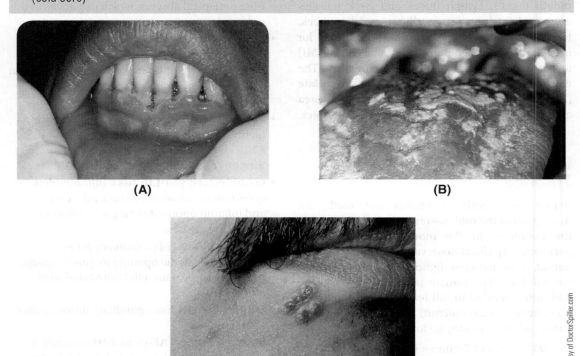

(A)

(B)

(C)

Courtesy of DoctorSpiller.com

- ○ **recurrent herpes:** reappears on the lip area (*labialis*) throughout life (see Figure 7-2C).
- ○ **herpes genitalis:** lesions occurring on male/female genitalia; called HSV-2; sexually transmitted.
- **cheilosis** (key-**LOH**-sis; cheilo = *lips,* osis = *condition*): inflammation of the lip, particularly at the corners of the lips. Primary causes include candidiasis, vitamin B deficiency, or lack of vertical dimension at the commissures because of ill-fitting dentures.
- **mucocele** (**MYOU**-koh-seal): soft nodule commonly found on the lower lip, caused by trauma to accessory salivary gland.
- **circumvallate papillae:** large, mushroom-shaped papillae on the posterior dorsum area of

the tongue; considered to have developmental cause.

- **glossitis** (glah-**SIGH**-tiss = *tongue inflammation*): inflammation of the tongue from various reasons, topical and systemic.
- **geographic tongue:** flat, irregular, red lesions on the dorsum of the tongue.
- **hairy tongue:** black or dark brown projections resembling hairs arising from the tongue dorsum; may be caused by medications or drug treatment.
- **fissured tongue:** deep crack in center of tongue dorsum; considered a developmental cause.
- **ankyloglossia** (**ang**-keh-loh-**GLOSS**-ee-ah): shortness of the lingual frenum; tongue tied.

Oral Cancer

Some lesions of a suspicious nature can be detected in the mouth and are examined more closely with excision and biopsy to determine if they are malignant or premalignant. A malignancy is a cancerous tumor with the ability to infiltrate and spread to other sites. Conditions that should be investigated are:

- **leukoplakia** (**loo**-koh-**PLAY**-key-ah; leulos = *white,* plax = *plate*): white patches on oral tissues, particularly the tongue that may become malignant (see Figure 7-3A).

- **erythroplakia** (ah-rith-row-**PLAY**-key-ah; erythros = *red,* plak = *plaque*): red tissue patch on oral mucosa of palate, or mouth floor; may be precancerous.

- **neoplasm** (**NEE**-oh-plazm = *new tissue*): all unusual or abnormal tissues, which should be tested to determine if the condition is benign or malignant. Some common neoplasms are:

  ○ **fibroma** (fie-**BROH**-mah; fibr = *fiber,* oma = *tumor*): benign tumor of connective tissue.
  ○ **granuloma** (gran-you-**LOH**-mah = *granular tumor*): benign tumor of lymph and skin cells.
  ○ **sarcoma** (sar-**KOH**-mah = *tumor of flesh/ tissues*): a malignant skin tumor arising from underlying tissues.
  ○ **hemangioma** (he-**man**-jee-**OH**-mah): benign tumor of dilated blood vessels.
  ○ **neurofibroma** (new-roh-fie-**BROH**-mah): neoplasm of nerve sheath cell; may be single or multiple nodules.

- **lymphoma** (lim-**FOH**-mah): new tissue growth within the lymphatic system.

- **carcinoma** (kar-sih-**NO**-mah = *tumor of connective tissue*): malignant tumor of epithelial origin that may infiltrate and **metastasize** (meh-**TASS**-tah-size = *move*) (see Figure 7-3B).

- **nicotine stomatitis:** malignant leukoplakia of the hard palate, caused by smoking.

- **AIDS:** acquired immunodeficiency syndrome; related symptoms include gingival lesions, thrush, swollen glands, and herpes lesions. There may be indications of Kaposi sarcoma (skin lesion cancer).

Diagnostic Tests

Many tests are being developed to assess body conditions for present and future disease. In addition to the visual, X-ray, and palpation testing of the oral exam, many dental offices provide a commercial test for oral cancer that may provide areas for monitoring or biopsy sampling. Some tests are listed here:

- **epithelian color variation (VELscopeVx):** hand-lamp device that illuminates a blue spectrum light causing a fluorescent mouth glow; abnormal tissue cells lack the ability to absorb, thereby standing out for observers and photo recording.

Figure 7-3 (A) Leukoplakia, (B) carcinoma of the lip

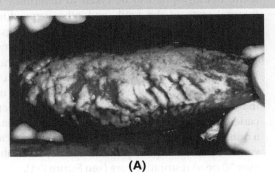
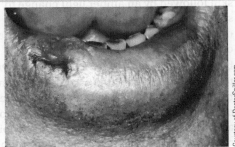

Courtesy of DoctorSpiller.com

(A) (B)

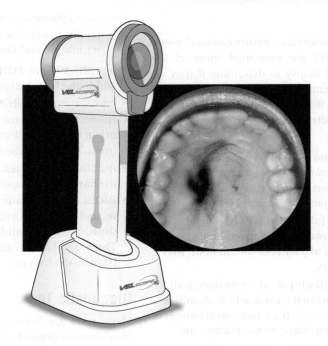

- **chemical-luminescent method (Vizilite Plus):** patient rinses with 1% acetic acid solution for 30–60 seconds, and a light stick is activated and inserted into the mouth to view illuminated suspect areas, which are then marked with a blue dye and photographed.
- **fluorescence and reflection method (Identifi 300):** with patient and doctor wearing tinted eyeglasses, the handheld light device is placed into the mouth for visual examination. When the tissues have absorbed the white rays, the lamp color is changed to violet rays for a blue reflection of abnormal skin followed by an amber light change to show vasculation of the area. Suspected dysplasia is charted, followed by appropriate observance or treatment.
- **brush cytology (Oral CDx):** similar to a PAP test, a collection of cells in a suspicious area is rubbed with a disposable brush that is wiped onto a prepared and coded glass slide, wrapped, and sent for laboratory analysis. Microscopic results are forwarded to the dentist for proper treatment, monitoring, or planning.

- **oral cancer risk (Oral DNA Labs):** test to identify type(s) of HPV present and risk profile for each as high, low, or uncertain to determine need for monitoring or referral. Patient gargles saline solution and empties mouth into collection tube that is sent to lab for oral DNA-PCR analysis.

EXAMINATION OF THE TEETH

During the initial visit, the dentist will examine and chart or record the present conditions of the teeth. Radiographs will be taken to determine the internal state of the teeth and other procedures. After the tooth surfaces have been cleaned, a visual and physical tooth examination will be performed. The operator may use an explorer to detect carious lesions, defects, and tooth flaws or may search for decay with a laser caries detector handpiece unit that measures the fluorescence level of undetected caries. After probe placement, the machine registers a number. The scale value of 10–15 requires no care, values of 15–30 require preventive care, and values over 30 need restorative care (see Figure 7-4).

Figure 7-4 Laser probe machine for caries detection

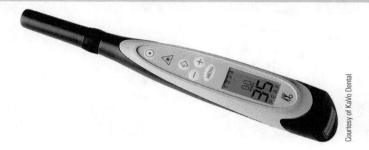

Courtesy of KaVo Dental

Dental Caries

Dental **caries** (**CARE**-eez = *tooth decay*) is known as decay or carious lesions. One cause of decay is the *Streptococcus mutans* bacteria, which produce acid to destroy tooth tissues through decalcification and demineralization of the enamel tissue and matrix, and can later move deeper to other tissue structures. Assorted types of dental decay include:

- **incipient caries:** beginning decay.
- **rampant caries:** widespread or growing decay.
- **recurrent caries:** decay occurring under or near repaired margins of tooth restorations.
- **arrested caries:** decay showing no progressive tendency.

Destruction of tooth surfaces by dental decay varies according to the size and position of the decay. Dental caries are classified into three types:

- **Simple cavity:** decay involving one surface of the tooth, usually on the occlusal surface, the lingual surface of maxillary incisors, or fissured buccal or lingual surfaces of the mandibular posterior teeth.
- **Compound cavity:** decay involving two surfaces of a tooth, usually charted as mesio-occlusal (MO), disto-occlusal (DO), or any other two surfaces.
- **Complex cavity:** decay involving more than two surfaces, usually charted as mesiocclusodistal (MOD) or any other three or more surfaces.

Cavity Classification System

Dr. G.V. Black (1836–1915) developed a system to categorize carious lesions based on the type of tooth affected (anterior or posterior) and the location of the lesion (lingual, buccal, occlusal). The six classes of carious lesions, according to G.V. Black, are depicted in Figure 7-5.

Class I

This includes decay on the occlusal, buccal, or lingual surfaces of the molars and premolars, and one surface decay on facial or lingual surfaces of the anterior teeth.

Class II

These cavities occur only in the posterior teeth involving the mesial and/or distal surfaces.

Class III

This decay occurs only on the anterior teeth, and involves the mesial or distal surfaces, but it does not involve the incisal edge.

Class IV

This decay occurs only on the anterior teeth involving the mesial or distal surface and the incisal edge.

Class V

These cavities appear on the facial or lingual surfaces of the posterior or anterior teeth at the cervical third of the tooth near the gingiva.

Figure 7-5 Cavity classification: (A) Class I caries, (B) Class II caries, (C) Class III caries, (D) Class IV caries, (E) Class V caries, (F) Class VI caries

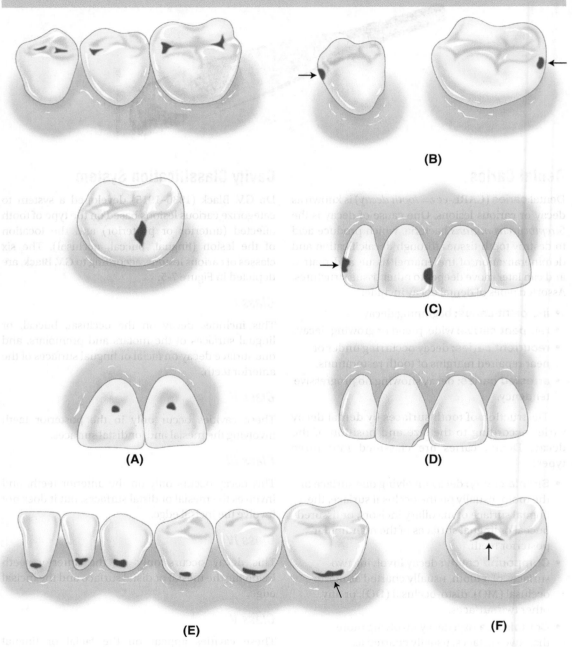

(B)

(C)

(A)

(D)

(E)

(F)

Class VI

This class is found on the occlusal cusps of the posterior teeth or incisal edges of the anterior teeth. This is considered severe attrition, which can lead to decay.

Periapical Abscess

A **periapical** (**pear**-ee-**APE**-ih-kahl = *around the tooth apex*) **abscess** is also called a *gum abscess*. An abscess results from necrosis (death) of pulp tissues. The three stages of pulp irritation are:

- **hyperemia** (high-per-**EE**-mee-ah = *over, blood*): an increase in blood and lymph vessels, as a result of irritation from decay.
- **pulpalgia** (pul-**PAL**-jee-ah; pulp = *inner tooth tissue*, algia = *pain*): tooth pain or toothache resulting from irritation and infection in the pulp chamber.
- **pulpitis** (pul-**PIE**-tis = *inflammation of the pulp*): inflammation and swelling of pulp tissue, leading to necrosis or death of the pulp.

Miscellaneous Maladies

In addition to dental caries and periapical abscesses or pulpal irritations, common dental maladies that may be observed during the dental examination are:

- **abrasion** (ah-**BRAY**-shun = *scraping from*): wearing away of tooth structure from abnormal causes such as malocclusion or bad habits.
- **attrition** (ah-**TRISH**-un = *rubbing against*): wearing away of tooth structure from normal causes such as usual tooth chewing or **mastication** (mass-tih-**KAY**-shun = *the act of chewing*).
- **erosion** (ee-**ROE**-zhun = *gnawing away*): wearing away or destruction of tooth structure as a result of disease or chemicals such as stomach acid from bulimia vomiting; also termed *acid etching* from reflux or purging.

- **ankylosis** (ang-kill-**OH**-sis = *stiff joint*): tooth fixation, retention of a deciduous tooth past the exfoliation time, or retention of permanent teeth that are fixed in the tooth socket because of an absence of periodontal ligaments; may be a result of heredity, disease, or constant trauma.
- **avulsion** (ah-**VULL**-shun = *pull away from*): tearing or knocking out; forcible removal of tooth.
- **bruxism** (**BRUK**-sism = *grinding of teeth*): grinding of teeth, especially during sleep or from bad habits.
- **malocclusion** (**mal**-oh-**CLUE**-zhun; mal = *disorder*): imperfect occlusion, or irregular meeting of teeth; malposition of teeth.
- **abfraction** (ab-**FRACK**-shun): loss of tooth surface in the cervical area, caused by tooth grinding and compression forces, resulting in hypersensitivity of the area.
- **torus palatinus** (**TORE**-us pal-ah-**TEEN**-us; plural is *tori*): bony overgrowth or elevations in the roof of the mouth.
- **torus mandibularis** (**TORE**-us man-dib-you-**LAIR**-us): bony growths usually in anterior lingual area; interfere with denture fit (see Chapter 14, Oral and Maxillofacial Surgery).

CHARTING METHODS

Tooth charting is a visual recording of existing oral conditions of the teeth and oral tissues. The findings are recorded in an electronic tooth chart or on paper charts in a form drawn as an anatomical replication or shown in a geometric diagram. Each facility records or "charts" conditions in its own fashion, using coded letters and marks to designate areas of interest. Colors, particularly red and blue, are often used to note treated and untreated areas. The completed chart is a written legal record (see Figure 7-6).

Assorted styles of charts are used in this process. All charts number the teeth for abbreviation and

Figure 7-6 (A) Perio chart, (B) charting symbols

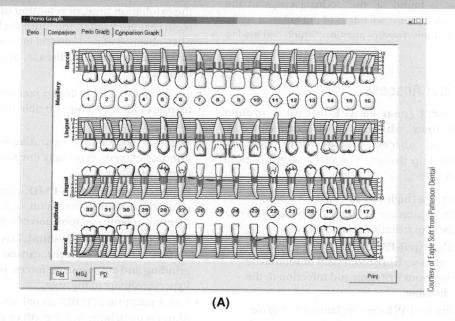

(A)

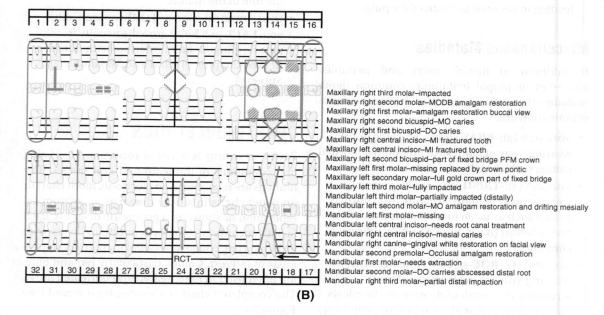

Maxillary right third molar–impacted
Maxillary right second molar–MODB amalgam restoration
Maxillary right first molar–amalgam restoration buccal view
Maxillary right second bicuspid–MO caries
Maxillary right first bicuspid–DO caries
Maxillary right central incisor–MI fractured tooth
Maxillary left central incisor–MI fractured tooth
Maxillary left second bicuspid–part of fixed bridge PFM crown
Maxillary left first molar–missing replaced by crown pontic
Maxillary left secondary molar–full gold crown part of fixed bridge
Maxillary left third molar–fully impacted
Mandibular left third molar–partially impacted (distally)
Mandibular left second molar–MO amalgam restoration and drifting mesially
Mandibular left first molar–missing
Mandibular left central incisor–needs root canal treatment
Mandibular right central incisor–mesial caries
Mandibular right canine–gingival white restoration on facial view
Mandibular second premolar–Occlusal amalgam restoration
Mandibular first molar–needs extraction
Mandibular second molar–DO carries abscessed distal root
Mandibular right third molar–partial distal impaction

(B)

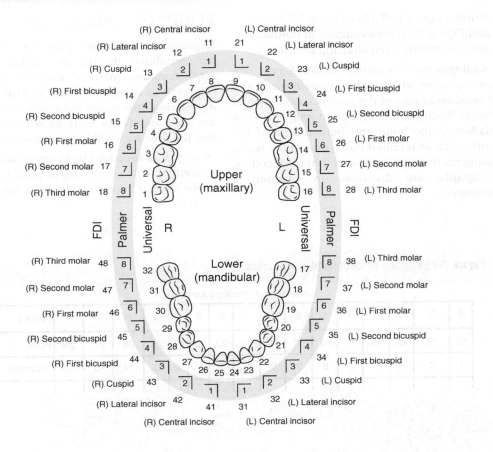

(R) Central incisor   (L) Central incisor
(R) Lateral incisor   11   21   (L) Lateral incisor
          12   22
(R) Cuspid 13   23 (L) Cuspid
(R) First bicuspid 14   24 (L) First bicuspid
(R) Second bicuspid 15   25 (L) Second bicuspid
(R) First molar 16   26 (L) First molar
(R) Second molar 17   27 (L) Second molar
(R) Third molar 18   28 (L) Third molar

Upper (maxillary)

FDI   Palmer   Universal   R   L   Universal   Palmer   FDI

Lower (mandibular)

(R) Third molar 48   38 (L) Third molar
(R) Second molar 47   37 (L) Second molar
(R) First molar 46   36 (L) First molar
(R) Second bicuspid 45   35 (L) Second bicuspid
(R) First bicuspid 44   34 (L) First bicuspid
(R) Cuspid 43   33 (L) Cuspid
(R) Lateral incisor 42   32 (L) Lateral incisor
          41   31
(R) Central incisor   (L) Central incisor

organization. There are three generally accepted methods of tooth numbering used in charting tooth conditions, as shown in Figure 7-7A and Figure 7-7B:

- **Universal:** Each adult tooth has a number from 1 to 32, and the deciduous teeth range from A to T. Assessment begins at the maxillary right third molar (1), progresses along the arch to the maxillary left third molar (16), then down to the mandibular left third molar (17), and back around to the mandibular right third molar (32). The deciduous teeth follow the same pattern using letters instead of numbers.

- **Palmer:** Teeth are numbered 1–8 with a bracket indicating quadrant location. Each central incisor is tooth 1, and the quadrant signal indicates which quadrant. Deciduous teeth are lettered A (central incisor) to E (second molar) with a quadrant indicating bracket.

- **Federation Dentaire Internationale (FDI):** Teeth are numbered in the same manner as the Palmer method but with no quadrant sign. Instead of brackets, a number prefix of 1 to 4 indicates the quadrant. The deciduous prefix quadrant numbers are 5 to 8. (See Figure 7-7A and Figure 7-7B for examples of methods and commonly used charting symbols.)

Radiographs, commonly called X-rays, are normally taken at the initial appointment and are considered part of the patient's usual dental records. Radiology examination may discover maladies in the bone and hard tissues of the mouth, such as retained roots, unerupted teeth, missing tooth buds, cysts, and other difficulties. Radiographs are discussed in Chapter 9, Radiology.

ALGINATE IMPRESSIONS

Impressions of the patient's teeth may be completed during the initial visit. The most common material used to make teeth impressions is **alginate** (**AL**-jin-nate = *seaweed, agar-based impression material*). Several terms are used to describe working with this material and the process of taking impressions:

- **negative reproduction:** impression of the teeth in which each cusp or protrusion in the tooth is now a dent in the impression material.

Figure 7-7 Examples of teeth numbering systems

Permanent Maxillary Arch

8	7	6	5	4	3	2	1	1	2	3	4	5	6	7	8	Palmer
18	17	16	15	14	13	12	11	21	22	23	24	25	26	27	28	FDIS
1	2	3	4	5	6	7	8	9	10	11	12	13	14	15	16	Universal

Right · Left

32	31	30	29	28	27	26	25	24	23	22	21	20	19	18	17	Universal
48	47	46	45	44	43	42	41	31	32	33	34	35	36	37	38	FDIS
8	7	6	5	4	3	2	1	1	2	3	4	5	6	7	8	Palmer

Permanent Mandibular Arch

(*Continues*)

Figure 7-7 (*Continued*)

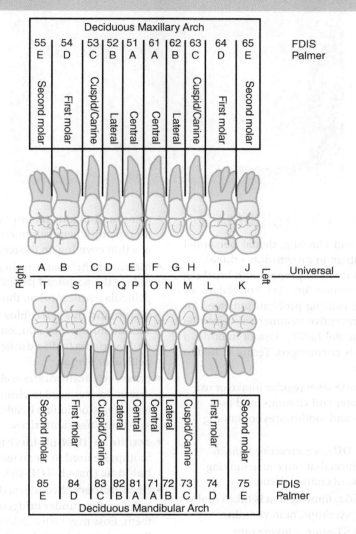

Deciduous Maxillary Arch

	55	54	53	52	51	61	62	63	64	65	FDIS
	E	D	C	B	A	A	B	C	D	E	Palmer
	Second molar	First molar	Cuspid/Canine	Lateral	Central	Central	Lateral	Cuspid/Canine	First molar	Second molar	

	A	B	C	D	E	F	G	H	I	J	Universal
Right	T	S	R	Q	P	O	N	M	L	K	Left

	Second molar	First molar	Cuspid/Canine	Lateral	Central	Central	Lateral	Cuspid/Canine	First molar	Second molar	
	85	84	83	82	81	71	72	73	74	75	FDIS
	E	D	C	B	A	A	B	C	D	E	Palmer

Deciduous Mandibular Arch

- **positive cast:** a gypsum reproduction of the patient's mouth; also called a **study model** (see Figure 7-8). This reproduction may be used for diagnosis or preparation of treatment plans. A reproduced cast has two parts:
  - **anatomical portion:** part of the cast that reproduces the teeth and gingiva.
  - **art portion:** part of the cast that is added to make an esthetic base support.

- **bite registration:** a piece of wax material, impression material injection, or commercial pad that is placed into the patient's mouth; when the patient bites down, the material registers the occlusion pattern that is used to put the models together to imitate the patient's normal bite position.

- **articulation** (are-**tick**-you-**LAY**-shun; articulatus = *jointed*): placement of positive casts into the patient's bite or articulating position.

Figure 7-8 Study model

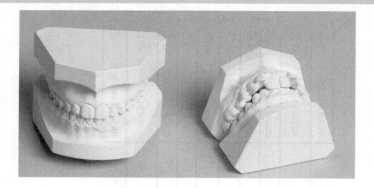

HOME PREVENTIVE TECHNIQUES

After examination and charting, dental personnel may instruct the patient in **prevention education**, including demonstrations of proper tooth brushing and flossing, information on diet correction, or whatever a specific existing problem indicates for home treatment. Preventive treatment also may be performed in the dental facility. Use of fluoride, a tooth strengthener, is encouraged. Terms related to fluoride use include:

- **regulated fluoride use:** regular intake or use of fluoridated water and vitamins, and uses of mouthwashes and toothpastes containing fluoride.
- **fluorosis** (floor-**OH**-sis = *excessive fluoride ingestion*): condition that can cause molting and discoloration of enamel tissue.
- **systemic fluoride:** fluoride that is taken orally, in the water supply, drops, or in vitamins.
- **ingestion** (in-**JEST**-shun = *taking into gastrointestinal tract*): taking a substance into the gastrointestinal tract.
- **topical fluoride:** fluoride that is placed on the tooth surfaces, such as liquids, gels, and pastes.

Miscellaneous Prevention Aids

Dental personnel also may recommend the use of additional home prevention aids to eliminate decay and gingival problems:

- **rinse:** anti-plaque mouth rinses containing therapeutic chemicals may reduce the amount of a thin covering on the teeth called plaque.
- **mouthwash:** breath-freshening rinses may reduce the **acquired pellicle** (**PEL**-ih-kal; pellicula = *little skin*) on the tooth surfaces.
- **disclosing dyes:** red/blue food coloring or a sodium fluorescein solution that is placed on tooth surfaces to disclose or stain the acquired pellicle or plaque.
- **powered toothbrushes:** electric or battery-driven devices used to clean the teeth; may have single or double heads, with or without self-contained dentifrices.
- **dentifrice** (**DEN**-tih-friss): tooth powder or toothpaste used to clean teeth and prevent **halitosis** (hal-ah-**TOE**-sis), that is, bad breath.
- **floss holders/threaders:** devices used to hold or insert floss under bridgework and between teeth; floss may be waxed, unwaxed, colored, flavored, or plain, and available in thin, regular, and extra thick rope or tape style.
- **interdental brushes/picks:** handles that hold small brush tips to be inserted between the teeth and into sulcus areas. Some small battery-powered floss and interdental appliances have been developed to perform this work.
- **wooden picks/flat balsam wedges:** used to stimulate interproximal gingival tissue circulation.

- **water irrigation machines:** electric water spray devices with pulsating tips to power rinse interproximal areas and bridgework gaps.

Diet Plans

Diet modification lessons may be presented after the patient completes a **diet evaluation form**, which is the patient's diet diary of food eaten over a period of a few days. Meals and snacks with fewer **cariogenic** (care-ee-oh-**JEN**-ick; carie = *decay*, genic = *start*) or caries-forming properties may be suggested, along with instructions on how to balance the diet, in keeping with the dietary guidelines of the United States Department of Agriculture (USDA) MyPlate program.

DENTAL FACILITY PREVENTIVE PRACTICES

The dental facility may provide some professional decay-prevention procedures throughout the patient's treatment (explained in more detail in Chapter 17, Pediatric Dentistry):

- **fluoride application:** professional application of fluoride in the form of liquid, gel, foam, or varnish to tooth surfaces. The fluoride is placed on cleaned tooth surfaces, timed, and removed. After 30 minutes or more, the fluoride is rinsed off.
- **sealant application:** placement of gel or liquid acrylic material on clean and prepared (acid-etched) occlusal surfaces of teeth to cover and protect tooth surfaces; sealant may be clear or tinted, auto-cured or self-cured, or may require ultraviolet light to set or become hard.
- **selective adjustment:** deep occlusal pits or fissures eliminated by selective abrasive or grinding of some enamel surfaces, thereby lessening the chances of deep carious lesions. This procedure is also called **enamoplasty**.

Review Exercises

Matching

Match the following word elements with their meanings.

1. _____ incipient caries	A. decay of more than two surfaces	7. _____ complex cavity	G. candidiasis of oral mucosa
2. _____ dysphagia	B. examine by touch	8. _____ ausculate	H. beginning decay
3. _____ cheilosis	C. tooth position relationship	9. _____ erythoplakia	I. listen to movement
4. _____ cellulitis	D. red precancerous patch	10. _____ lesion	J. infection in the pulp chamber
5. _____ ingestion	E. difficulty in swallowing	11. _____ articulation	K. grinding of teeth, especially in sleep
6. _____ palpate	F. infection in cellular or connective tissue	12. _____ thrush	L. inflammation of the lips
		13. _____ philtrum	M. taking a substance into the gastrointestinal tract

14. _____ pulpalgia
    N. injury, wound, or altered tissue or infected patch

15. _____ bruxism
    O. median groove on the external edge of the upper lip

Definitions

Using the selection given for each sentence, choose the best term to complete the definition.

1. Foods that encourage the development of dental caries may be termed:
   a. sugar-coated
   b. dentocarious
   c. cariogenic
   d. caries

2. The system of tooth numbering associated with a different number from 1 to 32 for a tooth is:
   a. Universal
   b. Palmer
   c. Federation Dentaire Internationale
   d. National

3. Which of the following is not considered a decay-prevention procedure?
   a. tooth whitening
   b. sealant application
   c. selective adjustment
   d. enamoplasty

4. Loss of tooth surface in the cervical area from grinding and compression is:
   a. avulsion
   b. abfraction
   c. ankylosis
   d. attrition

5. An impression of the lower dentition is considered to be in which reproduction state?
   a. articulated
   b. positive
   c. neutral
   d. negative

6. Another word for widespread decay is:
   a. rampant caries
   b. recurrent caries
   c. arrested caries
   d. incipient caries

7. The selective removal of some occlusal and pit surfaces of teeth is called:
   a. ingestion
   b. articulation
   c. ausculation
   d. enamoplasty

8. Pus from an abscess may escape from the subgingival area into the mouth through a/an:
   a. abscess drain
   b. fibroid
   c. fistula
   d. sulcus

9. Inflammation of the pulp tissue, leading to necrosis, is called:
   a. hyperemia
   b. pulpalgia
   c. pulpitis
   d. septicemia

10. The tearing out or forcible removal of a tooth is:
    a. abrasion
    b. avulsion
    c. attrition
    d. alienation

11. The wearing away of tooth tissue through normal occlusion and wear is:
    a. abrasion
    b. avulsion
    c. attrition
    d. alienation

12. Which of the following is not considered to be a lesion?
    a. dental decay
    b. ANUG
    c. Bell's palsy
    d. caries

13. Inflammation extending into connective tissue is:
    a. cellulitis
    b. gingivitis

c. glossitis

d. pulpititis

14. A viral disease that forms painful vesicles or watery pimples that burst and crust is:
    a. leukoplakia
    b. carcinoma
    c. herpes simplex
    d. thrush

15. Canker sores occurring throughout the mouth are also called:
    a. aphthous ulcers
    b. herpes simplex
    c. epulis
    d. fistulas

16. ANUG (acute necrotic ulcerative gingivitis) is also called:
    a. trench mouth
    b. periodontal abscess
    c. thrush
    d. trismus

17. Kaposi sarcoma is a cancer disease linked with:
    a. tobacco rubbing
    b. ANUG patients
    c. AIDS patients
    d. cigar smoke

18. An inflamed condition of a salivary gland is called:
    a. palsy
    b. trismus
    c. sialoadenitis
    d. dysphagia

19. Which of the following tumors would be considered malignant?
    a. carcinoma
    b. fibroma
    c. granuloma
    d. neoplasm

20. Which of the following decay-preventive measures is not considered home therapy?
    a. brushing and flossing
    b. fluoride rinsing
    c. sealant application
    d. dyes

Building Skills

Locate and define the prefix, root/combining form, and suffix (if present) in the following words.

1. **periapical**
   prefix _____
   root/combining form _____
   suffix _____

2. **glossitis**
   prefix _____
   root/combining form _____
   suffix _____

3. **malocclusion**
   prefix _____
   root/combining form _____
   suffix _____

4. **enamoplasty**
   prefix _____
   root/combining form _____
   suffix _____

5. **asymmetric**
   prefix _____
   root/combining form _____
   suffix _____

Fill-Ins

Write the correct word in the blank space to complete each statement.

1. Decay that involves two surfaces of a tooth is called a/an _____ cavity.

2. An increase in the pulp's blood and lymph vessels is called _____.

3. Decay occurring under or near the margins of a restoration is called a/an _____ cavity.

4. Another name for an aphthous ulcer is a/an _____.

5. The disease _____ is a degeneration of or a pressure on the fifth cranial nerve.

6. The disease _____ appears as red patches on oral tissue and may become malignant.

7. Tooth fixation, due to heredity, disease, or constant trauma, is called _____.

8. A fungus disease that causes white patches or ulcerated tissues is _____.

9. _____ is the imperfect meeting of teeth or improper occlusion.

10. An application of a/an _____ is the placement of a clear or tinted acrylic material to the occlusal surfaces of newly erupted teeth.

11. Toothbrush, floss, floss threader, disclosing solution, water irrigation, perio picks, and the like are examples of _____ prevention aids.

12. Bell's palsy is a sudden, temporary paralysis affecting the _____.

13. _____ herpes occurs in young children in the mouth or on the lips.

14. _____ is the loss of tooth surface in the cervical area caused by tooth grinding and compression forces.

15. The term _____ is used when a cancerous tumor moves to another site and infiltrates the area.

16. Disorders in the joint union of the temporal and mandible bones are termed _____ dysfunction.

17. Difficulty in swallowing or deglutition is called _____.

18. The _____ portion of a study cast is the section that contains the teeth and gingival areas.

19. The charting system that numbers the teeth 1–8 and uses brackets to designate quadrants is termed the _____ method.

20. Red, blue, or fluorescent solutions used to dye or color plaque and acquired pellicle are called _____ solutions or pills.

Word Use

Read the following sentences and define the boldfaced words.

1. The **cellulitis** caused such a swelling of the face that the patient's eye was almost totally closed.

   _____

2. The office manager is careful to use the proper code for a **compound cavity** restoration when filing the insurance form.

   _____

3. The patient with **glossitis** complained of much discomfort at meals and throughout the day.

   _____

4. The assistant included the **bite registration** with the impressions when she prepared the lab shipment.

   _____

5. The dentist carefully read the laboratory report of the **leukoplakia** biopsy that was sent last week.

   _____

CHAPTER 8 | PAIN MANAGEMENT AND PHARMACOLOGY

✓ Learning Objectives

On completion of this chapter, you should be able to:

1. Discuss the meaning of pain and ways to relieve and control pain.

2. Explain the means of administering local anesthesia, and identify the necessary equipment and injection sites.

3. Explain the conditions for using general anesthesia, the methods used, stages of sedation, and the terms used.

4. Define the study of drug agents, explain the difference between generic and brand names, and name the regulatory bodies that are concerned with drugs.

5. Discuss how the body reacts when processing drugs and the effects of drugs on the body systems.

6. List and identify the various forms in which drugs are delivered.

7. Identify the assorted routes, and give examples of drug administration.

8. Describe and explain the different parts of a drug prescription and the federal drug regulatory bodies that control drugs.

9. List and explain the assortment and classification or families of the common drugs.

DESCRIPTION OF PAIN AND METHODS TO RELIEVE DISTRESS

Pain has been described as a physical or mental suffering or distress with a variety of sources. Pain may come from emotional factors, or it may be a

Vocabulary Related to Pain Management and Prevention

This list contains selected new and important word parts and terms from this chapter. Take the time to learn these word parts and their meanings. You may use the list to review these terms and practice pronouncing them correctly. When you work with the audio for this chapter, listen to the word, repeat it, and then place a checkmark in the box. Proceed to the next boxed word and repeat the process.

(hyphen before word means it's a suffix, hyphen after word means prefix, no hyphen means root word.)

Word Parts	Meaning	Word Parts	Meaning
-ant	promoting action or process	ligament	tough fibrous band of tissue
anti-	against	-or	agent
-ary	pertaining to	osse	bone
coagul	clot	-ous	pertaining to
constrict	tighten	rhythm	pattern
intra-	within, inside	vas/o	vessel

Key Terms

- ☐ acetaminophen (ah-seat-ah-MIN-oh-fen)
- ☐ addiction (ah-DICK-shun)
- ☐ adrenocorticosteroid (ah-dren-oh-kor-tih-koh-STARE-oyds)
- ☐ analgesia (an-al-JEE-zee-ah)
- ☐ anaphylaxis (an-ah-fah-LACK-sis)
- ☐ anesthesia (an-es-THEE-zee-ah)
- ☐ angina pectoris (an-JIGH-nah PECK-tor-ris)
- ☐ antagonism (an-TAG-oh-nizm)
- ☐ anticoagulant (an-tie-koh-AGG-you-lant)

(Continued)

Vocabulary Related to Pain Management and Prevention *continued*

Key Terms *continued*

- **antihistamine**
  (an-tie-**HISS**-tah-mean)
- **antihyperlipid**
  (an-tie-high-per-**LIP**-id)
- **antihypertensive**
  (an-tie-high-per-**TEN**-sive)
- **arrhythmia** (ah-**RITH**-me-ah)
- **biofeedback**
  (bye-oh-**FEED**-back)
- **carpule** (**CAR**-pule)
- **cognitive** (cog-nah-**TIVE**)
- **diuretic** (dye-you-**RET**-ick)
- **efficacy** (**EFF**-ah-kah-see)
- **enflurane** (**EN**-floh-rane)
- **enteral** (**EN**-ter-al)
- **enteric** (en-**TEAR**-ic)
- **excretion** (ecks-**KREE**-shun)
- **halothane** (**HA**-loh-thane)
- **hematoma**
  (he-mah-**TOE**-mah)
- **hemostasis**
  (he-moe-**STAY**-sis)
- **hyperkinetic**
  (**high**-per-ka-**NET**-ick)

- **hyperthermia**
  (high-pur-**THER**-mee-ah)
- **hypokinetic**
  (**high**-poh-ka-**NET**-ick)
- **hypoxia** (high-**POX**-ee-ah)
- **ibuprofen** (eye-byu-**PRO**-fen
  or eye-**BYU**-pro-fen)
- **idiosyncrasy**
  (**id**-ee-oh-**SIN**-krah-see)
- **infiltration** (in-fil-**TRAY**-shun)
- **interpulpal** (in-ter-**PUHL**-pal)
- **intolerance** (in-**TOL**-er-ance)
- **intraligamentary**
  (in-tra-**lig**-ah-**MEN**-tah-ree)
- **intraosseous**
  (in-tra-**OSH**-ee-us)
- **intraperitoneal**
  (**in**-trah-**per**-ih-toh-**NEE**-al)
- **intrathecal** (**in**-trah-**THEE**-kal)
- **isoflurane**
  (eye-soh-**FLUR**-ane)
- **metabolism**
  (mah-**TAB**-oh-lizm)
- **naproxen** (nah-**PROX**-en)

- **opioid** (**OH**-pee-oyd)
- **parenteral** (par-**EN**-ter-al)
- **paresthesia**
  (**par**-ah-**THEE**-sis)
- **pharmacokinetics**
  (**far**-mah-koh-kah-**NEH**-ticks)
- **pharmacology**
  (**far**-mah-**KOL**-oh-jee)
- **potency** (**POH**-ten-see)
- **prophylactic**
  (proh-fah-**LACK**-tik)
- **proprietary**
  (pro-**PRY**-ah-ter-ee)
- **salicylate** (suh-**LIS**-uh-late)
- **sedation** (sah-**DAY**-shun)
- **synergism** (**SIN**-er-jizm)
- **teratogenic**
  (**ter**-ah-toh-**JEN**-ic)
- **therapeutic**
  (ther-ah-**PYOU**-tick)
- **topical** (**TAH**-pih-kol)
- **trismus** (**TRIZ**-mus)
- **vasoconstrictor**
  (vas-oh-con-**STRICT**-or)

reaction to injury, illness, or body sickness. Each person has an individual **threshold of pain** (*ability to withstand pain*) that is either **hypokinetic** (**high**-poh-kih-**NET**-ick; hypo = *under,* kinetic = *energy),* which is associated with high tolerance for pain, or **hyperkinetic** (high-per-kih-**NET**-ick; hyper = *over,* kinetic = *energy*), which is a low tolerance for pain. The patient's concept of the intensity of pain is so important that it is termed the **fifth vital sign.** Patients are requested to describe their pain in levels from 1 to 10 to determine a mean level.

Pain and anxiety are controlled and managed by applying our current knowledge of medicine and techniques. There are two main ways to control conscious pain:

- **anxiety abatement:** control of emotional and stress factors through psychological methods such as:

  - **stress reduction:** voice calming, concerned movement, thoughtful, caring manners, soft setting.
  - **relaxation methods:** guided imagery; suggestions of happy times, relaxing places; patient thoughts dwell on suggested happy thoughts or scenes.
  - **deep-breathing exercises:** patient concentrates on breathing and muscle movement; oxygenates blood stream and brain oxygen supply.

- **distraction technique:** discuss patient hobbies, family, and accomplishments to divert attention from dental treatment.
- **biofeedback principles:** use of memory, reasoning, judgment, and perception applied to uncomfortable situations; patient concentrates on reducing tension progressively from toe to head with relaxing suggestions.
- **cognitive behavioral therapy:** psychotherapeutic therapy using counseling to discover patient's thoughts that are causing behavior stress in dental (or other) situations; learning to control body functions; may include hypnosis.

- **conscious sedation** (sah-**DAY**-shun): relaxation of mental and physical distress without loss of consciousness. Relief of pain without the loss of consciousness is accomplished through the following:
  - **premedication:** medicine to depress the central nervous system (CNS) administered prior to treatment by mouth, by intramuscular injection, or by intravenous injection. Some antianxiety classifications of medications, with examples are:

    benzodiazepines (ben-zoh-dye-**AZ**-eh-peens): Xanax, Ativan, Librium, Valium, Halcion, and Serax.

    barbiturates (bar-**BIT**-you-rates): Nembutal, Surital, Seconal, Amytal, Luminal, and Mbaral.

    hypnotic: chloral hydrate, Equanil.
  - **T.E.N.S. (transcutaneous electrical nerve stimulations):** device to send small electrical impulses to nerve endings to block pain signals. Electrodes are applied to selected spots on the patient's head while the patient holds an activator. When distressed, the patient pushes the hand control, which signals the electrode to give off small sensations that confuse the nerve endings from carrying pain messages to the brain.
  - **analgesia** (an-al-**JEE**-zee-ah): relaxation and sedation without loss of consciousness by inhalation of a combination of nitrous oxide and oxygen gas. A smaller concentration formula will permit sedation, and the same gases in stronger concentrations will cause loss of consciousness and general anesthesia. Analgesic drugs are classified according to nonnarcotic drugs or nonopioid drugs (substances that have an effect on the peripheral nerve endings) or narcotic drugs or **opioid** (**OH**-pee-oyd) drugs (substances that depress the central nervous system [CNS] providing an altered perception of pain).

Examples of nonnarcotic or nonopioid drugs are:

- **acetaminophens** (ah-seat-ah-**MIN**-oh-fens): carefully used in proper doses as an aspirin replacement for young children and adults; has analgesic and antipyretic (an-tee-pye-**RET**-ick = *lower fever*) qualities (e.g., Tylenol).
- **salicylate** (suh-**LIS**-uh-late): used as an analgesic, antipyretic, and anti-inflammatory; may be helpful in preventing **myocardial infarction (MI).** Supplied as regular aspirin (Bayor, Empirin), powdered crystals, **enteric-coated** (en-**TARE**-ick = *to the intestinal tract*; Ecotrin), or with buffer chemicals added to reduce stomach upset (Alka-Seltzer, Ascriptin).
- **nonsteroid anti-inflammatory:** analgesic, antipyretic, and anti-flammatory; **ibuprofen** (eye-bee-**PRO**-fen or eye-**BEE**-pro-fen) group (Advil, Motrin), or **naproxen** (na-**PROX**-en) family (Naprosyn, Anaprox).

Examples of narcotic or opioid drugs are:

- **Morphine** (more-**FEEN**)
- **Methadone** (**METH**-ah-dohn), **Dolophine** (**DOE**-low-feen)
- **Meperidine** (**MEP**-er-ah-dine), **Demerol** (**DEM**-uh-rawl)
- **Dihydromorphinone** (dye-high-droh-**MORE**-fone), **Dilaudid** (dye-**LAW**-did)
- **Oxycodone** (ox-ee-**KOH**-dohn), Percodan, **Percocet** (**PER**-koh-set), Roxipin, Tylox
- **Pentazocine** (pen-**TAZ**-oh-seen), **Talwin** (**TALL**-win)
- **Codeine** (**KOH**-deen; Tylenol 3, **Empirin 3**, **EM**-puh-rin)
- **Propoxyphene** (pro-**POX**-suh-feen), **Darvon** (**DAR**-von)

LOCAL ANESTHESIA

Local **anesthesia** (an-ess-**THEE**-zee-ah) (derived from two Greek words: an = *without* and athesia = *feeling*) is given while the patient is fully conscious. It blocks nerve endings from transporting pain messages to the brain. It can be differentiated as:

- **topical** (*in a specific place*) **analgesia:** application of topical anesthetics to pain sites, to minor operative procedure areas, and to places about to receive injections. Anesthetics in the form of creams, liquids, sprays, gels, and ointments are used to desensitize nerve endings and work only on mucous tissue. Two topical sprays used on skin tissue are *benzocaine* and *lidocaine*.
- **local** (*limited to one place*) **anesthesia:** loss of sensation in a selected area.

Methods of Administration of Local Anesthesia

Local anesthesia is administered in several different ways:

- **infiltration** (**inn**-fill-**TRAY**-shun = *passing into*) **anesthesia:** directed into the tissue near the nerve ending of the operative site; used for minor treatment, root planning, gingivectomy, and some tissue surgery.
- **regional or field anesthesia:** around the nerve ending for anesthesia of a block of two or three teeth apices.
- **block anesthesia:** injection into a nerve bundle to enable anesthesia to a wider area, such as the mandibular quadrant of teeth or palatal into the palate.
- **intraosseous** (in-trah-**OSS**-ee-us = *into the bone structure*): directly into the spongy bone for a single tooth or multiple teeth in the same quadrant. It may be used for a patient who does not desire a fat lip or tongue. The perforation for the injection is made with a needle in the slow handpiece and placed directly into the cortical plate of the bone.
- **interpulpal** (in-ter-**PUHL**-pahl): injecting directly into the pulp chamber using a long needle.

- **intraligamentory** (in-trah-ligg-ah-**MEN**-tah-ree; intra = *within,* ligamentory = *ligament*): also called *periodontal ligament injection;* done mainly in the mandibular arch for one or two teeth in the same quadrant. The needle is placed into the sulcus along the long axis of the tooth using a pressure syringe (see Figure 8-1A).
- **electronic-controlled local anesthesia ("The Wand"):** computer-controlled anesthetic-delivery system for subcutaneous or intramuscular local anesthetic and nerve blocks, consisting of a sterile disposable handpiece component and a computer control unit. The solution is delivered through a small needle in the connected handpiece and is controlled by an operator's foot pump. The computer regulates the amount and flow of the solution at a precise pressure dependent upon the tissue thickness and resistance. It is effective for all standard types of anesthetic injections plus dense palatal and periodontal ligament injection sites (see Figure 8-1B).

Equipment Used for Local Anesthesia

Most local anesthetic injections are delivered using the following basic equipment:

- **anesthetic syringe:** two types—plain and aspirating. The aspirating syringe has a harpoon on the plunger end to penetrate the rubber plunger in the 1.8 mL carpule and provide suction to draw back the solution. It is the syringe of choice because it is used to determine if the needle penetration has been placed in the proper site.
- **needle:** size gauges 25, 27, and 30; the higher the number, the thinner the needle. The length of the needle typically is 1 inch for infiltration, or 1-5/8 inch for deeper penetration, such as a block injection. The **bevel** of the needle is the slant at the entry tip, and the **lumen** of the needle is the hole in the needle's shaft for solution to pass through.
- **carpule** (**CAR**-pule): also called *cartridge;* glass vial containing the anesthetic solution to be placed by the syringe; labeled with contents

> **Figure 8-1** Two additional methods for delivering local anesthesia: (A) periodontal ligament injection syringe; (B) electronic-controlled unit with a local anesthesia injector ("The Wand")

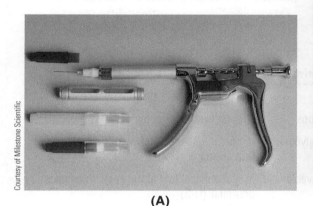

Courtesy of Milestone Scientific

(A)

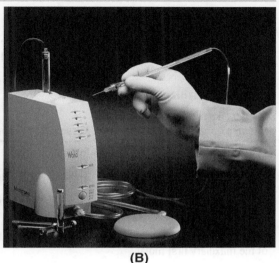

(B)

and has an aluminum cap, color-coded rubber plunger, and a diaphragm for puncture.

- **anesthetic solution:** either of two types:
  - ○ **ester:** alcohol-based solution, such as procaine or propoxycaine.
  - ○ **amide:** water-based solution, such as lidocaine, prilocaine, articaine.

A **vasoconstrictor** (vas-oh-kahn-**STRICK**-tore; vaso = *vessel,* constrictor = *tightener*) is a chemical (epinephrine) that is added to the anesthetic solution to constrict blood vessels, which allows less bleeding and longer anesthesia through **hemostasis** (hee-moh-**STAY**-sis; hemo = *blood,* stasis = *stationary*). Epinephrine is added in various intensities from 1 drop of epinephrine to 50,000 drops of anesthetic solution (1:50,000, 1:20,000, 1:100,000, 1:200,000) or none added at all. The color of the carpule's rubber plunger signifies the epinephrine concentration.

Complications with Local Anesthesia

Complications arising with local anesthesia include the following:

- **allergy:** a reaction to the anesthesia.
- **anaphylactic shock:** a reaction to the medication, delivery, or amount of anesthesia.
- **hematoma** (he-mah-**TOE**-mah): blood swelling or bruise.
- **trismus** (**TRIZ**-mus): grating or tonic contracting of the jaw or muscle rigidity.
- **paresthesia** (**par**-ah-**THEE**-zee-ah): abnormal feeling occurring after anesthesia has worn off.

Common Local Anesthetics

Some local anesthetics commonly used in the dental office are:

- **Lidocaine** (**LYE**-doh-kane; Xylocaine, Octocaine)
- **Benzocaine** (topicals) (**BEN**-zoh-kane; Hurricaine, Solarcaine)
- **Tetracaine** (**TEH**-trah-kane; Pontocaine)
- **Procaine** (**PROH**-kane; Novocain)
- **Propoxycaine** (proh-**POCKS**-ih-kane; Ravocaine)
- **Mepivacaine** (meh-**PIV**-ah-kane; Carbocaine, Polocaine, Isocaine)

- **Bupivacaine** (boo-**PIV**-ah-kane; Marcaine)
- **Prilocaine** (**PRIL**-oh-kane; Citanest)

Injection Sites for Local Anesthesia

Because anesthetic solution is to be placed into the oral tissues to produce a loss of sensation, the dental personnel have to be aware of the location of these sites for the placement of topical anesthetic material. Proper placement provides better anesthesia and uses less solution. Injection sites are named after the specific nerve area that provides sensation. See Tables 8-1 and 8-2, as well as Figure 8-2, for these nerve areas (labeled U-1 through U-6 and L-1 through L-5).

Table 8-1 Maxillary Arch Injections

Teeth or Tissue to Receive Local Anesthesia	Nerve Branch Involved	Injection Site Location
Individual teeth	Infiltration areas	Apex of tooth, near the mucobuccal fold
Maxillary quadrant	Maxillary nerve block	Over the distal root of the maxillary molar (U-1)
Centrals, laterals, and canines	Anterior superior alveolar	In mucobuccal fold between the canine and first premolar (U-2)
Premolars and mesial root of the maxillary first molar	Middle superior alveolar	In mucobuccal fold at the apex of the second premolar (U-3)
Remaining maxillary molars and buccal molar tissues	Posterior superior alveolar	In mucobuccal fold at the apex of the second molar (U-4)
Anterior block from canine to canine	Nasopalatine block	On palate near the incisive papilla (U-5)
Hard palate	Greater anterior palatine	Palate near the second molar and greater palatine foramen (U-6)

Table 8-2 Mandibular Arch Injections

Teeth or Tissue to Receive Local Anesthesia	Nerve Branch Involved	Injection Site Location
Individual teeth	Infiltration areas	Near apex of individual teeth
Mandibular quadrant	Inferior alveolar nerve	Posterior to the retromolar pad inside the mandibular ramus (L-1)
Molar buccal tissues	Buccal nerve block	On the buccal side, distal to most posterior tooth (L-2)
Lingual tissue, side of tongue, molars to mid-quadrant	Lingual nerve block	Mandibular posterior lingual area, near mandibular ramus (L-3)
Premolars, canine in quadrant	Mental nerve block	Between apices of mandibular premolars in mucobuccal fold (L-4)
Premolars, canines, laterals, centrals, lips, mucous membranes	Incisive nerve block	Anterior to the mental foramen in the mucobuccal fold (L-5)

Figure 8-2 Injection sites for local anesthesia: (A) maxillary arch, (B) mandibular arch

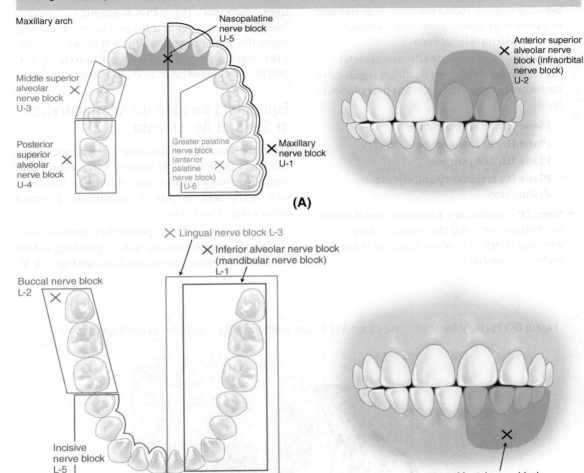

Maxillary arch

Nasopalatine
nerve block
U-5

Middle superior
alveolar
nerve block
U-3

Posterior
superior
alveolar
nerve block
U-4

Greater palatine
nerve block
(anterior
palatine
nerve block)
U-6

Maxillary
nerve block
U-1

Anterior superior
alveolar nerve
block (infraorbital
nerve block)
U-2

(A)

Lingual nerve block L-3

Inferior alveolar nerve block
(mandibular nerve block)
L-1

Buccal nerve block
L-2

Incisive
nerve block
L-5

Mental nerve block
L-4

Mandibular arch

(B)

GENERAL ANESTHESIA

General anesthesia is the lack of pain and sensation in which the patient loses consciousness. Although the patient is capable of performing the auto-reflexes, the central nervous system has been temporarily depressed and does not respond to pain or sensations. General anesthesia may be administered by injection or inhalation methods. The method used most commonly in the dental office is the inhalation of nitrous oxide and oxygen gas sedation.

Stages of Sedation

The four stages of anesthesia are:

- **Stage I – analgesia:** a loss of sensation but conscious and able to carry on a conversation.

- **Stage II – excitement:** loss of consciousness; the patient may experience **delirium** or become violent. Blood pressure may rise and/or become irregular, breathing increases, and muscle tone heightens.
- **Stage III – surgical anesthesia:** skeletal muscles relax, breathing becomes regular, eye movement stops. This stage has four planes or levels:
  - **Plane I:** light surgery stage
  - **Plane II:** moderate stage of surgery
  - **Plane III:** deep surgery
  - **Plane IV:** respiratory and circulatory dysfunction
- **Stage IV – medullary paralysis:** not desired; breathing center and vital function stop working; death may occur if patient is not revived immediately.

Other complications occurring with general anesthesia may be nausea, temporary dizziness from **hypoxia** (high-**POCK**-see-ah = *oxygen insufficiency in lungs and tissues*), drug interaction, organ dysfunction, and **malignant hyperthermia**, a reaction that may cause high fever, muscle rigidity, and fluctuations of heart and blood pressure rates.

Equipment Needed for Administration of General Anesthesia

Most facilities that administer general anesthesia will have large tanks of nitrous oxide (blue) and oxygen (green) gases in a centrally located area, used with equipment to provide anesthesia. Relevant terminology is as follows:

- **anesthesia unit:** equipment that receives and delivers gases by means of tubing and regulation devices to control anesthetic flow (see Figure 8-3).

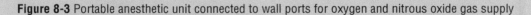

Figure 8-3 Portable anesthetic unit connected to wall ports for oxygen and nitrous oxide gas supply

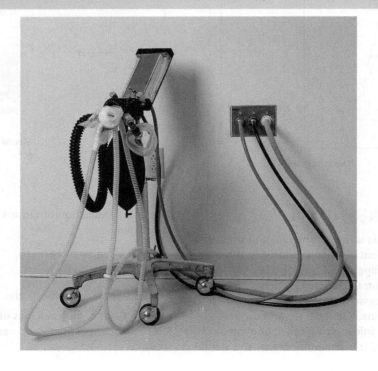

- **pressure gauges:** indicate the amount of gas pressure present within the cylinder tanks.
- **regulators:** control the amount of gases coming from the central supply to the anesthesia stand.
- **flowmeters:** control the amount of gas from the anesthesia unit to the patient.
- **nasal mask:** placed over patient's nose to present gas into the body.
- **reservoir bag:** may be used for hand-forced induction pressure of gases and a **monitor** to observe patient breathing rate and force.

During the administration of general anesthesia, the operatory/treatment room contains some important items:

- **blood pressure equipment:** stethoscope and sphygmomanometer to monitor blood pressure.
- **emergency tray:** a tray or box containing syringes and equipment necessary to deliver drugs or medicines for medical emergencies, such as vasodilators, anticonvulsives, stimulants, antihistamine, and so forth. An assortment of airway devices, such as endotracheal and nasopharyngeal tubes; a laryngoscope for viewing the larynx area; and suction equipment are also needed.
- **emergency plans and numbers:** emergency transportation and phone numbers.
- **defibrillator:** mechanical device to restore heart contractions.
- **oximeter:** monitoring equipment used to determine oxygen saturation in the blood.
- **patient records and history:** current records of patient with history and condition.

If nitrous oxide and oxygen gases are not used to obtain general anesthesia, other available volatile liquids include ether, chloroform, **halothane** (**HAL**-oh-thane; Fluothane), **enflurane** (**EN**-floh-rane; Ethrane), and **isoflurane** (eye-soh-**FLUR**-ane; Forane).

General anesthesia agents given intravenously include opioids (Sublimaze, Sufenta, Alfenta), barbiturates (Pentothal, Brevital, Surital), and benzodiazepines (Valium, Versed), which are primarily used for sedation and preanesthesia. An intramuscular general anesthetic is **ketamine** (**KEET**-ah-meen; Ketalar).

PHARMACOLOGY AND THE SCIENCE OF DRUGS

The use of drugs and medicines in operative treatment and the care of the patient require knowledge of drug agents and body reactions. The study of drugs and their effects is termed **pharmacology** (**far**-mah-**KAHL**-oh-jee). Each drug has a registered US-patented name called the **brand** or **proprietary name**, and a **generic name**, the official name given by the US Adopted Name Council. Drugs are regulated by the Food and Drug Administration (FDA), Drug Enforcement Administration (DEA), and the Federal Trade Commission (FTC).

The following books are excellent sources of information regarding drugs and medicinal products:

- *Physician's Desk Reference* (PDR)
- *United States Pharmacopedia*
- *The Pill Book*
- *The Dental Therapeutic Digest*

DRUG INTERACTIONS WITH BODY FUNCTIONS

Although drugs enter the body by various methods, each undergoes the same processing of the body organs and systems. Effectiveness of a drug depends on bodily processes involved in taking in (absorbing), distributing, using (metabolizing), and removing drugs from the body:

- **absorption:** process in which fluids are transferred from the administration site by the circulating body fluids.
- **distribution:** process of dividing and delivering the absorbed drug to the desired site.
- **metabolism** (mah-**TAB**-oh-liz-um): process of physical and chemical changes that enable the body to use the drug.

- **excretion** (ecks-**KREE**-shun): process of elimination of waste products from the body.

Effects of Drugs on the Body

Drugs produce a variety of effects on the body, defined as follows:

- **adverse effect:** response to a drug that is not desired because it is too intense, too weak, toxic, possibly allergic, and so on; also called a *side effect*.
- **addiction** (ah-**DICK**-shun): compulsive, uncontrollable dependence on a drug to the extent that cessation causes severe physiological and emotional reactions.
- **allergy:** specific body reaction to a drug, also termed *hypersensitivity*; can be the result of an antibody harbored in the patient's body.
- **anaphylaxis** (an-ah-fil-**ACK**-sis): a life-threatening allergic reaction to a drug that may produce an immediate or a delayed body reaction; called anaphylactic shock.
- **antagonism** (an-**TAG**-oh-nizm): opposite or contrary action of a drug.
- **dependence:** physical (chemical) or psychological (desire) need to use a drug despite related problems that may accompany it.
- **drug interaction:** effect resulting from the combination of two or more drugs at one time.
- **idiosyncrasy** (**id**-ee-oh-**SIN**-krah-see): unusual and abnormal drug response that may be genetic in nature or a result of an immune disorder.

- **intolerance** (inn-**TAHL**-er-ance): inability of the body to endure a drug or the incapacity of a drug to achieve a desired effect because of long-term use.
- **overdose:** effect from excessive drug dosage. A toxic dose results in systemic poisoning, and a lethal dose results in death.
- **side effect:** reaction from a drug that is not the desired treatment outcome.
- **secondary effect:** an indirect effect or consequence resulting from drug action.
- **synergism** (**SIN**-er-jizm): harmonious action of two drugs to produce a desired effect. A drug may be added to enhance the properties of the original drug.
- **teratogenic** (**tare**-ah-toh-**JEN**-ick; terato = *monster*, genesis = *production*): drug effects on a fetus, for example, thalidomide producing short limbs, or tetracycline affecting tooth color.

DRUG FORMS AND METHODS OF DISTRIBUTION

Drugs are supplied in various forms. Some medicines are prepared in more than one shape or form, and other drugs are available in only one specific preparation. A drug may be given in an injection to begin immediate protection and then have its action sustained by the ingestion of the same drug in pill form. The various methods of distribution of drug preparations are listed in Table 8-3.

Table 8-3 Methods of Distribution of Drug Preparations

Form	Method of Distribution	Example
Aerosol spray	Drug solution suspended in and delivered by a propellant	Inhaler, nasal spray
Capsule	Drug encased in gelatin shell, dissolves in the stomach	Antibiotic (e.g., Ampicillin)
Cream, balm	Oil and water suspended emulsion	Hydrocortisone, lip balm
Elixir	Sweetened, aromatic, hydroalcoholic solutions	Phenobarbital elixir

(Continues)

Table 8-3 (*Continued*)

Form	Method of Distribution	Example
Emulsion	Mixture of two liquids not mutually soluble	Laxative preparations
Intradermal implant	Pellets or drug pack implanted under skin for sustained slow release	Estrogen (e.g., Norplant)
Lozenge or troche	Solid medicinal mass of drug, flavored for holding in mouth and slow dissolving of mass	Cough suppressant, irritated throat desensitizer
Micropump	Implanted device with timed release of drug	Insulin
Ointment	Medicine suspended in fatty substance, cream	Topical anesthetic (e.g., Betadine)
Pill	Compressed mass of drug powder	Analgesic (e.g., Tylenol caplet)
Solution	Liquid containing dissolved drug	Otic solution
Spirit	Volatile substance solution in alcohol	Camphor, ammonia
Suppository	Medicated disc-shaped or cone-shaped, wax-based form to be inserted into rectum or vagina for release	Glycerin suppository
Suspension	Solution of liquid drug by mixing with but not dissolving in	Fluoride solution
Syrup	Drug mixed in sugary solution	Cough syrup
Tablet	Small, disc-like mass of medicine powder	Antibiotic (e.g., Ceclor)
Tincture	Diluted alcoholic solution of drug	Iodine tincture
Transdermal patch	Membrane-backed patch containing drug dose, applied to skin for slow release	Tobacco cease patch (e.g., Nicoderm)

ROUTES FOR DRUG ADMINISTRATION

The route and method of drug administration affects the action of a medication. The **onset**, or start, of the drug effect and the length of its effect—its **duration**—depends on its method of entry into the body. Intravenous (IV) is the quickest method, and rectal entry is the most ineffective method. The **potency** (**POH**-ten-see = *strength*) and the **efficacy** (**EFF**-ah-kah-see

= *intensity*) of a drug also are affected by the route of administration. Drugs may be taken in the gastrointestinal tract by the oral or rectal route. These methods are termed **enteral** (**EN**-ter-al = *into the intestines*), and other methods, such as injections, bypass the GI system and are called **parenteral** (par-**EN**-ter-al = *opposite the intestines*).

The various ways of drug administration are presented in Table 8-4.

Table 8-4 Methods of Drug Administration

Abbreviation	Route of Administration	Method of Administration
PO	Oral route	Swallowing, ingesting medication
IV	Intravenous	Injection within a blood vessel
IM	Intramuscular	Injection into a muscle
SC, SQ	Subcutaneous	Injection into subcutaneous tissue
ID	Intradermal	Injection into the skin epidermis
IH	Inhalation	Breathing in of drugs, NO_2, gas
SUPPOS	Rectal	Insertion into rectum, suppository
IT	Intrathecal (**in**-trah-**THEE**-kal)	Within the spinal canal
	Intraperitoneal (in-trah-**per**-ih-toh-**NEE**-al)	Within the peritoneal cavity
	Topical	On the surface
	Sublingual, buccal	Under the tongue or side of cheek
	Transdermal patch	Applied to skin
	Drug implant	Surgical implant (stent) under skin

DRUG PRESCRIPTION CONTENT

Some drugs can be purchased at the drugstore or the health and beauty section of the supermarket. These drugs are termed over-the-counter (OTC). Other drugs require a prescription to obtain and are carefully monitored by local, state, and federal government.

Government Control of Drugs

Federal drug laws regulate how drugs are dispensed. The following were early drug laws:

- **Food, Drug, and Cosmetic Act (1906):** FDC regulation of interstate drug business.
- **Harrison Narcotic Act (1914):** control over narcotics and those prescribing narcotics.
- **Food, Drug, and Cosmetic Act (1938):** control of drug safety and effectiveness.
- **Durham-Humphrey Law (1952):** labeling of drugs.
- **Drug Amendments (1962):** changes to FDC laws to require testing, reporting of adverse effects, use of generic names, and effects of drug.
- **Drug Abuse Control Amendments (1965):** control of potential abuse drugs such as barbiturates and amphetamines.

In 1970, the **Controlled Substances Act** replaced all previous control acts and set the schedule for drugs. Table 8-5 lists the schedules or classifications of controlled substances.

The Drug Prescription

Most drug prescriptions look alike (see Figure 8-4). They may differ in the color or type of stationary and the type style, but the standard drug prescription must contain the following:

Heading   Name, address, and telephone number of the prescriber

Superscription   Name, address, age of patient, date, and Rx symbol.

Body	Rx symbol (abbreviation of Latin recipe, take thou)	Closing	Signature of prescriber
	Inscription: Drug name, dose form, and amount of drug.		DEA number
			Refill instructions
	Subscription: Directions to the pharmacist.		
	Transcription or signature: Directions to the patient.		

Table 8-5 Schedules of Controlled Substances Act, 1970

I	Heroin, marijuana, LSD, hallucinogens, opiates, GHB (date rape), Ecstasy, Ibogaine	High potential for abuse No accepted medical use Experimental use, research
II	Morphine, amphetamine, secobarbital, codeine, methadone, opium, oxycodone, cocaine	High potential for abuse By prescription only, no refill
III	Stimulants, sedatives, anabolic steroids, barbiturates, hydrocodone/codeine/NSAID combinations	Moderate potential for abuse Prescription may be phoned No more than five refills in six months
IV	Depressants, diazepam (Valium, Darvon), Xanex, Librium, Ambien, Talwin	Less potential for abuse Same prescription requirements as schedule III drugs
V	Mixtures with limited opiates, cough syrups	Least potential for abuse, may include a few over-the-counter (OTC) drugs
All	Prescriptions for controlled-substance drugs require prescriber's DEA number (Drug Enforcement Administration identification number assigned to the prescriber)	

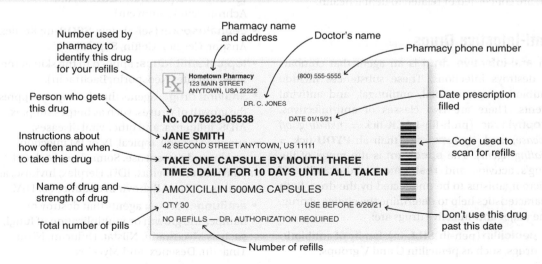

141

Figure 8-4 Example of a standard drug prescription

```
Superscription        Lester Payne, D.D.S.
                      1000 Central Avenue
                      Anytown, US 12345
                        1-867-555-5667


For _____ Date _____

Address _____ Age _____


Rx
Inscription      Name and amount of drug  =  Drug X tabs xx mg.
Subscription     Directions to the pharmacist = Dispense xx tabs.
Transcription    Directions to the patient =   sig: 1 tab. as needed

                                    _____ D.D.S.


                      D.E.A. #12345
```

CLASSIFICATION AND TYPES OF DRUG AGENTS

Drugs are classified according to their chemical content, drug manufacturer, and their intended effect or purpose. The following subsections list some drug families that have not been mentioned but are concerned or related to dental health.

Anti-Infective Drugs

An **anti-infective drug** is an agent that combats or destroys infections. These substances include antibiotic, antimicrobial, antifungal, and antiviral agents. There are two classes of anti-infectives, **prophylactic** (proh-fih-**LACK**-tick = *warding off disease*) and **therapeutic** (thair-ah-**PYOU**-tick = *healing agent*). The **spectrum** is the range of the drug's activity, and **resistance** is the ability of microorganisms to be unaffected by the drug. Both characteristics help to determine the choice of drug. The major anti-infective drugs are:

- **penicillin** (pen-ih-**SILL**-in): family of antibiotic drugs, such as penicillin G and V groups.

- **ampicillin** (am-pih-**SILL**-in; Polycillin, Omnipen).

- **amoxicillin** (ah-mocks-ih-**SILL**-in; Amoxil, Larotid).

- **erythromycin** (eh-rith-roe-**MYE**-sin; E-mycin, ERYC, Erycette).

- **tetracycline** (teh-trah-**SIGH**-klean; Achromycin V, Sumycin).

- **cephalosporin** (sef-ah-low-**SPOR**-in; Kerflex, Anspor, Cecelor, Ceftin, Suprax).

- **topical antibiotics:** applied to the skin at the infection site (Neosporin, Bacitracin).

- **antiviral drugs:** agents that destroy or suppress the growth of viruses, such as herpes simplex, AIDS, influenza, and other viral diseases; supplied for oral, topical, IV or IM injection, cream, and aerosol use. Some dental-related antivirals are Zovirax, IDU, Herplex, Invirase, as well as AZT and Retrovir in treatment of HIV.

- **antifungal drugs:** agents that destroy or hamper the growth or multiplication of fungi, such as Mycostatin, Nilstat, Diflucan, Nizora, Tinactin, Desenex, and Mycelex.

Cardiovascular Drugs

Cardiovascular drugs are agents employed for treatment of a variety of diseases of the heart and blood vessels:

- **anticoagulants** (an-tie-koh-**AGG**-you-lants): delay or prevention of blood clots, coagulation (Heparin, Coumadin, Dicumarol).
- **antihyperlipids** (an-tie-high-per-**LIP**-ids): decrease or prevent high blood plasma lipid, cholesterol (Questran, Lipid, Colestid, Lopid, Zocor, Lipator).
- **antihypertensives** (an-tie-**high**-per-**TEN**-sives): lower or decrease high tension (Lopressor, Inderal, Capoten, Vasotec, Tenex, Apresoline, Prinvil, Procardia).
- **antihypertensive with diuretic** (dye-you-**RET**-ick): drugs to increase secretion of urine (Aldactone, Dyazide, Ser-Ap-Es, Lasix).
- **angina pectoris** (an-**JYE**-nah **PECK**-tore-iss = *condition of pain or pressure around the heart*): treated with nitroglycerin, amyl nitrate (Cardizem).
- **arrhythmia** (ah-**RITH**-mee-ah = *absence of rhythm*): treated with Rythmol, Inderal, Tonocard, and Enkaid.

Allergy Drugs

Drugs used to treat allergies and other maladies related to the immune system are classified as:

- **adrenocorticosteroids** (ah-dren-oh-**kor**-tih-koh-**STARE**-oyds; *byproducts secreted from the adrenal cortex*): drugs to treat inflamed conditions, allergies, and emergencies (Kenalog, Kenacort, Valisone, Hexadrol, Nasonex).
- **antihistamines** (**an**-tie-**HISS**-tah-means): drugs that counteract the effects of histamine (Benadryl, Dramamine, Chlor-Trimeton, Dimetane, Vistaril, Claritin, Clarinex, Zyrtec).

Anti-Inflammatory Agents

Anti-inflammatory drug agents are used to relieve inflammation from arthritis and inflammatory conditions. They include Celebrex, Clindoril, Feldene, Tolectin, Nalfon, and Indocin.

Antidepressant Agents

Antidepressant drugs, used to treat depression, include SSRI (Selective Serotonin Reuptake Inhibitors) such as Prozac, Zoloft, Paxil, Luvox, Celexa, Wellbutrin, Effexor, and Rameron.

Anticonvulsant Agents

Drugs used to control convulsions and seizures include Phenobarbital, Dilantin, Zarontin, Valium, and Ativan.

Review Exercises

Matching

Match the following word elements with their meanings.

1. _____ drug potency	**A.** hole or opening in the anesthetic needle	3. _____ arrhythmia	**C.** glass vial holding anesthetic solution
2. _____ quadrant	**B.** drug name, dose form, and amount on an Rx	4. _____ inscription	**D.** strength of a drug
		5. _____ bevel	**E.** slanted cut at end of needle tip
		6. _____ carpule	**F.** oral route for drug administration

7. _____ PO

G. one-fourth area of the mouth

8. _____ IV

H. absence of rhythm

9. _____ anesthesia

I. relaxation and sedation without loss of consciousness

10. _____ Rx

J. *recipe, take thou*

11. _____ elixir

K. without feeling

12. _____ lumen

L. sweetened, aromatic water or alcohol solution

13. _____ vasoconstrictor

M. intravenous delivery of a drug

14. _____ analgesia

N. undesirable reaction from a drug

15. _____ drug side effect

O. added to anesthetic to prolong effects

Definitions

Using the selection given for each sentence, choose the best term to complete the definition.

1. Which stage of general anesthesia is termed the *excitement stage*?
   a. Stage I
   b. Stage II
   c. Stage III
   d. Stage IV

2. The name, address, and age of patient information is in which part of the prescription?
   a. heading
   b. body
   c. salutation
   d. closing

3. Harmonious action of two drugs to produce a desired effect is termed:
   a. idiosyncrasy
   b. synergism
   c. addiction
   d. dependence

4. Which of the following anesthetic needles would be the thinnest?
   a. 25 gauge
   b. 26 gauge
   c. 27 gauge
   d. 30 gauge

5. A water-based anesthetic, such as lidocaine, is a member of which family?
   a. amide
   b. ester
   c. opiate
   d. petroleum

6. The efficacy of a drug is also known as the drug's:
   a. strength
   b. duration
   c. administration
   d. intensity

7. A drug used to lower or decrease blood pressure is termed a/n:
   a. antihistamine
   b. anticoagulant
   c. antibiotic
   d. antihypertensive

8. A monitoring device that indicates the amount of oxygen level in the blood is called a/n:
   a. oximeter
   b. defibrillator
   c. sphygmomanometer
   d. thermometer

9. An injection into a nerve bundle to enable anesthesia to a wider area is called:
   a. topical anesthesia
   b. field anesthesia
   c. block anesthesia
   d. general anesthesia

10. A vasoconstrictor is added to anesthetic solution to obtain which result?
    a. dilation of blood vessels
    b. decrease blood supply to the area
    c. maintain current blood temp
    d. increase blood flow in the area

11. Medication given prior to surgery is termed:
    a. surgery-medication
    b. post medication

c. surface medication

d. premedication

12. Local anesthesia that is administered by needle placement into the tooth sulcus with a pressure syringe is called which type of anesthesia?

   a. intrapulpal
   b. intraosseous
   c. infiltration
   d. intraligamentory

13. Which of the following is not found in a dental anesthetic carpule?

   a. harpoon
   b. aluminum cap
   c. diaphragm
   d. rubber plunger

14. Anesthetic injections at the apex of the individual tooth are which type of anesthesia?

   a. infiltration
   b. block
   c. general
   d. intrapulpal

15. The process of dividing and circulating an absorbed drug throughout the body is called:

   a. healing
   b. metabolism
   c. distribution
   d. absorption

16. An anesthetic complication, such as grating or tonic concentration of the jaw is:

   a. trismus
   b. allergy
   c. hematoma
   d. shock

17. The loss of sensation but conscious and able to carry on a conversation is termed:

   a. anesthetic
   b. general anesthesia
   c. antibiotic
   d. analgesia

18. If anesthesia of the side of the tongue is desired, which of the following nerves would be injected?

   a. maxillary middle superior alveolar
   b. maxillary greater palatine nerve

c. mandibular mental nerve block

d. mandibular lingual nerve block

19. The study of drugs and their effects is called:

   a. therapeutics
   b. pharmacopedia
   c. formulary
   d. pharmacology

20. A reaction to general anesthesia that causes high fever, muscle rigidity, fluctuations of the heart, and irregular blood pressure rates would be:

   a. malignant hypothermia
   b. malignant hyperthermia
   c. medullary paralysis
   d. delirium majoris

Building Skills

Locate and define the prefix, root/combining form, and suffix (if present) in the following words.

1. **intraosseous**
   prefix _____
   root/combining form _____
   suffix _____

2. **vasoconstrictor**
   prefix _____
   root/combining form _____
   suffix _____

3. **arrhythmia**
   prefix _____
   root/combining form _____
   suffix _____

4. **intraligamentary**
   prefix _____
   root/combining form _____
   suffix _____

5. **anticoagulant**
   prefix _____
   root/combining form _____
   suffix _____

Fill-Ins

Write the correct word in the blank space to complete each statement.

1. Anesthesia that is placed on a specific area, prior to injection, is called _____ anesthesia.

2. The mechanical device that sends electrical impulses to nerve endings to block pain signals is termed _____.

3. A/an _____ anesthetic injection is placed directly into the pulp.

4. A/an _____ is added to an anesthetic solution to constrict the blood vessels, allowing a longer time of anesthesia effectiveness.

5. Another word that indicates the drug's strength is _____.

6. The symbol for intradermal applications of a drug is _____.

7. A blood swelling or bruise that may be a complication of local anesthesia is called a _____.

8. The process of eliminating waste products from the body is _____.

9. A periodontal ligament injection is also called a/an _____ injection.

10. _____ is an abnormal feeling occurring after anesthesia has worn off.

11. Injection of local anesthetic to the anterior superior alveolar nerve branch will result in lack of sensation to the canines, laterals, and _____.

12. The moderate surgical anesthesia plane is the Stage _____ degree of anesthesia.

13. The reaction from a drug that is not the desired treatment outcome is a _____.

14. The glass vial that contains the anesthetic solution used in the syringe during injection anesthesia is called the _____.

15. To anesthetize the mandibular premolars and canine in the same quadrant, the operator must inject near the _____ block area.

16. The physical or psychological need or desire for a drug is termed _____.

17. The _____ anesthetic syringe is considered the choice syringe to enable the dentist to draw back during the injection to test the proper site penetration.

18. A/an _____ is placed over the patient's nose during the application of general anesthesia.

19. _____ is considered by many to be the fifth vital body sign.

20. An injection placed around the nerve ending that will desensitize two or three teeth apices is a/an _____ anesthetic injection.

Word Use

Read the following sentences and define the boldfaced words.

1. When placing drugs in storage, the assistant must take precautions to ensure that the **potency** of the drug will not be affected.

   _____

2. The recently ordered **defibrillator** has been delivered and is being readied for use.

   _____

3. One of the most dreaded emergencies in the dental office is an **anaphylactic** attack.

   _____

4. The dental personnel make it a practice to use **anxiety abatement** in dealing with every patient.

   _____

5. The doctor prescribed an antibiotic as a **prophylatic** medicine for the patient prior to surgery.

   _____

CHAPTER 9 | RADIOGRAPHY

✔ Learning Objectives

On completion of this chapter, you should be able to:

1. Define the principle of radiant energy, and discuss how these X-rays, or Roentgen rays, are generated.

2. Identify the perils of radiation, and describe the various effects on the body.

3. Explain the various factors for measuring radiation, and discuss their relevance to the biological effects of radiation exposure.

4. List and give examples of acceptable methods for radiation protection in the dental facility.

5. Discuss the composition of conventional film packets. Describe the various types of dental radiographs available and the qualities necessary for diagnosis using radiographs.

6. Identify the methods used to expose conventional and digital dental radiographs.

7. Describe the methods used to produce a processed dental radiograph.

8. Explain the procedure used to display the acquired digital image and the types of enhancements available.

9. Discuss the types of radiograph mounts and the methods used to store processed films. Explain the procedure for the storage and transfer of digital radiographs.

10. List and describe the common radiographic errors and the causes of each.

11. Understand terms related to 3D cone beam computerized tomography.

Vocabulary Related to Radiography

This list contains selected new and important word parts and terms from this chapter. Take the time to learn these word parts and their meanings. You may use the list to review these terms and practice pronouncing them correctly. When you work with the audio for this chapter, listen to the word, repeat it, and then place a checkmark in the box. Proceed to the next boxed word and repeat the process.

(hyphen before word means it's a suffix, hyphen after word means prefix, no hyphen means root word.)

Word Parts	Meaning	Word Parts	Meaning
cephal/o	head	lucent	through
e-	without	metric	measuring
graphy	picture	radio	reception of signals
kilo-	measurement, 1,000	volt	unit of measure
lamina	layers		

Key Terms

- ❏ anode (ANN-ode)
- ❏ aperture (AP-er-chur)
- ❏ cathode (KATH-ode)
- ❏ cephalometric (seff-ah-loh-MEH-trick)
- ❏ cephalostat (SEFF-ah-loh-stat)

- ❏ collimator (KAHL-ih-may-tore)
- ❏ coulomb (COO-lum)
- ❏ diaphragm (DYE-ah-fram)
- ❏ dosimeter (doh-SIH-meh-ter)
- ❏ edentulous (ee-DENT-you-luss)

- ❏ electromagnetic (ee-lect-tro-mag-NET-ick)
- ❏ elongation (ee-long-GAY-shun)
- ❏ erythema (air-ih-THEE-mah)
- ❏ filament (FILL-ah-ment)
- ❏ foreshortening (for-SHORE-ten-ing)

(Continued)

Vocabulary Related to Radiography *continued*

Key Terms *continued*

- ❏ **Frankfort** (**FRANK**-furt) **plane**
- ❏ **kilovolt** (**KILL**-oh-volt)
- ❏ **latent image**
- ❏ **laminagraphy** (lam-in-**AUG**-rah-fee)
- ❏ **milliampere** (mill-ee-**AM**-peer)
- ❏ **panoramic** (pan-oh-**RAM**-ick)
- ❏ **phantom** (**FAN**-tum)
- ❏ **phosphors** (**FAHS**-fors)

- ❏ **polytomography** (**poly**-toe-**MAGH**-roh-fee)
- ❏ **pseudocolor** (**SUE**-doh-**cull**-er)
- ❏ **radiant** (**RAY**-dee-ant)
- ❏ **radiology** (ray-dee-**AWL**-oh-gee)
- ❏ **radioloucent** (**RAY**-dee-oh-**loo**-cent)

- ❏ **radiopaque** (**RAY**-dee-oh-payk)
- ❏ **teleradiography** (tell-ih-**RAY**-dee-aug-roh-fee)
- ❏ **tomogram** (**TOE**-moe-gram)
- ❏ **tomography** (toe-**MAGH**-rah-fee)
- ❏ **volumetric** (vol-you-**MET**-rick)
- ❏ **voxel** (**VOX**-el)

DEFINITION AND PRODUCTION OF X-RAYS

X-rays are **radiant** (**RAY**-dee-ant) energy waves that are produced, charged, and emitted from a common center in the dental radiation tube. These highly active, penetrating electromagnetic waves of charged electrons are tiny energy bundles or waves of photons with extremely short wavelengths that are used to penetrate matter and expose photographic film surfaces. When first discovered by Wilhelm Conrad Roentgen (**RENT**-gen) in 1895, they were termed X-rays, but in many places today they are called *Roentgen rays* in his honor. The resulting film image is called a radiograph. This type of radiant energy is considered "hard" radiation, as contrasted with "soft" radiation, such as microwaves, remote controls, or digital clocks.

How X-Rays Are Generated

The **X-ray tube**, also known as a *vacuum tube*, produces X-rays (see Figure 9-1). The vacuum tube contains these seven elements of note:

- **cathode** (**KATH**-ode = *negative pole*): electrode in the X-ray tube that is the electron source.

- **filament** (**FILL**-ah-ment = *fine thread*): tungsten coil in the cathode focusing cup that heats up to generate the electrons.

- **anode** (**ANN**-ode = *positive pole*): the target for the electron cloud that converts the electron force into photons.

- **focal spot:** target area on the anode where rays are projected to make the primary beam, or *central* beam; the smaller focal spot produces a better image.

- **aluminum filter:** aluminum disks that are placed between the collimator attachment and the exit window of the tube to absorb weak radiation.

- **collimator** (**KAHL**-ih-**may**-tore = *to align*): a lead device inside the X-ray tubehead used to restrict the size and shape of the X-ray beam, helping to avoid stray radiation.

- **aperture** (**AP**-er-chur = *opening* or *port*): opening in the lead collimator disk that regulates the size of the primary beam.

- **PID:** stands for *position indicating device*; it has lined walls to assist collimation. The operator uses the PID to help align the X-ray beam with the beam alignment device.

Control Factors in X-Ray Generation

The production and the generation of X-rays in the tube head are affected by regulating conditions that are set on the control panel. Each of the following factors affects the outcome of the radiation:

- **milliampere control** (**mil**-ee-**AM**-peer = *thousand of an ampere* [electric current], abbreviated as mA): mA describes the quantity of the electrons that control the amount of X-rays produced for the primary beam. An increase in milliamperage increases the *amount of electrons* available and darkens the overall radiograph.

- **kilovolt power** (**KILL**-oh volt = *1000 volt unit*, abbreviated as kVp): kVp describes the quality of the X-ray beam and controls the force that attracts the electrons to the anode. kVp helps to determine the penetrating power and the energy of the X-rays.

- **exposure time:** duration of the interval during which current will pass through the X-ray tube; this period may be stated as fractions of a second or *impulses* (60 pulses to a second). The amount of exposure that a patient actually receives is measured in milliampere seconds (mAs) (mA × Exposure time = mAs).

- **target–film distance** (source–film distance, or focus–film distance): distance of the film surface from the source of radiation (target or focal spot).

- **target–object distance** (source–object distance or focus–object distance): distance between the anode target and the object to be radiographed.

Figure 9-1 Internal view of the X-ray tube head that produces radiation used to expose films and pixels

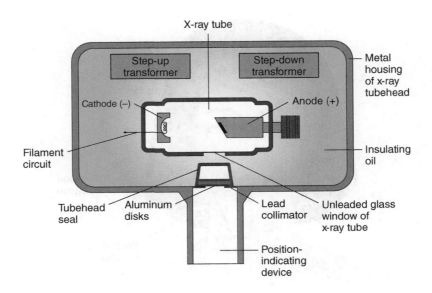

X-ray tube

Step-up transformer

Step-down transformer

Metal housing of x-ray tubehead

Cathode (−)

Anode (+)

Filament circuit

Insulating oil

Tubehead seal

Aluminum disks

Lead collimator

Unleaded glass window of x-ray tube

Position-indicating device

- **film speed:** A (slowest) to F (fastest) speed; faster speed film requires less radiation exposure time for the patient.

Types of X-Ray Radiation

There are four types of X-ray radiation generated during radiography (see Figure 9-2):

- **primary radiation:** central ray of radiation emitting from the tube head and PID. Primary radiation is the desired radiation and is used to expose radiographic film.
- **secondary radiation:** once the primary beam interacts with matter.
- **scattered radiation:** radiation deflected from its path during its passage through matter; may be deflected or diffused in all directions, becoming attenuated (weakened) or another form of secondary radiation.

- **leakage radiation:** any radiation other than the useful beam produced from the tube head. A faulty or broken tube head may be the source of stray radiation.

PROPERTIES OF ROENTGEN RAYS

Roentgen rays are considered hazardous and dangerous to the body tissues. X-radiation is made possible by producing ions. An **ion** (**EYE**-on = *going*) is a particle that carries an electrical charge. This unbalanced atom particle may attempt union with body cell atoms, causing *ionizing radiation,* or a change in cell structure that has a variety of effects such as:

- **sensitivity:** ability of X-rays to penetrate and possibly ionize. The reproductive cells (*genetic*) are more radiosensitive than the radioresistant body tissue (*somatic*) cells.

Figure 9-2 Examples of different types of radiation

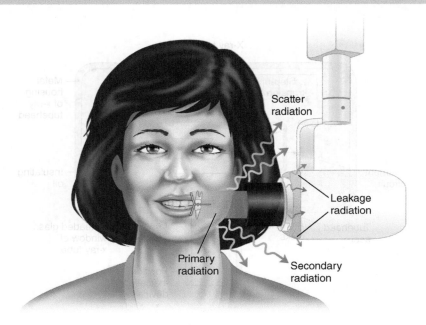

Scatter radiation

Leakage radiation

Primary radiation

Secondary radiation

Younger cells are more sensitive than older, thicker cells.

- **cumulative effect:** long-term outcome of radiation. Repetition increases and intensifies the ionizing effect on cells for a buildup of damage. The **latent period** of exposure is the time interval between the exposure and the effect or detection.
- **mutation** (myou-**TAY**-shun) **effect:** abnormal growth or development due to radiation causing a genetic change.

TYPES OF EXPOSURE

There are two types of X-radiation exposure that will damage the body cells:

- **acute radiation exposure:** radiation occurring from a massive short-term ionizing dose, such as an accidental exposure or explosion of radiation material.
- **chronic radiation exposure:** accumulated radiation cell damage from continual or frequent small exposures absorbed over a period of time (thus the need for questioning the patient as to when the last X-ray was taken).

MEASUREMENT OF RADIATION ENERGY

Knowledge of radiation energy levels and their biological effects can be useful to the X-ray operator's safety awareness. These terms are used to measure radiation effects and uses, both laboratory and biological:

- **Roentgen (R)** (international unit is *coulomb per kilogram* [C/kg]): the basic unit of exposure to radiation; the amount of X-radiation or gamma radiation needed to ionize 1 cc of air at standard pressure and temperature conditions (C/kg = 3880 roentgens).

- **rad (radiation absorbed dose)** (international unit is *Gray [Gy]*): the basic unit of absorbed radiation dose equal to 100 ergs (energy units) per gram of tissue or 1 rad = cGy.
- **rem (roentgen equivalent in man)** (international unit is *sievert [Sv]*): the unit of ionizing radiation needed to produce the same biological effect as 1 roentgen (R) of radiation.
- **rbe (relative biological effectiveness):** unit of measurement used to determine amount of biological absorption effects on body tissues by different types of radiation energy.
- **coulomb** (**COO**-lum): international electromagnetic measurement abbreviated as C; 1 C per kilogram (C/kg) is equal to 3880 roentgens.
- **maximum permissible dose (MPD):** highest rate of exposure permissible for the occupationally exposed person. The formula for calculating MPD:

MPD = (Operator's age − 18) × 5 rems/year or (Operator' age − 18) × 5 Sv/year

RADIATION PROTECTION

When exposing X-rays, the use of radiation safety apparel and devices is critical. Serious harmful effects can occur with the misuse of this energy. One such malady is **erythema** (air-ih-**THEE**-mah = *redness*) **dose**, which is radiation overdose that produces temporary redness of the skin.

Among the equipment and methods of protection against overexposure of X-radiation to the patient and the operator are:

- **ALARA** (*as low as reasonably achievable*): a policy of using the lowest amount of radiation exposure possible. Measures to accomplish this include proper exposure and protection aids, use of fast films, good techniques in exposure and developing, questioning the patient regarding recent exposure, and the correct calculations or control settings.

- **dosimeter** (doh-**SIH**-meh-ter = *giving measure*): operator's radiation-monitoring device with ionizing chamber or a device to indicate exposure and measure accumulated doses of radiation; available in the form of a film badge, pen, ring, and flashdrive.
- **lead apron/thyrocervical collar:** patient apparel with lead protection for genetic (sex) cells in the torso and the thyroid glands in the cervical area (Figure 9-3).
- **lead barriers, shields:** devices used by operators to block out scattered radiation.
- **phantom** (**FAN**-tum): practice mannequin containing tooth and head structures to imitate the actual condition. A popular model is **DXTTR**, affectionately called Dexter.

CONVENTIONAL RADIOGRAPHS

Conventional dental radiographs are composed of a celluloid base that supports an emulsion containing silver bromide, silver sulfide, and silver halide crystals. This emulsion is sensitive to light and radiation so that when exposed and processed, it will record a radiographic image. When film is exposed to X-rays, it forms an invisible image, termed **latent image**, on the film emulsion. Conventional film radiographs may be exposed within the oral cavity (intraoral) or outside the mouth (extraoral).

Most intraoral dental film packets contain one film, but they are also supplied in double film packets. There are several basic kinds, sizes, and speeds of conventional dental films (see Figure 9-4):

- **periapical film packet:** size 0 (pedodontic size), 1 (adult anterior), or 2 (adult anterior and posterior); used for the intraoral periapical view of the entire tooth or teeth

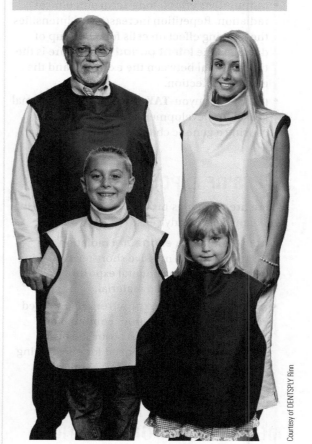

Figure 9-3 Aprons are available in various sizes and colors, with or without the protective collar

Courtesy of DENTSPLY Rinn

in a given area along with adjacent tissues and oral structures. This film may also be placed in a device or loop to expose an intraoral bitewing view and may be ordered in a double film packet, if desired.

- **bitewing film packet** (also called interproximal radiograph, size 3): film used to record crown and interproximal views of both arches while in occlusion; used intraorally with attached bite tab. Other film sizes may be adapted to accomplish this task.

Figure 9-4 Sample dental X-ray films showing sizes and numbers (Size 1, narrow anterior film, and size 3, long bitewing film are not shown)

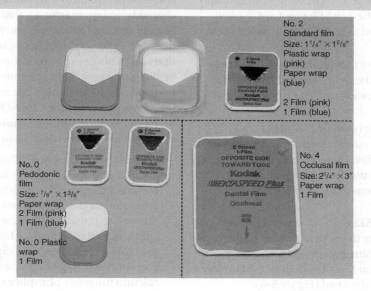

No. 2
Standard film
Size: 1¼" × 1⅝"
Plastic wrap (pink)
Paper wrap (blue)
2 Film (pink)
1 Film (blue)

No. 0
Pedodonic film
Size: ⅞" × 1⅜"
Paper wrap
2 Film (pink)
1 Film (blue)

No. 0 Plastic wrap
1 Film

No. 4
Occlusal film
Size: 2¼" × 3"
Paper wrap
1 Film

- **film speeds:** films are rated A to F according to the amount of exposure needed, with A needing the most time. Popular trade names for Kodak film are D–Ultra-speed, E–Ektavision, and F–Insight. Other manufacturers have similar trade names for films from A to F.

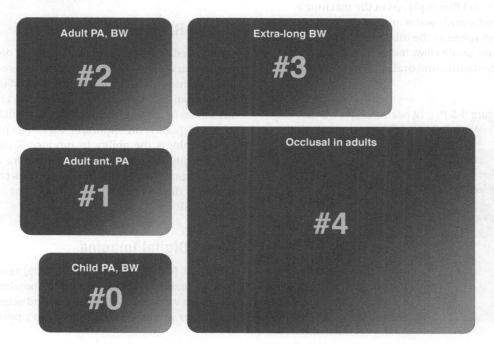

Adult PA, BW

#2

Extra-long BW

#3

Adult ant. PA

#1

Occlusal in adults

#4

Child PA, BW

#0

- **occlusal film packet:** size 4; film that may be used intraorally or extraorally to expose large areas (2¼" × 3"). These film packets may contain more than one film and are marked and color-coded to identify the amount of film enclosed.
- **extraoral films:** radiographs exposed outside the oral cavity; larger in size and loaded in a film cassette or wrapped for protection from light rays.
- **cephalometric** (**seff**-ah-low-**MEH**-trick; cephal = *head*, metric = *measure*) **films:** also called headplates. These extraoral radiographs of the head are used in orthodontic, oral surgery, and sometimes in prosthodontic dentistry.
- **cephalostat** (**SEFF**-ah-loh-stat): a device used to stabilize the patient's head in a plane parallel to the film and at right angles to the central ray of the X-ray beam. It is used for large radiographs of the head (Figure 9-5).
- **panoramic radiograph:** a special radiograph capturing a view of the entire dentition with the surrounding structures on one film. The extraoral film is placed in the machine's cassette and rotates around the patient at the same speed as the tube head rotation, providing a panoramic view. It is in popular use in orthodontics and oral surgery (Figure 9-6).

Panoramic and cephalographs (headplates) are completed using special mounted machines, while regular intraoral films are exposed at chairside using machines that are smaller and usually attached to the operatory wall. NOMAD is a portable, lightweight, battery-energized X-ray unit that is capable of exposing either conventional film or digital images. This machine needs no control panel because the settings are incorporated on the top of the portable unit. The NOMAD may be used in the dental office, mobile clinics, nursing homes, or in field areas as needed (Figure 9-7).

- **intensifying screen:** a lining of calcium tungstate phosphors or rare earth within the cassette that gives off a bluish light (calcium tungstate) or green glow (rare earth) when exposed to radiation. This combination of light and radiation forms a latent image on the film faster and reduces exposure time. The rare earth screen gives off more light than the calcium tungstate phosphor screen, which makes its exposure time shorter. Care is needed in the selection of the proper film with each type of intensifying screen.

Digital Radiographs

Digital radiography has transformed dentistry. Digital imaging eliminates chemical processing and hazardous wastes from chemicals and lead foil. Images can be electronically transferred to dental specialists or insurance companies without the loss of image quality. An important advantage of digital radiography is the ability to produce X-rays with significantly less radiation. The receptors used to create digital images are called: sensors (charged coupled devices CCD) and phosphor storage plates, PSP.

Direct Digital Imaging

The **CCD (charged coupled device)** sensor is a solid-state sensor that may or may not be wired to the computer workstation. The sensor and sensor wire are barrier wrapped and inserted into a positioning

Figure 9-5 Patient positioned for a lateral cephalometric radiograph

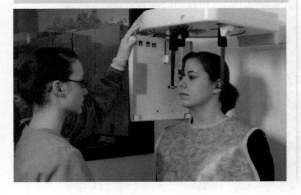

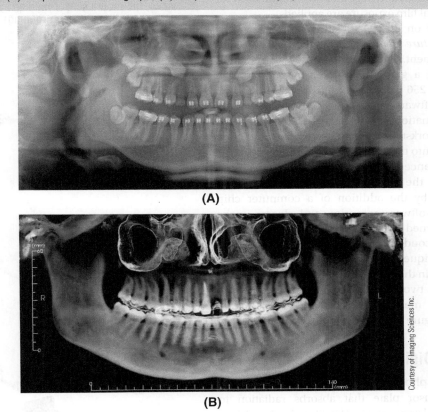

(A)

(B)

Courtesy of Imaging Sciences Inc.

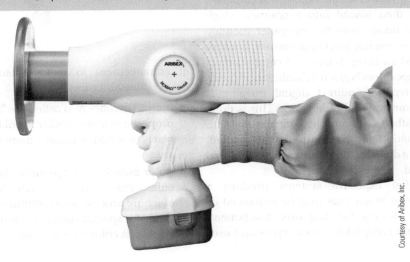

Courtesy of Aribex, Inc.

device for insertion and exposure in the mouth. The same placement and alignment technique used for conventional film exposure are applied.

Situated on the sensor surface is an array of **pixels** (*picture elements*) arranged in a line and row placement. Each pixel exposed to radiation is assigned a gray shade color number from 0 (black) to 256 (white) that is recorded in the program software. After the surface is exposed, the pixel information is transported to the computer program workstation for interpretation and then projected onto the monitor or computer screen.

An advanced and less-expensive technology system of the CCD digital sensor has been developed by the addition of a computer chip for better software reception and clearer image output. Termed the CMOS (complementary metal oxide semiconductor), this sensor works with the same technique and principles as the CCD and is considered in the same grouping and type of digital sensor. The two systems are interchangeable; the use of this method is considered direct digital imaging (Figure 9-8).

Indirect Digital Imaging

PSP, phosphor storage plate, is a cordless, indirect sensor plate that absorbs radiation to complete a latent image. The plate is placed in a barrier wrap, put in a positioning device, and then exposed using conventional exposure techniques. The plate is then placed into a scanner, which translates the image onto the computer monitor. These PSPs are reusable just like the sensor, because as it is scanned the image is erased. A comparison of the intraoral receptors is given in Table 9-1.

Another type of indirect digital imaging is digitizing a conventional radiograph. This is done by using a flatbed scanner. The conventional film image information may be captured, manipulated, and stored as a digital radiograph, and is considered to be digitized.

Both digital exposure systems produce a grayscale screen image that may be enhanced or modified for viewing for diagnosis, assessment, measuring, and comparison. Some types and uses

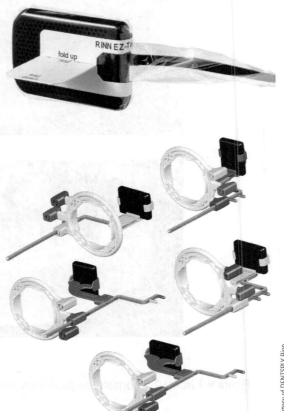

Figure 9-8 Sensor holder in barrier wrap (upper view), full-mouth sensor-holding system for various positions (lower grouping)

Courtesy of DENTSPLY Rinn

of enhancement to make anatomic structures more visible and viewable are:

- **magnification:** also called the "zoom in" property; machine ability to enlarge selected pixels to produce a larger, more visible viewing area.
- **color substitution:** pseudocolor enhancement; more appealing to patient. Machine process of substituting a selected color shade for specific digital shade numbers to produce a color screen image.

Table 9-1 Radiograph Image Receptor Comparison

Qualities	Film-Based	CCD (CMOS-APS)	PSP
Application	Indirect	Direct	Semi-direct
Radiation dose	Higher	Lower	Lower
Processing	Chemical	Computer	Scanner, computer
Image/view	Delayed, view box	Instant, screen	Delayed, screen
Enhancement	Fixed image	Multiple, color, size, measurement, density, brightness, assessment, alterations for both	Multiple, color, size, measurement, density, brightness, assessment, alterations for both
Life span	Single use	Sensor use	Sensor plate, reuse after reconditioning
Sterilization	One use	Barrier cover	Barrier cover
Storage	Mounted record	Electronic recovery or hard-copy printout	Electronic recovery or hard-copy printout

- **digital substitution:** technique used to determine small changes in image sequences. Use of before treatment and after treatment image comparisons may not be evident to the human eye but can be mathematically compared and evaluated. Follow-up of periodontal bone loss, implant bone regeneration, bone lesion progress, and caries development are only a few uses of this technique.

Another advantage of digital radiography is the ease of storage of the dental image and **teleradiography** (tell-ih-**RAY**-dee-**aug**-rah-fee), which is the ability to transfer the captured information to other sites and sources by the computer DICOM (Digital Imaging and Communications in Medicine) interchange.

Diagnostic Qualities for Dental Radiographs

Dental radiographs must exhibit certain qualities to be effective. The following list defines and explains relevant terminology related to radiography quality:

- **contrast:** variations in shades from black to white. A radiograph exhibiting many variations in shades is considered to possess long-scale contrast. Increased kilovoltage helps to produce this effect. A radiograph with high contrast has very few shades of gray, with mostly black and white areas. A radiograph with low contrast has many shades of gray, which is considered to be a more diagnostic image.
- **density/brightness:** the overall blackness or darkness of an image. An increase or decrease in density is accomplished by an increase or decrease in milliamperage and exposure time (mA/second).
- **detail:** point-to-point delineation or view of tiny structures in a radiograph image. Proper exposure, handling factors, and kVp selection provide good detail.
- **definition/smoothness:** outline sharpness and clarity of image exhibited on a radiograph. Movement of the film, patient, or tube head is the most common cause of poor definition or fuzzy outline called **penumbra**

(pen-um-**BRA, BRAE** plural; Latin is *paene* = nearly, *umbra* = shadow). Proper digital machine filtration of electronic **noise** (*low and high frequency components that hamper reception and computation of digital signals*) can improve the sharpness and smoothing of the digital image.

- **radiolucent** (**RAY**-dee-oh-**loo**-sent; radius = *ray*, lucent = *shine*): describes a radiograph that appears dark, or the ability of a substance to permit passage of X-rays, thereby causing the radiographic film to darken.
- **radiopaque** (**RAY**-dee-oh-**payk**; radius = *ray*, pacus = *dark*): the portion of the radiograph that appears light, or the ability of a substance to resist X-ray penetration, thereby causing a light area on the film.

TECHNIQUES FOR EXPOSING RADIOGRAPHS

The two basic techniques used by conventional and digital methods for exposure of intraoral radiographs are the bisecting angle and the parallel angle, as shown in Figure 9-9:

- **bisecting angle:** The central X-ray beam is directly perpendicular with an imaginary bisecting line of the angle formed by the plane of the film and the long axis of the tooth. This technique is also called the *short cone technique*.
- **paralleling:** The film packet is placed parallel to the long axis of the tooth and at a right (90-degree) angle to the central X-ray beam. This technique is also called the *extension cone* or *right-angle technique*.

Positioning Terms for X-Ray Exposure

Various positioning methods and angulations that affect the outcome of exposure are:

- **sagittal plane** (**SAJ**-ih-tol): also called midsagittal plane; imaginary vertical line bisecting the face into a right and left half;

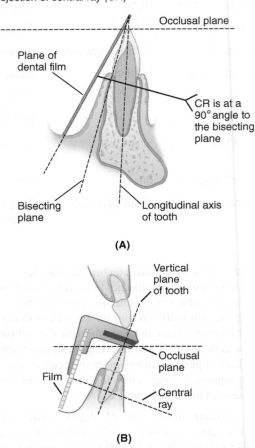

Figure 9-9 Two common methods of radiographic exposure: (A) bisecting angulation, (B) paralleling angulation

Projection of central ray (CR)

Occlusal plane

Plane of dental film

CR is at a 90° angle to the bisecting plane

Bisecting plane

Longitudinal axis of tooth

(A)

Vertical plane of tooth

Occlusal plane

Film

Central ray

(B)

important during exposure to determine positioning of the patient.

- **ala-tragus** (**ah**-la-**TRAY**-gus) **line:** imaginary line from the ala (wing) of the nose to the tragus (skin projection anterior to acoustic meatus), center of ear. This line is important for positioning the patient in the bisecting-angle technique.
- **Frankfort** (**FRANK**-furt) **plane:** imaginary line from the tragus of the ear to the floor of the orbit that is used to align the maxillary arch parallel

to the floor; used mostly for extraoral films. Many machines that expose large extraoral films and digital images have a stabilizing chin rest or an aiming light to ensure this directional position.

The angulation or positioning of the PID and the direction of the central beam are very important to the exposure technique. When exposing films and digital images for the bisecting technique, the operator follows the machine's positive and negative angle figures marked on the side of the tube head.

- **positive angulation:** angulation achieved by positioning the PID downward; also called *plus angulation*. Maxillary exposures are incisors (+40 degrees), cuspids (+45 degrees), bicuspids/premolars (+30 degrees), and molars (+20 degrees).
- **negative angulation:** angulation achieved by positioning the PID upward; also called *minus angulation*. Mandibular exposures are incisors (–15 degrees), cuspids (–20 degrees), bicuspids/premolars (–10 degrees), and molars (–5 degrees).
- **zero angulation:** angulation achieved by PID placement parallel to the floor.

Because films and sensors for paralleling exposure are placed in alignment devices, the operator follows the angulation designated by the positioning of the PID (cone head) to the aiming ring of the device. Both techniques must use proper horizontal and vertical angulations, or errors will be evident on the finished X-rays:

- **Horizontal angulation:** direction of the central X-ray beam in a horizontal plane (side to side). The central beam must be placed perpendicular to the film front and teeth alignment. The error observed with improper horizontal angulation is called *overlapping* or *cone cutting*.
- **Vertical angulation:** direction of the central X-ray beam in an up or down position. Improper vertical angulation results in *foreshortening* or *elongation* errors.

Positioning Devices

Positioning and holding devices are used to help produce a good radiograph:

- **PID:** position indicating device may be a *long cylinder* (12–16 inches) or a *short cylinder* (8 inches); may be a round or rectangular, open-ended tube. It is used to collimate and direct the central beam, and it also determines the target-surface distance.
- **film-holding instrument:** device used to place and retain the film or sensor in the oral cavity during exposure. Common sets are the *VIP* (*Versatile Intraoral Positioner*) by UpRad or the *Rinn BAI* for the bisecting angle technique; *XCP* (*extension cone paralleling device*) and *Rinn XCP-DS* for sensor use; and *Rinn XCP* for endodontic views. Locator or aiming rings are color-coded to designate area placement (Figure 9-10), such as:
  - blue = anterior placement
  - yellow = posterior placement
  - red = bitewing placement
  - green = endodontic placement

There are universal film-holding single blocks for digital imaging. One system, XCP ORA, contains only one ring with color-coded slots for arm inserts to be used in the particular exposure desired (anterior, posterior, or bitewing).

- **biteblock:** a device inserted between the teeth to hold the film during exposure; made of foam, wood, or plastic.
- **individual film holder:** a grip device, such as Rinn's Eezee-grip, that will hold one film or one sensor for exposure in the mouth. Mostly used in a small mouth or difficult areas, the loaded film holder is put into position and held by the patient's bite or finger pressure.
- **bite loop/tab:** paper tab or a celluloid circle placed around periapical film, enabling the film to be used in a bitewing position. This combination is used in place of a commercially manufactured interproximal film. Some bite loops are constructed to assist with stabilizing

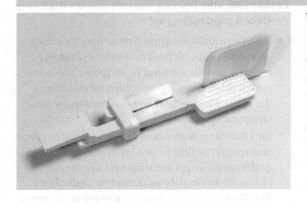
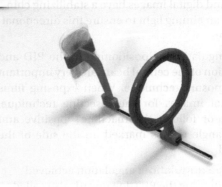
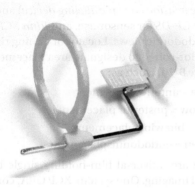
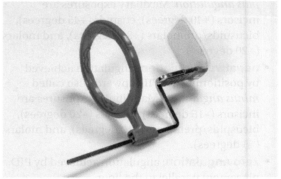

and holding the digital sensors in the film-holding device.

- **film-safe container:** a lead-lined container used to hold exposed films until processing; protects the film from exposure to scattered or secondary rays during exposure of films.

X-Ray Surveys

Although X-rays may be taken to diagnose a specific tooth area, most radiographs are taken in a survey or a combination of exposures. When conventional films are placed in a mount, side by side, or when digital images are aligned, these multiple exposures reveal the condition of a large area. The amount and placement of a survey of exposures depend on the nature of the dental visit and the problems encountered. The surveys are:

- **full mouth survey (FMS or FMX):** multiple exposures of the oral cavity showing crown and root area in a series of radiographic views. When arranged in proper sequence, these films or images give a survey or view of the condition of the entire mouth (Figure 9-11).

- **bitewing survey (BWS or BWX):** two- or four-film exposures of the posterior view to observe the crowns of maxillary and mandibular posterior teeth. Anterior bitewing exposure is also possible.

- **edentulous** (ee-**DENT**-you-luss = *without teeth*) **survey:** radiographic survey of a patient without teeth.

Figure 9-11 Digital presentation of a full-mouth series with accent view of lower right molar area

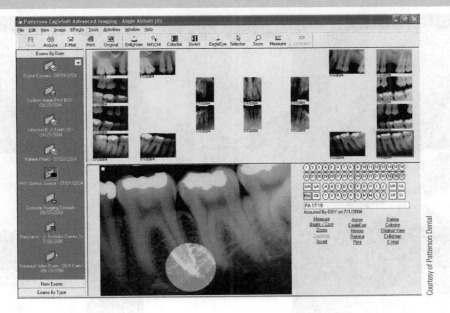

Courtesy of Patterson Dental

RADIOGRAPHIC FILM PROCESSING

After exposure of the dental film to radiation, the film must be processed or developed to present a picture of the existing conditions. **Radiograph processing** is a procedure for bringing out the latent image on a film and making the exposure permanent. The procedure involves developing, rinsing, fixing, washing, and drying. Processing may be completed in an automatic film processor or by manual methods in a processing tank. Following are terms related to film processing:

- **developing:** chemical process using the chemical elon to bring out contrast and another chemical, hydroquinone, to show contrast in films. The developer converts the exposed silver halide crystals to black metallic areas.
- **rinsing:** water bath used during manual processing, not automatic processing to remove chemical liquids from films during solution exchanges.
- **fixing:** chemical process that stops the developer action and "fixes" the image, making

it permanently visible. The fixer removes the unexposed silver halide crystals and creates the white or clear areas on the image.

- **hyposulfite** or **hyposulfite of sodium:** chemical in the fixer that removes exposed and unexposed silver halide crystals from the film emulsion.
- **drying:** procedure to dry films after the chemical and water baths.
- **safelight:** special light or filtered light that can remain on during the developing procedure in the dark room.
- **duplicating radiograph:** procedure utilizing duplicating film to make a duplicate exposure of a processed radiograph for purposes of insurance, referral, or records.

MOUNTING RADIOGRAPHS

After the dental conventional films have been processed, they must be viewed and stored. To hold the films in place for viewing and later for patient

161

Figure 9-12 Full mouth set of deciduous teeth with correct placement positioning

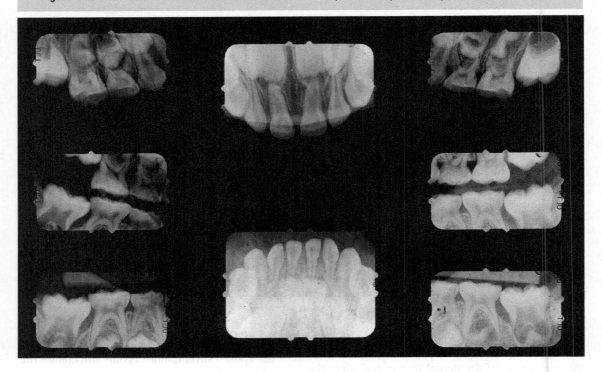

records, the films are mounted. **Mounting**, also called *carding*, of radiographs is a procedure to arrange the processed radiographs in a cardboard, plastic, or stiff carrier to present a view of the oral cavity. Mounts have preset window openings—horizontal for posterior views and vertical for anterior shots. A mount may be obtained with various window arrangements. Radiographs may also be presented in order such as the digital arrangement in Figure 9-12. Terms related to mounting radiographs are:

- **horizontal window:** preset window in the mount that is used to place posterior films.
- **vertical window:** preset window in the mount that is used for placement of anterior films.
- **bitewing window:** also called *interproximal* window; used to place bitewing exposures.
- **identification dot:** preset pressed or raised area on the surface of the film. The rounded or

convex view indicates the surface of the film that faced the radiation source (facial side). The convex or inward dot view on the film indicates that the film surface was placed away from the tube head or radiation source (lingual side).

- **view box:** a box or wall-mounted frame with fluorescent lights behind a frosted glass plate; used to view X-rays.

ASSORTED RADIOGRAPHIC ERRORS

When dental radiographs have not been exposed properly or handled in a clean manner, a faulty film will result. This may cause the radiograph to be unreadable and require additional radiation exposure for a patient in a makeup film. Included among the various radiographic errors seen in the dental facility are:

- **elongation** (ee-lon-**GAY**-shun): image of the tooth structure appearing longer than the actual size; caused by insufficient vertical angulation of the central ray (Figure 9-13).
- **foreshortening** (for-**SHORE**-ten-ing): tooth structures appear shorter than their actual anatomical size; caused by excessive vertical angulation of the central ray (Figure 9-14).
- **overlapping:** distortion of the film showing an overlap of the crowns of the adjacent teeth superimposed on neighboring teeth; caused by improper horizontal angulation of the central ray (Figure 9-15).

- **cone cutting:** improper placement of the central beam, which produces a blank area or unexposed area on the film surface caused by lack of exposure to radiation, such as when the PID is not centered properly on the film (Figure 9-16).
- **clear film:** A totally clear film indicates that no radiation has affected or exposed the film.
- **underdeveloping:** insufficient processing with weak chemicals or incorrect time or temperature that results in light, difficult-to-view films.
- **overdeveloping:** overprocessing that results in radiographs that are too dark and difficult to interpret.

Figure 9-13 An example of elongation of dental X-ray; the teeth images are longer than the actual teeth

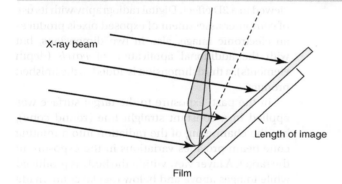
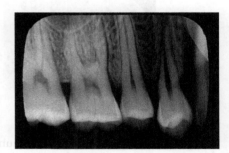

Figure 9-14 An example of foreshortening; the teeth images are shorter than the actual teeth

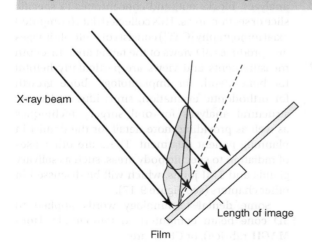
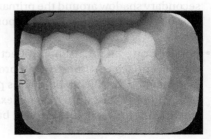

Figure 9-15 Overlapping error; the tooth crown images overlap each other for no clear definition

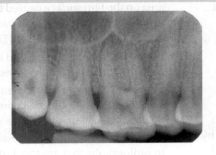
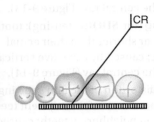

Figure 9-16 Cone-cutting example showing the film is white where the radiation did not expose

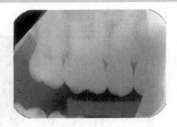

- **reticulation** (reh-**tick**-you-**LAY**-shun): crackling of film emulsion caused by wide temperature differences between processing solutions. Reticulation gives a stained glass window effect.

- **fog:** darkening or blemish of film that may be caused by old film, old or contaminated solutions, faulty safelight, scattered radiation, or improper storage of films.

- **penumbra:** poor definition, fuzzy outline, or secondary shadow around the primary form; may be caused by movement or exposure errors.

- **herringbone effect:** fishbone effect on the film surface resulting from improper placement of the film. Radiographs placed in the mouth in a backward position exhibit a shadow impression of the lead foil backing in the visual image.

3D RADIOLOGY

Since the discovery of X-rays, radiographs have been viewed in a 2D effect. Digital radiography with its use of computer assessment of exposed pixels produces an electronic image, also in two dimensions, but with the additional application of *voxels* (depth elements), a third dimension is added to the finished product.

In the past, exposure to the target surface was applied in a constant straight line (round cone), but the channeling of the radiation into a rotating cone beam provides variations in the exposure to the target. A layer view within the body is produced while images above and below that layer are made invisible by blurring. This assorted information is sent to computer software, which measures, analyzes, blocks out, and concentrates in specific slice or section areas. This collected data (computed axial tomography [CAT]) consists of multiple images and produces 3D views of the target area. In-depth measurements and views are particularly helpful for bone depth for implantology, bone growth for orthodontic evaluation, sinus lifts, and many structural analyses for oral surgery techniques as well as providing more detail for the dentist in planning patient treatment. There are other uses of radiation to specific body areas, such as salivary glands and TMJ joints, which will be discussed in other chapters (see Figure 9-17).

Some dental terminology words applied to 3D cone beam computerized tomography (**toe-MAGH**-rah-fee), or CBCT, are:

Figure 9-17 3D i-CAT scan X-ray image

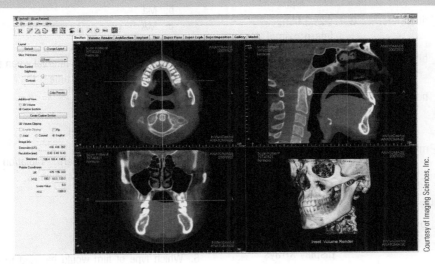

- **CBVT (cone beam volumizing tomography):** another term for CBCT.
- **tomography** (toe-**MAGH**-rah-fee; *tomas-GK. = section, slice or part, graphy = measured record*): the act of gathering and data measurement of a slice or section under view; imaging by sections.
- **tomogram** (**TOE**-moe-gram = *image produce*): the finished image product in a tomography procedure.
- **polytomography** (**poly**-toe-**MAGH**-rah-fee): several slices or sections of the tooth or body.

- **laminagraphy** (lam-in-**AUG**-rah-fee = *body section radiography*): same as tomography; technique in which tissue image is collected and measured in slices or sections.
- **voxel** (**VOX**-el = *picture element giving image depth or volume*): the exposure of voxels instead of pixels produces a 3D effect in the image:
  - **axial view** = *top to bottom view.*
  - **sagittal view** = *side to side view.*
  - **coronal view** = *front to back view.*
  - **volumetric view or study** = *addition of depth produces a 3D image with added volume.*

Review Exercises

Matching

Match the following word elements with their meanings.

1. _____ anode   **A.** size 4 film (2¼" × 3")

2. _____ ion   **B.** headplate

3. _____ erythema   **C.** particle carrying electrical charge

4. _____ accelerator   **D.** digital sensor used for immediate image

5. _____ voxel   **E.** digital imaging by slice or sections

6.	_____ CCD	**F.**	right-angle method of film exposure
7.	_____ dosimeter	**G.**	size 3 film, interproximal
8.	_____ bitewing	**H.**	solution used to swell film emulsion
9.	_____ horizontal window	**I.**	safety device to register absorbed radiation
10.	_____ midsagittal plane	**J.**	imaginary vertical line bisecting face
11.	_____ paralleling technique	**K.**	positive pole in X-ray tube
12.	_____ tomography	**L.**	light window or frame used to display X-rays
13.	_____ view box	**M.**	redness of skin, reaction to X-ray exposure
14.	_____ occlusal	**N.**	mounting space for posterior film
15.	_____ cephalometric X-ray	**O.**	3D digital depth element

Definitions

Using the selection given for each sentence, choose the best term to complete the definition.

1. The controlling factor in the production of electrons available for radiographs is:
   a. timer
   b. kilovolt power
   c. milliampere control
   d. timer switch

2. The tube head area where the central beam or primary ray is projected is the:
   a. focal spot
   b. filament
   c. target plane
   d. primary target

3. The abbreviation for the term *milliampere* is:
   a. MilA
   b. Ma
   c. MA
   d. mA

4. The time or duration of interval when the current will pass through the X-ray tube is the:
   a. latent time
   b. processing time
   c. exposure time
   d. count-up time

5. The effect of long-term radiation outcome or exposures repetition is known as:
   a. cumulative effect
   b. sensitivity effect
   c. mutation effect
   d. latent effect

6. Which type of film would be used to view the tooth crowns, roots, and surrounding tissues of a single arch?
   a. headplate
   b. periapical
   c. interproximal
   d. bitewing

7. A size 4 radiograph packet would contain which film?
   a. occlusal
   b. interproximal
   c. panoramic
   d. periapical

8. Which of the following is not considered a basic safety precaution in exposure of radiographs?
   a. dosimeter
   b. safelight
   c. lead barrier/screen
   d. lead apron/collar

9. Variations of black and white colors on a radiograph are considered an example of:
   a. fog
   b. detail
   c. definition
   d. contrast

10. If the PID is aimed in an upward position, it is considered to be which angulation?
    a. zero
    b. horizontal

c. negative

d. positive

11. A cone-cutting exposure error is the result of which improper angulation?

    a. vertical

    b. horizontal

    c. sagittal

    d. zero

12. The basic unit of exposure to radiation is:

    a. ALARA

    b. MPD

    c. rad

    d. R

13. The ability of X-rays to penetrate and possibly ionize body tissues is termed:

    a. sensitivity

    b. cumulative effect

    c. mutation effect

    d. chronic radiation

14. The central ray of radiation emitted from the tube head is termed:

    a. scattered radiation

    b. stray radiation

    c. secondary radiation

    d. primary radiation

15. The color of a Rinn positioning device film holder used for anterior teeth is:

    a. red

    b. blue

    c. yellow

    d. green

16. The technique used in digital imaging to determine small changes in image sequences is termed:

    a. digital substitution

    b. color substitution

    c. magnification

    d. zoom-in technique

17. The ability to transfer captured digital data from one area to another is known as:

    a. tomography

    b. laminagraphy

    c. volumizing

    d. teleradiography

18. An axial 3D digital dental view displays data in what direction?

    a. top-to-bottom view

    b. side-to-side view

    c. front-to-back view

    d. circular view

19. When tooth structures on a dental film appear longer than the actual tooth size, the error is termed:

    a. cone cutting

    b. foreshortening

    c. reticulation

    d. elongation

20. In chemical processing of dental films, which is the proper solution sequence?

    a. developer, water bath, fixer, water bath

    b. fixer, water bath, developer, fixer

    c. water bath, fixer, developer, water bath

    d. developer, fixer, water bath

Building Skills

Locate and define the prefix, root/combining form, and suffix (if present) in the following words.

1. **radiolucent**

   prefix _____

   root/combining form _____

   suffix _____

2. **kilovolt**

   prefix _____

   root/combining form _____

   suffix _____

3. **laminagraphy**

   prefix _____

   root/combining form _____

   suffix _____

4. **cephalometric**

   prefix _____

   root/combining form _____

   suffix _____

5. **edentulous**

   prefix _____

   root/combining form _____

   suffix _____

Fill-Ins

Write the correct word in the blank space to complete each statement.

1. X-rays, also known as Roentgen rays, are a source of _____ energy.

2. The tungsten coil in the cathode-focusing cup that generates the electrons is called the _____ _____.

3. Radiation that leaks from a faulty tube head is termed _____ radiation.

4. A lighted, wall-mounted glass window or frame used to look at X-rays is called a/an _____ _____.

5. A/an _____ is the finished image product of a 3D slice or section of body tissue.

6. Radiographs exposed outside the oral cavity are called _____ films.

7. A/an _____ effect is the abnormal growth or development that may occur from genetic changes due to radiation.

8. Poor definition or fuzzy outline of form that may be caused by movement is known as _____ _____.

9. A safety device that measures the amount of absorbed radiation during exposure of dental X-rays is called a/an _____.

10. A/an _____ dental film is size 0.

11. The temporary skin redness occurring as a result of radiation overdose is called _____ _____.

12. A/an _____ film is a larger size dental film (2¼" × 3").

13. A/an _____ colored film positioning device indicates use in the posterior region.

14. A lead apron and thyrocervial collar is considered protection for the _____.

15. The digital CCD sensor data produces _____ _____ on the monitor/screen.

16. A/an _____ is another word for a 2D computer picture element.

17. The variations from black to white in an X-ray film is called _____.

18. Maxillary X-ray exposures are made with the PID in a/an _____ angulation.

19. A radiographic survey of a patient without teeth is considered a/an _____ survey.

20. Metallic objects, such as restorations or crowns appearing as white areas, are said to be _____ _____.

Word Use

Read the following sentences and define the boldfaced words.

1. Many orthodontists require a **panoramic** and headplate film of the patient before beginning treatment.

   _____

2. **Radiolucent** areas in a dental X-ray or a digital image indicates bone loss.

   _____

3. Storage of digital films requires less space and record keeping than the conventional films, which need **mounting** and cross filing.

   _____

4. The dental staff pays particular care to **ALARA** principles when dealing with radiation.

   _____

5. Each dental operator who exposes radiographs should have a personal **dosimeter**.

   _____

✔ Learning Objectives

On completion of this chapter, you should be able to:

1. Discuss the purpose of dental restorations and their classifications, and identify the steps of the dental restoration procedure.

2. List the various methods employed to maintain a dry mouth area during dental preparations.

3. Name the steps in preparing a restorative site prior to placing the restorative materials.

4. Discuss the necessity for matrix placement, and identify the various types of matrix retainers and their uses.

5. Identify and describe the assorted dental cements, liners, and base materials used in tooth restorations.

6. Understand and define terminology commonly used in dental restorative procedures.

7. Discuss the various types and properties of dental restorative materials used in tooth restorations.

8. Identify the methods used to complete, finish, and refine the tooth restoration.

OPERATORY AND PROCEDURE AREA

Restoration of the patient's teeth is the most common treatment associated with the dental office. The purpose of a dental restoration is to do the following:

- Remove the **carious lesion** (**CARE**-ee-us **LEE**-zhun = *decay area*).

- Prepare the site for a restorative material of choice with the needed bases and liners.

Vocabulary Related to Tooth Restorations

This list contains selected new and important word parts and terms from this chapter. Take the time to learn these word parts and their meanings. You may use the list to review these terms and practice pronouncing them correctly. When you work with the audio for this chapter, listen to the word, repeat it, and then place a checkmark in the box. Proceed to the next boxed word, and repeat the process.

(hyphen before word means it's a suffix, hyphen after word means prefix, no hyphen means root word.)

Word Parts	Meaning	Word Parts	Meaning
bride	debris	-ic	pertaining to
de-	down, loss, without	-ment	action or state of
ex-	without	re-	return, back again
fine	unblemished, pure, high quality	stabiliza	firm, solid, steady
gene	to become	therm	temperature
homo-	same		

Key Terms

- ☐ **adhesive** (ad-**HEE**-siv)
- ☐ **amalgam** (ah-**MAL**-gum)
- ☐ **amalgamation** (ah-**mal**-gah-**MAY**-shun)
- ☐ **anneal** (ah-**NEAL**)
- ☐ **articulating** (are-**TICK**-you-lay-ting)

- ☐ **burnish** (**BURR**-nish)
- ☐ **composite** (cahm-**PAH**-zit)
- ☐ **condensation** (kon-den-**SAY**-shun)
- ☐ **debridement** (deh-**BREED**-ment)
- ☐ **dissipate** (**DISS**-ih-pate)

- ☐ **embrasure** (em-**BRAY**-zhur)
- ☐ **esthetic** (ehs-**THET**-ick)
- ☐ **exothermic** (**ecks**-oh-**THER**-mick)
- ☐ **galvanic** (gal-**VAN**-ick)
- ☐ **homogenous** (hoh-**MAH**-jeh-nus)

(Continued)

Vocabulary Related to Tooth Restorations *continued*

Key Terms *continued*

- ❏ **increment** (**IN**-kreh-ment)
- ❏ **infiltration** (in-fill-**TRAY**-shun)
- ❏ **instrumentation** (in-strew-men-**TAY**-shun)
- ❏ **insulation** (in-sue-**LAY**-shun)
- ❏ **invert** (in-**VERT**)
- ❏ **isolation** (eye-so-**LAY**-shun)
- ❏ **laminated** (**LAM**-i-nate-ed)
- ❏ **ligature** (**LIG**-ah-tchur)

- ❏ **luting** (**LOO**-ting)
- ❏ **manipulation** (muh-**nip**-you-**LAY**-shun)
- ❏ **matrix** (**MAY**-tricks)
- ❏ **mylar** (**MY**-lar)
- ❏ **palliative** (**PAL**-ee-ah-tiv)
- ❏ **polymerization** (pahl-if-mer-ih-**ZAY**-shun)
- ❏ **protective** (proh-**TECK**-tiv)

- ❏ **protocol** (**PROH**-toe-kahl)
- ❏ **solubility** (sahl-you-**BILL**-ih-tee)
- ❏ **spherical** (**SFEAR**-ih-kul)
- ❏ **translucency** (trans-**LOU**-sen-cee)
- ❏ **trituration** (try-chur-**AY**-shun)
- ❏ **veneer** (veh-**NEAR**)
- ❏ **viscosity** (viss-**KAHS**-ih-tee)

- Restore the tooth to its normal function and **esthetic** (ehs-**THET**-ick = *pertaining to beauty*) appearance.

Choice of the procedure and the materials used depend on the condition and site of the tooth involved. Dental caries are classified according to their area and amount of surface decay covering the tooth, as shown in Table 10-1 and illustrated previously in Chapter 7, Examination and Prevention.

Regardless of the type of restoration needed, the procedural routine is the same. The first step is making sure the patient is comfortable and experiences a pain-free procedure. Various levels of anesthesia are used for dental treatment. The level of anesthesia is decided according to the patient's individual needs, and the type of treatment required. Pain management associated with dental treatment was explained in detail in Chapter 8, Pain Management and Pharmacology.

Table 10-1 Classification of Caries

Classification	Type of Carious Lesion	General Surfaces Involved
Class I	Pits and fissures	Occlusal surfaces of posterior teeth
		Posterior buccal and lingual fissures
		Lingual fissure (cingulum pit) of maxillary incisors
Class II	Interproximal of posteriors	Proximal walls and some occlusal surfaces of posterior teeth
Class III	Interproximal of anteriors	Proximal surfaces and walls of anterior teeth
Class IV	Interproximal of anteriors with incisal edge involved	Anterior proximal walls, including the incisal edges or surfaces
Class V	Smooth surfaces, cervical areas	Gingival third of tooth; common in canines
Class VI	Decay or abrasions of chewing surfaces	Decay or abrasion of anterior teeth incisal edges or occlusal edges of posteriors

ISOLATION OF THE OPERATIVE SITE

The operative site must be isolated throughout the restoring process. Site isolation provides the operator with a clear view and a dry area for the proper use of dental materials. Oral evacuation by a dryfield isolator (Figure 10-1) or saliva ejector and the high volume evacuation tip removes saliva and cooling water from handpieces. Cotton rolls may be applied to strategic sites to control fluids. Absorbent pads, called "dry angles," may be situated over the parotid gland in the cheek to absorb the flow of saliva.

Isolation helps to control tongue interference common among young patients and nervous patients, and it also helps prevent aspiration or swallowing of small dental items, such as crowns, clamps, and amalgam debris. To assure total tooth isolation, a dental dam may be applied.

Figure 10-1 Dryfield isolator in place

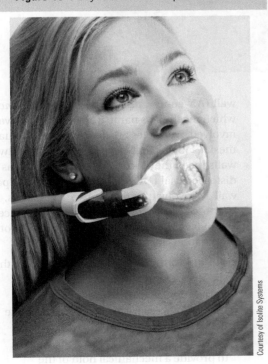

Courtesy of Isolite Systems

DENTAL DAM

A dental dam (also called rubber dam) is a material placed on the teeth for certain dental procedures. The dental dam serves two main functions:

- **isolation** (**eye**-so-**LAY**-shun = *separate or detach from others*): the tooth or teeth to receive treatment are isolated and exposed for the procedure, presenting better viewing and access.
- **barrier** (**BARE**-ee-er = *an obstacle or impediment*) control: the dam material protects against infection to the operative site and microorganisms, leaving the patient's mouth, damage from caustic materials, and accidents to adjacent tissues.

Items needed for placement of the dental dam are noted, pictured, and explained in Chapter 13, Endodontics. After the dam is prepared and placed into the mouth, the following steps are taken to ensure proper protection:

1. Place the **ligature** (**LIG**-ah-tchur = *banding or tying off*). Small pieces of floss or dam material are placed into the proximal areas to assist with control and retention of the dam material in the mouth.
2. **Invert** (in-**VERT** = *turn inward or reverse*) the material. This seals the edges of the dam material to the tooth surface and prevents moisture from escaping into the work area.
3. **Stabilize** (**STAY**-bill-ize = *condition of fixing, steadying, or firming*) the dam clamp. Ligatures, softened wax, or other materials may be placed about the dam clamp to assist the dam clamp in maintaining a firm seating.

Also, quick dams, lip and cheek retractors, props, and absorbent pads are available to the dentist for isolating a site that does not require controlling moisture and maintaining a sterile field, such as endodontic preparations. These dams are smaller, with or without a frame, and are set into the mouth. They are used mostly for a single tooth prep or for general isolation (see Figure 10-2).

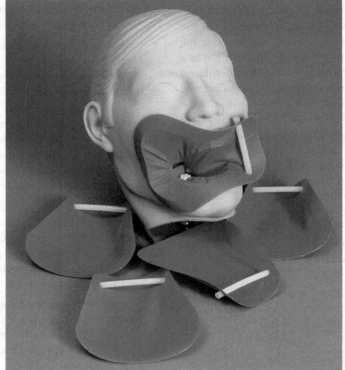

Courtesy of Aseptico, Inc.

PREPARATION OF THE RESTORATIVE SITE

Each caries-affected tooth requires special attention. The method, procedure, and choice of restorative materials for the affected tooth must be custom planned and adapted. The basic **protocol** (**PROH**-toe-kahl = *steps or method to follow*) for returning a decayed tooth to a restorative level involves three steps:

1. Remove caries and perform **debridement** (deh-**BREED**-ment = *removal of damaged tissue*) using rotary burs or diamonds in handpieces, abrasion, laser, or mechanical methods, as well as hand **instrumentation** (in-strewmen-**TAY**-shun = *use of instruments*).
2. Prepare tooth form to receive and retain restorative materials. To obtain the proper forms, preparations must be made in the **axial**

wall (**AX**-ee-al = *pertaining to the long line*), which receives its name from the surface wall involved. Examples are distal, buccal, lingual, mesial, labial, gingival, and pulpal. When two walls meet, they form a **line angle**, such as a disto-occlusal (DO) restoration. If the pulpal wall is involved with the two axial walls, a **point angle** is formed, and three surfaces are involved, such as distobuccopulpal. Tooth preparations include several prep forms:

- **outline form:** tooth cuts used to prepare the size, shape, and placement of restoration.
- **convenience form:** the cut of tooth material necessary for access to complete the cavity preparation.
- **retention form:** undercut of the walls to provide a mechanical hold of the restorative material.

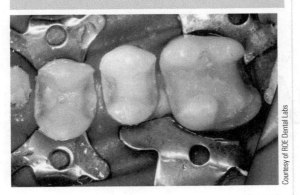

Figure 10-3 Teeth prepared for restoration of two bicuspid inlays and one molar onlay reconstruction

Courtesy of ROE Dental Labs

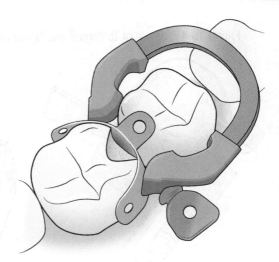

- **resistance form:** preparation cuts to ensure that the restored natural tooth can withstand trauma and pressure use of the tooth.

See Figure 10-3 for an example of prepared teeth.

3. Finish and **refine** (ree-**FINE** = *make new again*) of the tooth walls and surfaces in preparation to receive the restorative material. Extensive loss of tooth surface may require placement of a matrix to restore the original shape, and a combination of materials of liners and bases may be used to fill the preparation. When filled, the material is placed, anatomy formed, smoothed, polished, and checked for occlusion.

MATRIX PLACEMENT

After a tooth wall has been removed in a tooth preparation, it must be replaced. To hold the shape and form of the original wall and to prevent an **overhang** of restorative material, the dentist may use a **matrix** (**MAY**-tricks = *mold or shaping*), such as a Tofflemire, AutoMatrix, T-strip, or a retaining clamp-holding device such as the V3 sectional matrix system:

- **Tofflemire** (tauf-il-**MIRE**) **matrix:** a retainer device and assorted stainless steel bands to fit and be tightened around the tooth. Wedges made of wood, resin, or celluloid for passage of ultraviolet light are placed at the base of the matrix to stabilize and provide **embrasure**

(em-**BRAY**-zhur = *opening*) areas with nearby teeth (see Figure 10-4).

- **AutoMatrix:** presized, cone-shaped circle bands with locking ends that are tightened and locked after being placed on the tooth; visibility may be better because no retainer is necessary to hold the band.

- **T-strips:** stainless steel strips that are shaped like a T. The strip is circled with the T ends flapped over to retain the shape and hold the band on the tooth. Wedges are also used to provide embrasure space and stabilization. T-strips are commonly used in pediatric dentistry.

- **Ivory retainer/sectional matrix:** these systems are used mostly on posterior teeth. The strip does not circle the tooth but only replaces a wall. The retainer holds a stainless steel strip that is placed between the prep and the contact wall of the adjacent tooth. The strip is tightened, and a wedge is used for space and to assist with retention.

- **V3 system or sectional matrix systems:** the artificial wall band is set into a special forceps, carried into the mouth, placed around the preparation, and released to grasp and hold the matrix against the prep; wedges are placed in the embrasure for support, stabilization, and to maintain cervix space.

Figure 10-4 Example of Tofflemire matrix retainer with band and wedges in place

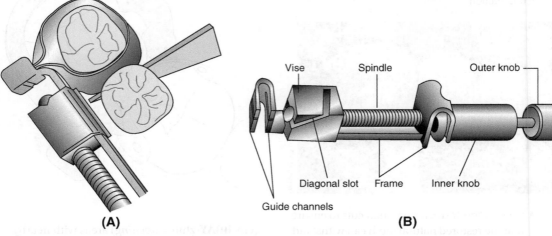

(A) (B)

- **Mylar** (**MY**-lar = *celluloid*) **matrix strips and crown forms:** used with anterior or tooth-shaded materials. The strips are placed around the tooth restoration and held in place by a clip or finger pressure until the restoration is set or light cured. Crown forms are filled with restorative material and placed on the preparation until the material has set.

CEMENTS, LINERS, AND BASE MATERIALS

Each dental material is chosen for its unique characteristic. Some materials may be used as a luting agent, pulp capping, base, or core buildup depending on which consistency is prepared. Some materials are obtained in a powder-liquid, two-paste, capsule, light, or self-cure ability. The selection of a particular material is determined by the preparation site, involvement, and physical makeup of the prepared tooth. Manufacturer's instructions for dosage, preparation, and use should be carefully followed. Among several popular material choices for protecting or preparing materials are:

- **varnish:** copal or resin gum in a suspension of organic solvents (acetone, ether, or chloroform); used to cover the cut edges of

tooth surfaces and seal the dentinal tubules against leakage under all restorations except composites and resins. Universal varnish that does not contain the organic solvents may be used under all restorations.

- **liner:** thin coating that provides a barrier against chemical irritation; usually a varnish material or a liquid suspension of calcium hydroxide or glass **ionomer** (eye-**AHN**-oh-mer) cement.

- **acid etchant:** phosphoric acid solution used to prepare the cavity margins to provide retention for the bonding and restorative materials. Etching makes the enamel surface more porous, creating enamel tags, and removes the smear layer of bacterial and tooth debris matter. When prepared, the enamel looks chalky white.

- **bonding agent:** material used to unite some restorative agents to the tooth surface and underlying materials; may be self-curing liquids or light-cured.

- **base:** barrier against chemical irritation. Bases will also provide thermal isolation, resist condensation forces, and are able to be contoured and shaped. A base may be calcium hydroxide, zinc-oxide eugenol (ZOE), or ZOE with ethoxybenzoic acid (EBA) added for strength, zinc phosphate, polycarboxylate, or glass ionomer. Each has its own characteristics.

- **cement:** a thicker material that can be used as a temporary or permanent restorative material; for example, glass ionomer cement may serve as a cement or a restoration material; self-cured or light-cured. Cements also may be used to retain pins or posts in a deep preparation.
- **retention pin:** metallic pin that is cemented into a drilled hole in the tooth prep. The exposed end of the pin will be incorporated into the restorative material.
- **core post:** titanium/stainless steel posts of various sizes that are cemented into a root canal of a tooth that has been endodontically treated (*the pulp of the tooth has been removed*). A core buildup of restorative material is placed over the extending post end. Figure 10-5 illustrates a pin and post.

Purposes of Liners, Bases, and Cements

Some materials are placed into cavity preparations prior to the restorative material of choice. These liners, bases, and cements are chosen for a specific purpose, such as the following:

- **insulation** (in-sue-**LAY**-shun = *to set apart*): prevents transfer of heat, stress force, and galvanic shock (gal-**VAN**-ick = *electrical charge from chemical reaction of two dissimilar metal meeting through biting forces*).
- **palliative** (**PAL**-ee-**ah**-tive = *relieves or alleviate pain*): soothing; encourages growth or reparative dentin, also called **tertiary** (**TERR**-shee-air-ee = *later stage*) dentin.
- **protective** (proh-**TECK**-tiv = *shielding*): preparation seal or temporary restoration between treatment visits.
- **luting** (**LOO**-ting = *holding together*): retaining items in union; usually a temporary measure between treatments; may be permanent or intermediate up to a year.
- **cementation** (see-men-**TAY**-shun = *bonding or uniting of two or more items*): used to permanently unite or restore shape and purpose; also may be used to cement retention pins into the preparation.
- **laminated** (**LAM**-in-**ate**-ed = *thin plate or layer*): materials applied in thin layers to the tooth surface; may be cemented or light activated for permanency.

RESTORATION PLACEMENT TERMINOLOGY

Terms specific to the preparation, handling, insertion, or use of cementing and restorative agents include the following:

- **manipulation** (muh-**nip**-you-**LAY**-shun = *skillful operation or handling and use*): preparation and handling during use; each material requires a different method.
- **homogeneous** (hoe-**MAH**-jeh-nus = *same or alike in development*): describes a uniform mixture; some materials, such as cements, have to be blended.
- **trituration** (**try**-ture-**AY**-shun = *pulverize*): the mechanical blending and mixing of the mercury and alloy materials, also called

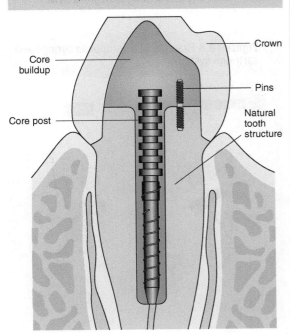

Figure 10-5 Example of restoration buildup using retention pin and core post

Crown

Core buildup

Pins

Core post

Natural tooth structure

amalgamation (ah-**mal**-gah-**MAY**-shun), the chemical act of blending the alloy and mercury mix for an amalgam restoration. This procedure is usually accomplished in a machine called an **amalgamator**.

- **mulling:** the further act of blending the amalgam material while it is in plastic form; performed in the amalgamator with the **pestle** (**PES**-toll) removed from the mixing capsule.

- **dissipate** (**DISS**-ah-pate = *to scatter or spread out*): to spread out over a larger area; some materials must be mixed over a large area to allow escape from the **exothermic** (**ecks**-oh-**THER**-mick = *give off heat*) reaction that is produced by the chemical union of the ingredients.

- **polymerization** (pahl-ee-**mare**-ih-**ZAY**-shun = *change of compound elements into another shape*): transforming material from a plastic (movable) shape to a hard substance through a curing process either automatically (self-curing) or using a light-source method.

- **bonding** (**BON**-ding = *uniting through microscopic cementation*): using acid materials called **etchants**; may be used to prepare a tooth surface for attaching to another material.

RESTORATIVE MATERIALS

A variety of materials and procedures are used in restoring the affected tooth to normal function, use, and beauty. An **amalgam** (ah-**MAL**-gum = *soft alloy mass containing mercury*) is a blend of various powdered alloy metals and liquid mercury mixed into a plastic (movable) form that soon hardens. Amalgam alloy may be supplied as **spherical** (**SFEAR**-ih-kul = *in the form of a sphere*) for better mixing or amalgamation and material flow, or the alloy may be supplied as lathe filings, which are small, irregular, metal grains. Amalgam is available in color-coded, single, double, or triple dose premeasured capsules. Some capsules include a pestle, a small metal or hard plastic cylinder that aids mixing. The alloy proportion in amalgam is mentioned before the mercury amount, such as 5:8

(five parts alloy to eight parts mercury). The choice of the dental alloy composition (silver, copper, tin, and zinc percentages) depends on the qualities of the material the dentist wants to use. Other relevant terms are:

- **cement:** plastic material that can unite or bond materials. The choice of cement depends on the **solubility** (**sahl**-you-**BILL**-ih-tee = *capability of being dissolved*), **viscosity** (**viss-KAHS**-ih-tee = *resistance to flow, thick, semi-fluid*), and **adhesive** (ad-**HEE**-sive = *sticky or adhering*) quality of the material.

- **composite** (cahm-**PAH**-zit): resin material used in dental restorations; supplied in **macrofilled** (*large particles*), **microfilled** (*small particles*), and **hybrid** (*mixed particles*) and may be purchased in paste, syringe, or single-dose capsules (see Figure 10-6). Composites may be self-cured (auto) or light-cured, tintable, and capable of being effective in all types of restoration classifications and teeth adaptations, which will be discussed in Chapter 11, Cosmetic Dentistry.

- **gold foil:** foil sheet of gold material that is **annealed** (*placed in a flame for a heat*

Figure 10-6 Example of a composite syringe and cartridge system

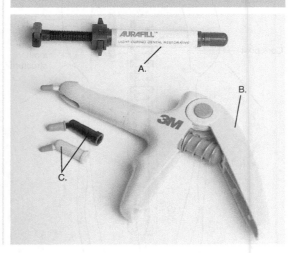

treatment to purify) to a clean and prepared surface for condensation into the prepared restorative site. Gold is also supplied in mat or powder form for direct insertion into tooth prep.

- **veneer** (veh-**NEAR** = *tooth-shaped layer*): thin resin composite or porcelain surface shields that are cemented or bonded onto the facial surface of a tooth. Veneer also refers to the thin surface facial covering on the porcelain veneer crown (PV).

Tooth crowns (caps) are restored using various materials, such as cast gold, porcelain facings, milled covers, and prepared resin toppings. Types of crown will be covered in Chapter 11, Cosmetic Dentistry, and construction will be discussed in Chapter 19, Dental Laboratory Procedures.

FINISHING METHODS

After the tooth has been prepared and has received the liner and bases as needed, the restorative material has to be inserted, condensed, and preliminarily carved. The matrix and dental dam (if used) are removed, and the final carving, articulation check, and polishing are completed. Several terms are specific to this procedure:

- **increment** (**IN**-kreh-ment = *increase or addition*): small amounts or doses of the materials that are placed into the preparation until filled.
- **condensation** (**kon**-den-**SAY**-shun = *to make thick*): the changed preparation as a result of the condenser or plugger instruments packing down the material into the preparation.
- **carving:** instrument shaping and cutting of condensed material to resemble original anatomical tooth surface.
- **burnish** (**BURR**-nish = *to smooth or rub*): to smooth the restoration surfaces toward the margins. Matrix strips may be burnished or rubbed into the proper shape. Burnishing also provides a shiny surface to gold.

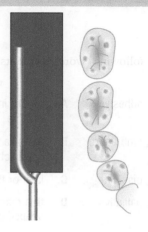

Figure 10-7 Articulating paper revealing high spots

- **articulating** (are-**TICK**-you-lay-ting) **paper:** colored strip of paper used to test results of the restored bite. The articulating paper is placed on the occlusal surfaces, and the patient bites down. When the paper is removed, the high spots are indicated by the marks that appear with carbon or colored traces to indicate where refinement is needed (see Figure 10-7).
- **laminated** (**LAM**-i-nate-ed = *thin plate or layer*): material applied in thin layers to the tooth surface; may be cemented or light activated for permanency.
- **HVE (high velocity evacuation):** fluid removal system used to maintain a clear, dry field of operation.

After placement, packing, and carving, then finishing burs, diamonds, wheels, abrasive strips, and polishes are used to smooth and refine the restoration. Amalgam material may not be polished for 48 hours, but many composite and resin materials are completely refined at the insertion appointment.

Review Exercises

Matching

Match the following word elements with their meanings.

1. _____ adhesive   **A.** to turn inward or reverse

2. _____ embrasure   **B.** to make thick or compact

3. _____ dissipate   **C.** later or third stage

4. _____ palliative   **D.** thin resin tooth-shaped layer

5. _____ manipulation   **E.** add in small amounts

6. _____ invert   **F.** sticky, adhering

7. _____ cementation   **G.** open space between contact point and gingiva

8. _____ increment   **H.** binding or tie-off material

9. _____ veneer   **I.** removal of damaged tissue

10. _____ burnish   **J.** to smooth or rub out

11. _____ esthetic   **K.** bonding or uniting of two or more items

12. _____ condensation   **L.** to scatter or spread out

13. _____ tertiary   **M.** skillful operation or handling and use

14. _____ ligature   **N.** relieving or easing pain

15. _____ debridement   **O.** pertaining to beauty

Definitions

Using the selection given for each sentence, choose the best term to complete the definition.

1. An example of a restorative material supplied in mat or sheet form and annealed before use is:
   a. composite
   b. gold foil
   c. amalgam
   d. zinc oxide

2. Which of the following metals is not used in an amalgam restoration?
   a. silver
   b. titanium
   c. tin
   d. copper

3. A Mylar matrix strip would be used for which type of restoration?
   a. Class II amalgam
   b. Class I amalgam
   c. Class V composite
   d. Class III composite

4. "Beauty," or the condition related to looking beautiful, refers to:
   a. veneers
   b. viscosity
   c. galvanics
   d. esthetics

5. Which of the following matrix devices is commonly used in pediatric dentistry?
   a. T-band
   b. Tofflemire
   c. Ivory
   d. AutoMatrix

6. Tooth cuts used to prepare the size, shape, and placement of a restoration are which form of cavity preparation?
   a. outline form
   b. retention form

c. resistance form

d. convenience form

7. The change of compound elements into another shape is a process called:
   a. trituration
   b. polymerization
   c. manipulation
   d. instrumentation

8. The ability or the capacity of being dissolved refers to the term:
   a. viscosity
   b. solubility
   c. malleability
   d. adhesive

9. Which of the following materials should not be polished for 48 hours after insertion?
   a. composite
   b. gold
   c. ZOE
   d. amalgam

10. The use of small dental instruments in operative dentistry is called:
    a. instrumentation
    b. manipulation
    c. handling
    d. transfer

11. During some dental procedures, a tooth area may need to be set aside or apart, this is called:
    a. injection
    b. infiltration
    c. inverting
    d. isolation

12. One of the important factors concerned with the cement use is its holding power called:
    a. solubility
    b. viscosity
    c. adhesiveness
    d. translucency

13. During an amalgam restoration, the material is placed into the prep in small loads called:
    a. macrofilled
    b. increments
    c. injections
    d. barriers

14. A carious lesion found on the proximal wall of an anterior tooth is classified as:
    a. Class I
    b. Class II
    c. Class III
    d. Class IV

15. A base that may be used to sedate and provide pain relief is described as:
    a. protective
    b. palliative
    c. homogeneous
    d. permanent

16. A permanent restoration containing powdered metal alloy and mercury is called:
    a. composite
    b. resin
    c. amalgam
    d. ZOE

17. An object or material used to tie off or bind is termed a:
    a. core post
    b. retainer
    c. ligature
    d. matrix

18. Copal varnish is not placed in a preparation about to receive which restorative material?
    a. ZOE cement
    b. gold foil
    c. amalgam
    d. composite

19. The mixing of amalgam material in an amalgamator after the pestle has been removed is termed:
    a. tituration
    b. manipulation
    c. instrumentation
    d. mulling

20. To scatter or spread out a mixture, allowing heat to be given off is termed:
    a. dissipate
    b. bonding
    c. mulling
    d. inverting

Building Skills

Locate and define the prefix, root/combining form, and suffix (if present) in the following words.

1. **stabilization**
   prefix _____
   root/combining form _____
   suffix _____

2. **debridement**
   prefix _____
   root/combining form _____
   suffix _____

3. **homogeneous**
   prefix _____
   root/combining form _____
   suffix _____

4. **refinement**
   prefix _____
   root/combining form _____
   suffix _____

5. **exothermic**
   prefix _____
   root/combining form _____
   suffix _____

Fill-Ins

Write the correct word in the blank space to complete each statement.

1. A carious lesion involving the interproximal of posterior teeth would be Class _____.

2. The band or tie-off used in dental dam placement and retention is called a/an _____.

3. Placing wax or compound around the wing of a dental dam clamp is a procedure used to fix or make steady and is called _____.

4. The basic steps or method to follow in a procedure is termed _____.

5. An electrical shock caused by the chemical reaction of two dissimilar metals meeting in a biting force is called _____ shock.

6. _____ paper is used to mark or indicate high areas on the surface of the restoration.

7. The skillful operation or handling and use of dental materials is called _____.

8. A _____ is a thin resin tooth-shaped layer that is placed on the facial side of a tooth.

9. A process called _____ is the instrumentation used to pack down or make restorative material thick in the preparation.

10. The Toffelmire matrix is used to prevent _____ of the amalgam material into the embrasure areas.

11. Restorative materials that are placed into the preparation in small amounts are called _____.

12. Composite material set up in two manners, self-cure and _____.

13. A cavity base material that relieves or alleviates pain is called _____.

14. _____ is a process of rubbing or smoothing off a material or metal surface.

15. Another term for a movable, workable amalgam is a _____ condition.

16. The small metal or hard plastic cylinder that is inside an amalgamator capsule is called a _____.

17. A metallic pin that is cemented in a large restoration preparation and used to help support that restoration is a _____ pin.

18. _____ is the term used to describe the capability of a material to be dissolved.

19. A hybrid composite restorative material is said to have _____-sized particles.

20. During the chemical setup or curing, some dental materials give off heat called a/an _____ action.

Word Use

Read the following sentences and define the meaning of the word written in boldface letters.

1. When placing a dental dam, it is important to properly **invert** the material.

   _____

2. The patient requested an **esthetic** restoration for her maxillary central incisor.

   _____

3. The dentist requested a piece of **articulating paper** after adjusting the bite.

   _____

4. To **dissipate** the heat, some materials must be spread out over the entire mixing slab.

   _____

5. It takes time for a new assistant to learn the proper **protocol** for each procedure.

   _____

CHAPTER 11 | COSMETIC DENTISTRY

✓ Learning Objectives

On completion of this chapter, you should be able to:

1. Define the meaning of cosmetic dentistry and the various applications in dentistry.

2. Describe the cosmetic procedures.

3. Cite reasons for tooth whitening and methods used to lighten tooth surfaces.

4. Discuss the procedures used to repair, or alter size, shape, and color of teeth by bonding or veneer applications.

5. Discuss the various types of cosmetic restorations, including inlays, onlays, and crowns.

6. Identify the different techniques used to correct damaged tissue and make an esthetic gum presentation.

7. Describe the assortment of dental implants and the use and necessity of implant dentistry.

8. Discuss accelerated orthodontics to improve the adult smile and mouth occlusion.

DEFINITION OF COSMETIC DENTISTRY AND RELATED AREAS

Beyond maintenance and reconstruction of the oral cavity, the modern dental patient desires an esthetic appearance. People seek dental care to improve their looks and turn to their dentist for cosmetic restorations and esthetic correction of diseased tissues, stains, genetic imperfections, accidents, and other maladies of the mouth.

Although most cosmetic dentistry procedures can be completed by the dentist, some require a

Vocabulary Related to Cosmetic Dentistry

This list contains selected new and important word parts and terms from this chapter. Take the time to learn these word parts and their meanings. You may use the list to review these terms and practice pronouncing them correctly. When you work with the audio for this chapter, listen to the word, repeat it, and then place a checkmark in the box. Proceed to the next boxed word, and repeat the process.

(hyphen before word means it's a suffix, hyphen after word means prefix, no hyphen means root word.)

Word Parts	Meaning	Word Parts	Meaning
dont	tooth	osse, oste	bone
endo-	within	-penia	few, decrease, deficiency
gingiv	gum tissue	perio-	around
muc/o	mucus lining	sub	below, under
ortho-	straight		

Key Terms

☐ **augmentation** (awg-men-**TAY**-shun)

☐ **endosseous** (en-**DOSS**-ee-us)

☐ **extrinsic** (ex-**TRIN**-sick)

☐ **intrinsic** (in-**TRIN**-sick)

☐ **mucogingival** (myou-koh-**JIN**-jah-vahl)

☐ **osseointegration** (**oss**-ee-oh-in-teh-**GRAY**-shun)

☐ **osteogenic** (oss-tee-oh-**JEN**-ic)

☐ **osteopenia** (ahs-tee-oh-**PEE**-nee-ah)

☐ **subperiosteal** (**sub**-pear-ee-**AHS**-tee-uhl)

☐ **transosteal** (trans-**AHS**-tee-al)

☐ **veneer** (va-**NEAR**)

team consisting of the dentist and other dental personnel such as a prosthodontist, oral surgeon, periodontist, and dental laboratory technician. Cosmetic techniques offered to improve patients' esthetic appearance and restore or provide a functional use include tooth whitening, bonding, veneer application, cosmetic restorations, periodontal adjustment, implants, and tooth movement. Major repair and reconstruction of the mouth and facial structures are covered in Chapter 14, Oral and Maxillofacial Surgery.

SMILE MAKEOVER

The first thing that comes to mind in cosmetic dentistry is a beautiful smile. Two terms for cosmetic mouth dentistry are *smile makeover*, the desire for an esthetic appearance and *full mouth reconstruction*, the need for repair of maladies from birth, disease, or dental-health issues. Some of the needs and treatments used in cosmetic dentistry are:

- **tooth appearance:** darker, rough-surface, pitted teeth may receive bleaching, whitening, resin surface application, veneer coverings, or crowns.
- **spacing and alignment:** gaps (diastemas, dye-ah-**STEE**-mah) in front teeth, peg-shaped teeth, overlapping teeth, and out-of-line teeth may receive bonding, veneers, crowns, surgical frenectomies, and orthodontic care.
- **smile harmony and balance:** chipped teeth, gummy smiles, tooth length, and uneven papillae may receive bonding, surgical contouring, or gingival augmentation.

- **missing and decayed teeth:** may receive restorations, inlays, onlays, crowns, implants, bridges, or partial dentures.
- **commercial smile enhancer:** sometimes called "Hollywood Smile" has been developed for total cosmetic use. **Snap-on Smile** is a full arch covering that can be placed on and off the teeth by the patient to offer immediate good looks. In cases where no major disease or structural problems exist, the dentist will take an impression and send it to the laboratory where a flexible, beautified cover is prepared for the patient to use when the occasion calls for an improved appearance or as desired. No tooth constructive or curative dentistry is performed. It is the patient's option when to wear the tooth covering. See Figure 11-1.

TOOTH WHITENING

The most common cosmetic procedure is the whitening or lightening of tooth surfaces. Aging, chemically stained teeth, such as the tetracycline brown band line, and genetic disposition are causes of **intrinsic** (in-**TRIN**-sick, *from within*) stain. Personal diet may cause teeth to look dark and unattractive with **extrinsic** (ex-**TRIN**-sick, *from the exterior*) stain. Whitening or bleaching of teeth surfaces can be completed in the dental office, at home, or a combination. Bleaching of teeth, as defined by the FDA, is the whitening of teeth beyond their natural color, such as lessening of brown bands, while tooth whitening is the restoration of natural tooth color.

Figure 11-1 Snap-on Smile, a cosmetic enhancer that may be placed and removed by the patient

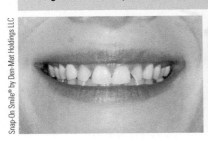 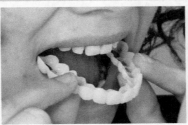 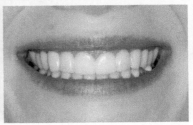

Snap-On Smile® by Den-Mat Holdings LLC

At the start of the procedure, the patient's present shade of tooth is photographed, recorded, and will be compared to the new shade after the whitening. Relevant terms to tooth whitening are:

- **shade guide:** handheld device with assorted and numbered tooth-shaded forms that are compared to the incisal two-thirds of the patient's incisors (Figure 11-2). Color types and levels include the following:
    - Reddish brown: up to five variant levels
    - Reddish yellow: up to four variant levels
    - Gray: up to four variant levels
    - Greenish gray: up to four variant levels
- **model impression:** a reproduction of the patient's teeth is made into a plaster/stone study model.
- **tray fabrication:** a plastic or celluloid tray is made to fit the study model cast and will be used to carry and hold chemicals for whitening.
- **gingival isolation:** painting or covering the patient's gingival areas with a liquid dam (mask) material to isolate the tissues from chemical damage; some systems also use face drapes, foil intraoral liners, and/or cheek retractors for the patients' protection, and provide protective glasses if about to use a curing lamp or laser setup.

- **tooth bleaching:** techniques and equipment vary according to the degree of lightening desired and the manufacturer's recommendations and instructions that differ in chemical strengths and application methods. Some techniques may require additional home care, but the basic methods are:
    - **acid brush:** 35% phosphoric acid solution applied to surfaces, particularly to tetracycline band lines on surfaces. The solution remains on the surface 15 seconds and then rinsed off; refreshened and reapplied up to three times as needed.
    - **tray method:** gel-, or paste-filled tray placed into the mouth over cleaned tooth surfaces; gel may be activated by diode-laser handpiece or activated by curing light up to three times.
    - **gel application:** a whitening gel containing a hydrogen peroxide or carbamide peroxide formula is applied directly to cleaned, isolated tooth surfaces, and may or may not be

Figure 11-2 Shade guides are moistened and matched to the natural tooth to determine the color, which is recorded in the patient's records.

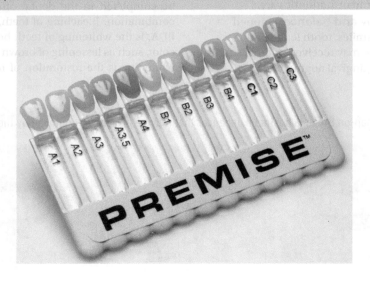

activated by bleaching, laser, or curing lights, as specified by the manufacturer; may be refreshed and reapplied as needed.

- **laser activation:** isolation of tissues, cleansing of tooth surfaces, and application of protective tissue covering and bleaching gel. Laser-light application for approximately an hour gives accelerated and more penetrating activation of the chemical gel material. Some patients are supplied DVD glasses for diversion during the wait.

- **pen-tip painting:** some commercial manufacturers have developed a pen that may be purchased at the drug store and used at home to paint the surfaces for whiter teeth. The pens contain some peroxide/bleaching material and do lighten teeth, but not as many shades as claimed.

- **tooth desensitization:** following bleaching, a desensitizing liquid, paste, or gel applied to tooth surfaces seals dentin tubules to minimize discomfort and reduce shade relapse. Some formulas that deter sensitivity and also remineralize the tooth include fluoride, calcium, and phosphate.

Following office lightening, the patient may be given a home tray and chemicals to complete the bleaching process. Assorted home bleach kits, strips, and gels are available, some from the dentist and others over the counter (OTC) at a local drugstore. Most contain a hydrogen peroxide or carbamide peroxide gel base that is placed in a tray, inserted in the mouth, and worn for a specified time, such as two to three hours, or overnight as directed. Professional whitening usually lasts a year, provided that the patient monitors his or her diet and does not smoke, both of which darken the tooth surfaces.

Tooth Bonding and Veneer Application

Tooth bonding and veneer application are alternatives to tooth whitening, particularly if the tooth surfaces are excessively stained or have other irregularities such as open spaces, broken edges, pitted surfaces, and abnormally shaped teeth.

Tooth Bonding

Tooth bonding involves applying a composite material that is mixed to a pliable dough form, applying it to a prepared tooth surface, and sculpting it into a tooth shape. The composite shade is chosen to match the existing tooth surface. The tooth is prepared by removing any present decay, followed by an abrasive roughening, and a gel etch. The surface is primed, the composite material is applied in layers, and the material is activated by a curing light. When shaped and finished, the composite is smoothed and polished (Figure 11-3).

Figure 11-3 A before-and-after example of tooth bonding

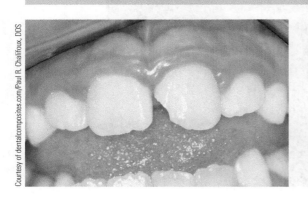
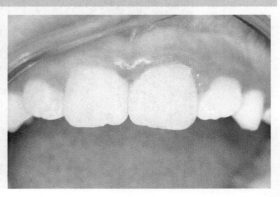

Courtesy of dentalcomposites.com/Paul R. Chalifoux, DDS

185

Veneer

In a **veneer** (veh-**NEAR**) **application**, a thin fabricated resin or porcelain cover is applied to the prepared tooth surface. Along with covering stained and affected teeth, the shape or color of the tooth may be altered. Depending on the severity and preparation needs of the teeth, veneers, also called laminates, can be applied using either of two methods:

- **Direct veneer application:** methods that can usually be completed in one visit include:
  - Similar to tooth bonding, a resin material is applied to tooth surfaces that have been roughened by air abrasion or rotary burs and wheels. The plastic material is cemented directly on the surface and then smoothed and polished.
  - Chair-side custom laminates can be made at the initial first visit with the use of a CAD/CAM technology. These laminates are prepared immediately, thereby eliminating the return second visit.
  - Lumineers, Durathins, or other premanufactured, "no prep" veneer coatings

can also be applied to facial tooth surfaces that need little or no surface removal (Figure 11-4).

- **Indirect veneer application (requires two visits):** At the first visit, the teeth are prepared by removing a small amount (0.5–1.0 mm) of enamel tissue. An impression is taken for fabrication of the porcelain veneers or laminates and sent to the laboratory. The dentist may or may not apply a temporary cover to last between visits. At the second visit, the teeth are cleaned, acid etched, and primed to receive the new laminates that are cemented on the tooth surface and light cured to set up. The porcelain veneers are cleaned and polished. Porcelain veneers usually are longer lasting and more expensive than direct veneer application. See Figure 11-5 for an example of a before-and-after veneer application.

COSMETIC TOOTH RESTORATIONS

Tooth restorations are completed using materials that resemble enamel tissue. Older amalgam fillings can be replaced using composite material to give the

Figure 11-4 Lumineers

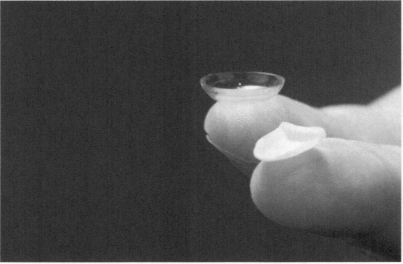

LUMINEERS by Den-Mat Holdings, LLC

Figure 11-5 Veneer photos. Diastema of the central incisors has been eliminated by the application of veneer coverings.

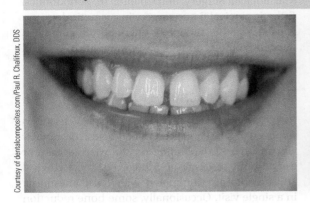
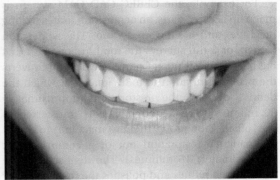

Courtesy of dentalcomposites.com/Paul R. Chalifoux, DDS

whole mouth a natural look. Restorative procedures include:

- **tooth restoration:** prepared tooth receiving white composite restorative material, instead of metallic amalgam or gold; replacement of existing amalgam fillings with composite.
- **inlay:** a solid-casted or milled restoration, involving some occlusal and proximal surfaces, that is cemented into a tooth preparation.
- **onlay:** a solid-casted or milled restoration that covers some occlusal tooth cusp and side wall area and is cemented onto the prepared site.
- **tooth crowns:** covering the crown surfaces of the tooth with artificial coverings. The type of crown applied depends on the extent of the tooth repair and is named by the area involved:
  - **full crown:** cast or milled restoration covering the entire crown area of a tooth (Figure 11-6).
  - **three-quarter crown:** cast or milled restoration covering all surfaces except the facial view.
  - **porcelain fused to metal crown (PFM):** full cast crown restoration with porcelain facing on exposed areas for cosmetic appearance.
  - **jacket crown:** thin metal cover with a porcelain facing for an anterior tooth.

Multiple crowns or combination restorations involving larger areas of the mouth are united in dental bridgework. This area of reconstruction is covered in Chapter 19, Dental Laboratory Procedures. The construction of cast restorations will also be discussed in Chapter 19. Although many cast restorations are made with gold or precious metals and covered with porcelain or resin to present an esthetic appearance, a new system of chairside ceramic restoration construction

Figure 11-6 Full crown

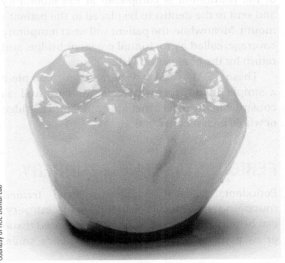

Courtesy of ROE Dental Lab

has been developed for immediate cosmetic restoration: CAD/CAM systems (computer assisted design/computer assisted machine).

For example, the CEREC CAD/CAM system is made up of three parts, an acquisition unit, a milling machine, and a software system. The acquisition camera or wand surveys the tooth preparation that has been covered by a reflective powder and converts the pixel information to a 3D image on which the dentist designs the restoration (approximately 30 minutes). The acquired data is transferred to the office laboratory milling machine to carve the patient's restoration out of a ceramic block (approximately 15 minutes). The dentist tests the fit, and then refines and polishes the restoration for bonding into the tooth preparation. The completed restoration is a solid ceramic block instead of a metal inlay, onlay, or crown with a porcelain esthetic covering. This method allows a one-trip restoration of tooth structure compared to other methods, where a provisional or temporary restoration must be prepared while the lab is fabricating the restoration.

Other systems work in the same manner, but imaging information may be sent from the camera capture in the patient's mouth to a company software design center for digital interpretation and construction of a working model. The dentist may receive and use this model, or it may be sent to a commercial lab chosen by the dentist. Construction of the restoration is completed at the laboratory and sent to the dentist to be placed in the patient's mouth. Meanwhile, the patient will wear temporary coverage, called a provisional crown or bridge, and return for the completion visit.

These CAD/CAM systems can complete a simple inlay or crown restoration as well as construct many pieces that are united into a bridge or whole arch reconstruction.

PERIODONTAL TISSUE SURGERY

Periodontal plastic surgery, also termed **mucogingival** (myou-koh-**JIN**-jih-vahl) **surgery**, can be performed as a treatment for diseased tissue or as a method to enhance the patient's smile.

Therapeutic periodontal treatment of gingival tissue will be discussed in Chapter 14, Oral and Maxillofacial Surgery, and Chapter 16, Periodontics. Esthetic gingival tissue surgery in cosmetic dentistry is used to either reduce or augment the gingiva as needed. Some examples and treatment of gingival cosmetic maladies are discussed next.

Gingival Reduction

In gingival reduction, excessive gingival tissue is removed by laser, periodontal knives, or bipolar electrosurgery. Depending on the case severity or the amount of tissue area involved, most gingival adjustments are completed with local anesthesia in a single visit. Occasionally, some bone reduction or augmentation may be required, which will require deeper anesthesia and surgical intervention. Reduction is used for the following:

- **crown lengthening:** exposing more tooth surface to eliminate a "gummy smile" (see Figure 11-7).
- **gingival contouring:** removing excessive tissue to obtain symmetry of the gingival crest.
- **exposing unerupted teeth:** removal of coronal tissue to expose tooth surface, such as slowly emerging mandibular third molars.
- **enlarged labial frenum:** condition where thick or enlarged labial frenum presents tissue growth between the mesial of central incisors, causing a space gap. A *frenectomy* (removal of excessive frenum tissue) will permit teeth to grow back together with minor tooth bracing.

Gingival Augmentation

Gingival augmentation builds up or reconstructs the gingiva to repair or replace tissue where needed. It involves the following:

- **soft tissue grafting:** transplanting mouth tissue from nearby gingival tissue or from the palate area to other sites.
- **interdental papilla regeneration:** replacing papilla tissue in interdental spaces.
- **gingival recession:** restoring the gingival crest to a natural height.

Figure 11-7 Before-and-after example of laser crown lengthening

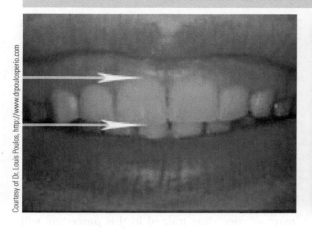 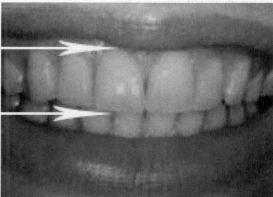

Courtesy of Dr. Louis Poulos, http://www.drpoulosperio.com

- **pocket depth reduction:** eliminating the pocket area and restoring the gingiva.
- **exposed roots covering:** replacing gingival tissue over exposed roots (Figure 11-8).
- **ridge augmentation:** building up gingiva and bone tissue in collapsed areas resulting from tooth extraction.

DENTAL IMPLANTS

Dental implants are titanium fixtures that are surgically installed in the jawbone and used to stabilize or serve as an anchor for a tooth, an appliance, or a denture. They may be used as an alternative to a fixed bridge or in areas where tooth replacement requires stability. Placement of an implant often requires a team cooperation of several specialists, such as an oral surgeon, a prosthodontist, and perhaps a periodontist.

Implants are surgically installed and remain in place for three to six months while the appliance and bone unite in a process called **osseointegration** (**oss**-ee-oh-inn-teh-**GRAY**-shun = *union of the bone with the implant device*). They are then uncovered, and the artificial device is attached. Implants will

Figure 11-8 Tissue replacement for exposed cuspid root

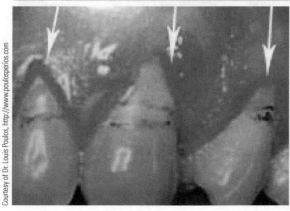 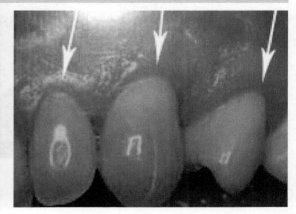

Courtesy of Dr. Louis Poulos, http://www.poulosperios.com

be discussed more in Chapter 12, Prosthodontics, and Chapter 14, Oral and Maxillofacial Surgery. Terms related to implants are:

- **root form implant—endosseous** (en-**DOSS**-ee-us = *within the alveolar bone*): screw-type device that is screwed or cemented into the alveolar bone; used for a single tooth or post implant (Figures 11-9A and 11-9B).
- **plate form implant:** used for the narrow jawbone; flat-plate style.
- **subperiosteal** (**sub**-pear-ee-**AHS**-tee-al) **implant:** implant plate or frame extending through the jawbone, placed under the periodontium, and stabilized on the mandible bone. It is used when bone height or width is insufficient; rests on top of the bone.
- **transosteal** (trans-**AHS**-tee-al) **implant:** larger plate stabilized on the lower border of the mandibular bone with posts extending

through the gingiva; used to anchor prostheses in difficult situations.

ACCELERATED ORTHODONTICS

Malocclusion can present an unattractive smile, and the desire for a better cosmetic appearance may cause a patient to seek accelerated orthodontic treatment. Most orthodontic treatments require two years or more to complete, and many adults desire a quicker treatment method. With accelerated orthodontics, the task can be accomplished in three to nine months, with retainers to be worn another six months.

A surgical orthodontic approach requiring a team of specialists trained in this procedure will be needed. It is a multiple-step process where the teeth are aligned and banded, sometimes after **rectification** (selective removal of interproximal

---

Figure 11-9 (A) Parts of implant with prosthesis, (B) radiograph showing implants in place

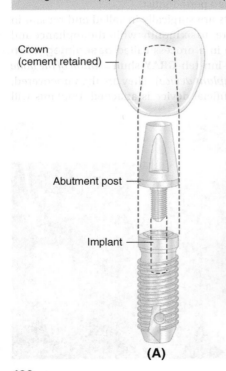

Crown (cement retained)

Abutment post

Implant

(A)

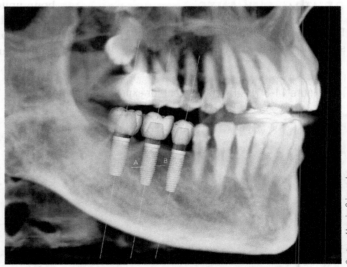

Courtesy of Imaging Sciences, Inc.

(B)

tooth tissue of multiple teeth) that provides space for tooth movement. This slimming or narrowing of teeth eliminates the need for extraction. A week after banding, the patient's gingiva is incised to expose the alveolar bone where a surgical drill is used to create holes or remove bone tissue in the alveolar crest to demineralize the bone, causing a condition called **osteopenia** (ahs-tee-oh-**PEE**-nee-ah = *lack of bone tissue*). A bone graft material mixed with an antibiotic is placed on the site, and the gingiva is replaced and sutured into place.

While the bone is in a weakened stage, movement progresses rapidly. Return visits and banding readjustments are more frequent than with the normal orthodontic treatment, and retainers are worn for six months or so after the bands have been removed, allowing total remineralization to finish.

Other cosmetic applications for orthodontic treatment include the following:

- **Invisalign™:** an orthodontic polyurethane tray method for tooth alignment using a series of clear, preformed, custom trays that apply pressure for tooth movement. Trays must be worn 20–22 hours per day, and when movement is finished, they must be worn at night. The trays are frequently changed (every two weeks) as movement or realignment occurs. Some tooth surface-slimming adjustment may be made after the impression, X-rays, photos, and records are sent to the Invisalign lab for 3D model planning and tray fabrication.

- **orthodontic enameloplasty:** removing small amounts of enamel walls to acquire enough room to cause a slight correction movement; usually performed in a small area or trouble spot.

- **lingual banding:** placement of brackets and bands on the lingual tooth surfaces so they are not easily viewed.

More conventional methods of orthodontic treatment are discussed in Chapter 15, Orthodontics.

Review Exercises

Matching

Match the following word elements with their meanings.

1. _____ full mouth makeover	**A.**	tooth stain from internal sources	
2. _____ inlay	**B.**	a thin resin or porcelain shell covering	
3. _____ transosteal implant	**C.**	protective gingival tissue covering when tooth bleaching	
4. _____ tooth whitening	**D.**	tooth stain from external sources	
5. _____ jacket crown	**E.**	lightening of teeth to natural color	
6. _____ osseointegration	**F.**	a cast restoration for a tooth cusp and proximal walls	
7. _____ tooth bleaching	**G.**	implant placed through the jawbone	
8. _____ onlay	**H.**	necessary repair for mouth maladies	
9. _____ intrinsic stain	**I.**	periodontal plastic surgery	
10. _____ root form implant	**J.**	anterior tooth metal covering with porcelain covering	

11. _____ mucogingival surgery	**K.**	casted cover on some occlusal surface and side walls	
12. _____ gingival augmentation	**L.**	union of bone with implant device	
13. _____ veneer	**M.**	lightening of tooth beyond the normal color	
14. _____ extrinsic stain	**N.**	a buildup of gingiva to replace tissue where needed	
15. _____ gingival isolation	**O.**	screw-type device inserted into the jawbone	

Definitions

Using the selection given for each sentence, choose the best term to complete the definition.

1. A prepared restoration that is placed on a tooth prep involving some occlusal cusps and proximal wall is a:
   a. full crown
   b. jacket crown
   c. onlay
   d. inlay

2. Tooth whitening completed by the application of phosphoric acid is which method?
   a. acid brush
   b. tray application
   c. gel rub
   d. air polish

3. Which procedure is considered gingival augmentation?
   a. gingival contouring
   b. crown lengthening
   c. exposing root surfaces
   d. interdental papilla regeneration

4. Tooth stain from genetic, aging, or chemical enamel reactions is which type of stain?
   a. intrinsic
   b. extrinsic
   c. environmental
   d. regional

5. Tooth stain from diet, personal tooth care, or smoking is which type of stain?
   a. intrinsic
   b. extrinsic
   c. environmental
   d. regional

6. Implant placement would be considered proper treatment for which condition?
   a. missing tooth
   b. gummy smile
   c. fractured tooth edge
   d. full embrasure

7. The last step in office power tooth bleaching is:
   a. gel application
   b. desensitizing
   c. tray fabrication
   d. model impression

8. A tooth diastema (open gap) can be corrected using which technique?
   a. tooth bonding
   b. gingival augmentation
   c. acid etching
   d. tooth restoration

9. Invisalign is the term applied to which orthodontic procedure method?
   a. lingual banding
   b. clear bracket use
   c. customized tray
   d. metal braces

10. Which of the following is considered to be a laminate?
    a. implant post
    b. dental dam
    c. die pattern
    d. veneer

11. A cast restoration involving the entire tooth surface that is cemented onto the tooth preparation is called:
    a. inlay
    b. onlay
    c. full crown
    d. jacket crown

12. The FDA requires a whitening of tooth surface beyond the natural color to occur for:
    a. tooth whitening
    b. veneer placement

c. tooth bleaching

d. color tone

13. The method of applying gel whitening material directly to the tooth surfaces is termed:
    a. acid wash
    b. tray coverage
    c. strip placement
    d. gel application

14. Protection of the gingival tissue during the application of chemicals in power bleaching is completed by which method?
    a. liquid dam mask
    b. cotton roll application
    c. oral evacuation
    d. tooth bonding

15. An example of an alignment and spacing problem would be which of the following?
    a. chipped tooth
    b. peg-shaped lateral
    c. pitted tooth surface
    d. gummy smile

16. Soft tissue grafting is considered which type of periodontal surgery?
    a. gingival stabilization
    b. gingival reduction
    c. gingival desensitizing
    d. gingival augmentation

17. Which of the following implant devices is placed through the jawbone?
    a. root form implant
    b. plate form implant
    c. subperiosteal implant
    d. transosteal implant

18. Mouth impressions are taken for construction of which of the following:
    a. implant post
    b. tray fabrication
    c. brush well
    d. dental dam pattern

19. The demineralization and lessening of the alveolar bone in accelerated orthodontics creates a condition termed:
    a. osteogenesis
    b. osseointegration

c. osteopenia

d. osteoporitis

20. Which type of crown would be used mainly on anterior teeth?
    a. bracket crown
    b. jacket crown
    c. three-quarters crown
    d. full crown

Building Skills

Locate and define the prefix, root/combining form, and suffix (if present) in the following words.

1. **mucogingival**
   prefix _____
   root/combining form _____
   suffix _____

2. **endosseous**
   prefix _____
   root/combining form _____
   suffix _____

3. **subperiosteal**
   prefix _____
   root/combining form _____
   suffix _____

4. **osteopenia**
   prefix _____
   root/combining form _____
   suffix _____

5. **orthodontic**
   prefix _____
   root/combining form _____
   suffix _____

Fill-Ins

Write the correct word in the blank space to complete each statement.

1. The procedure of removing small amounts of enamel wall to permit orthdontic tooth movement is known as _____.

2. The union of bone with a titanium dental implant device is known as _____.

3. A/an _____ crown is a thin metal-casted restoration with a porcelain covering placed on an anterior tooth.

4. The orthodontic treatment method of moving teeth by using customized activation trays is known as _____.

5. _____ is the term given to the surgical removal of gingiva to expose more enamel surface and reduce a "gummy" smile.

6. When power-bleaching teeth with chemicals, the gingiva is protected by _____.

7. A/an _____ is taken to prepare a study model for fabrication of a bleaching tray.

8. A/an _____ is used to compare tooth colors and obtain the restoration color for a patient.

9. A dental implant is usually constructed using _____ metal.

10. Another term for periodontal plastic surgery is _____ surgery.

11. In the Invisalign tray treatment plan, the patient is required to wear the tray for _____ hours a day.

12. The white or tooth-colored material of choice used for an anterior restoration is _____.

13. A/an _____ implant is used for a patient with a narrow jawbone.

14. The placement of orthodontic bands on the back surfaces of the anterior teeth is termed _____ banding.

15. _____ may be used to change the color and shape of the anterior teeth or to cover badly stained teeth.

16. A full-casted crown that is covered by a porcelain covering is known as a/an _____ crown.

17. Repairing a chipped tooth by using a composite material in a dough consistency to build up the tooth surface is a process called tooth _____.

18. Another name for a dental veneer is a dental _____.

19. _____ stain is tooth stain caused by smoking or frequently drinking coffee or tea.

20. _____ is a term applied to the condition of the alveolar bone after receiving the surgical bur treatment in accelerated orthodontics.

Word Use

Read the following sentences and define the meaning of the word written in boldface letters.

1. The last step of a tooth-whitening procedure is **tooth desensitization**.

   _____

2. Certain medicines can cause **intrinsic** staining of newly forming teeth.

   _____

3. Mrs. Swartz chose **veneers** to enhance the color and shape of her teeth.

   _____

4. When matching tooth colors to a **shade guide**, the guide should be moist so that it reflects light like the natural tooth surfaces do.

   _____

5. The assistant made an appointment for **gingival augmentation** to address Mr. Peterson's gum recession.

   _____

✔ Learning Objectives

On completion of this chapter, you should be able to:

1. Examine the requirements for prosthodontic care, and define the terms *prosthesis* of fixed and removable prosthodontic appliances.

2. Describe the assorted materials used in prosthesis construction and their characteristics.

3. List and describe the function or purpose of the various types of fixed prosthodontics.

4. Define and describe the function or purpose of the various components used in removable dental prostheses.

5. Name and describe the various procedural steps and methods used to complete construction of fixed and removable dental prostheses.

6. Discuss the various types of dental implants and their necessity in dental prostheses application.

7. Describe additional devices and the conditions they are used to treat.

DIVISIONS IN THE FIELD OF PROSTHODONTICS

Prosthodontics is one of the nine recognized specialties of the ADA. A licensed graduate of dentistry is permitted to perform dental treatment in this area. Some dentists pursue post-graduate studies in this art, and others will complete the three extra years of training to be ABP (*American Board of Prosthodontics*) certified and limit their practice to prosthodontics. A few will continue with yet another

Vocabulary Related to Prosthodontics

This list contains selected new and important word parts and terms from this chapter. Take the time to learn these word parts and their meanings. You may use the list to review these terms and practice pronouncing them correctly. When you work with the audio for this chapter, listen to the word, repeat it, and then place a checkmark in the box. Proceed to the next boxed word, and repeat the process.

(hyphen before word means it's a suffix, hyphen after word means prefix, no hyphen means root word.)

Word Parts	Meaning	Word Parts	Meaning
alveol	tooth socket bone	implant	man-made device
colloid	suspended particles	hydro	water
dent	teeth	-ology	study of
e-	without	-ous	pertaining to
-ectomy	removal		

Key Terms

- ☐ **abutment** (ah-**BUT**-ment)
- ☐ **acrylic** (ah-**KRIL**-ick)
- ☐ **adjacent** (ah-**JAY**-sent)
- ☐ **alveolectomy** (al-vee-oh-**LECK**-toe-me)
- ☐ **alveoplastomy** (al-vee-oh-**PLASS**-toe-me)
- ☐ **bevel** (**BEV**-el)
- ☐ **cantilever** (**KAN**-tih-**lee**-ver)
- ☐ **catalyst** (**CAT**-ah-list)
- ☐ **centric** (**SEN**-trick)
- ☐ **chamfer** (**SHAM**-fur)
- ☐ **condylar inclination** (**KAHN**-dih-lahr in-klih-**NAY**-shun)
- ☐ **connector** (ku-**NECK**-tor)
- ☐ **coping** (**KOH**-ping)
- ☐ **ductility** (duck-**TILL**-ih-tee)

(Continued)

Key Terms *continued*

- **edentulous**
  (ee-**DENT**-you-luss)
- **elasticity** (ee-las-**TISS**-ih-tee)
- **elastomeric**
  (ee-las-toh-**MARE**-ick)
- **endosseous** (en-**DOSS**-ee-us)
- **extraction** (ecks-**TRACK**-shun)
- **extruder** (ecks-**TRUE**-dur)
- **hydrocolloid**
  (high-droh-**KOHL**-oyd)
- **imbibition** (im-bih-**BISH**-un)

- **impregnated**
  (im-**PREG**-nay-ted)
- **malleability**
  (mal-ee-ah-**BILL**-ih-tee)
- **polyether** (pohl-ee-**EE**-thur)
- **polysulfide** (pohl-ee-**SUL**-fide)
- **polyvinylsiloxane**
  (pohl-ee-**VINE**-uhl-sil-**OX**-ain)
- **pontic** (**PON**-tick)
- **porcelain** (**PORE**-sih-lin)
- **prosthesis** (prahs-**THEE**-sis)
- **protrusion** (proh-**TRUE**-zhun)

- **reduction** (ree-**DUCT**-shun)
- **retainer** (ree-**TAIN**-ur)
- **retrusion** (ree-**TRUE**-zhun)
- **shoulder** (**SHOL**-dur)
- **silicone** (**SILL**-ih-kone)
- **subperiosteal**
  (sub-pear-ee-**OSS**-tee-uhl)
- **tensile** (**TEN**-sill)
- **thermoplastic**
  (therm-oh-**PLAS**-tick)
- **transosteal**
  (trans-**OSS**-tee-ahl)

year of maxillofacial prosthetic training in correction of birth defects, TMJ disorders, cancer destruction, traumatic disfigurement, and difficult cases and obtain fellowships as maxillofacial prostheses specialists.

A **prosthesis** (prahs-**THEE**-sis; *plural = prostheses*) is a replacement for a missing body part. In the dental field, it may be a fixed or removable appliance that replaces removed or unerupted teeth. A **fixed appliance**, such as a cemented crown, is placed in the mouth and is not intended for removal. A **removable appliance** is placed in and out of the mouth at the patient's will. **Implantology**, *the science of dental implants*, involves the use of both fixed appliances and removable appliances in some instances.

TYPES AND CHARACTERISTICS OF PROSTHODONTIC MATERIALS

Assorted materials are used in the construction and repair of prostheses. Among the synthetic and precious or semi-precious metals used for appliance fabrication are:

- **noble metals:** the valuable alloys—gold (Au), palladium (Pd), platinum (Pt), and silver (Ag).

- **base metals:** chromium-cobalt or chromium nickel, which may be used alone or in a mixture with noble alloys. These alloys are further classified for insurance purposes as high noble, noble, and base according to their formulas:

  ○ **high noble alloy:** contains more than 60% of gold, palladium, and/or platinum (with at least 40% gold).

  ○ **noble alloy:** contains more than 25% of gold, palladium, and/or platinum.

  ○ **base metal alloy:** contains less than 25% of gold, palladium, and/or platinum.

- **porcelain** (**PORE**-sih-lin = *hard, translucent, ceramic ware*): shells, veneer covers, or facings fused to the surface of a metal crown to give the appearance of a natural tooth surface; often abbreviated **PFM** (porcelain fused to metal).

- **composite:** resin material used for tooth-colored replacement.

- **acrylic** (ah-**KRIL**-ick): synthetic resin material used in fabrication of appliance parts, as coverings for the metal frameworks, or as natural tissue replacement.

- **ceramic:** a hard, brittle material produced from nonmetallic substances fired at high temperatures; supplied in block shape for milling into crown and tooth forms.

- **titanium:** corrosion-resistant, lightweight, strong bio-compatible metal used in dental implants and posts.
- **zirconia (ZrO$_2$):** corrosion-resistant, bio-compatible material, similar to titanium; used for implants.

The choice of which material to use for an appliance depends on the characteristics of that material relevant to prostheses construction. Associated terms are:

- **hardness:** ability of a material to withstand penetration.
- **tensile** (**TEN**-sill) **strength:** capability of a material to be stretched.
- **elasticity** (ee-las-**TISS**-ih-tee): ability of a material to be stretched and then resume its original shape.
- **ductility** (duck-**TILL**-ih-tee): ability of a material to be drawn or hammered out, as into a fine wire, without breaking.

- **malleability** (**mal**-ee-ah-**BILL**-ih-tee): ability of a material to be pressed or hammered out into various forms and shapes.
- **elongation** (**ee**-long-**GAY**-shun): ability of a material to stretch before permanent deformation begins.

FIXED PROSTHODONTICS

Various fixed prosthodontic appliances are used in mouth restoration, from the singular crown to a full arched bridge. Related terms are:

- **inlay:** a solid-casted, or milled restoration, involving some occlusal and proximal surfaces, which is cemented into a tooth preparation (see Figure 12-1A).
- **onlay:** a solid-casted or milled restoration that covers some occlusal tooth cusp and side wall area and is cemented onto a prepared site (see Figure 12-1A).
- **crown:** a fabricated, tooth-shaped cover replacement for a missing crown area that is

Figure 12-1 (A) Laboratory preparation of two inlays on premolar teeth and a distal onlay on the molar tooth, (B) before-and-after example of laminated veneers on the anterior crowns

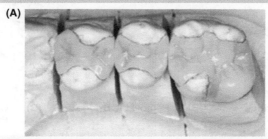

(A)

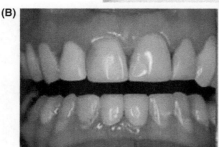

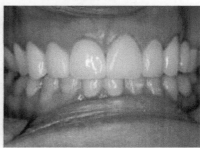

(B)

Courtesy of ROE Dental Labs

cemented onto the remaining prepared crown surfaces. Some of the types of crowns used in dentistry are:

- **full crown:** cast metal, tooth-shaped cover that replaces the entire crown area. Acrylic resin crowns may be used as a temporary crown cover during treatment.
- **jacket crown:** thin, preformed, metal shield used to cover a large area of anterior crowns; can be gold metal or metal covered with porcelain material to resemble tooth enamel.
- **dowel crown:** full crown cover with dowel pin extending into the root canal of a pulpless tooth; usually positioned on anterior teeth.
- **three-quarter crown:** similar to full crown, covering all of the crown except the facial surface of the tooth, which remains intact to present an esthetic, natural appearance.
- **pporcelain-fused-to-metal (PFM):** crown that has a complete capping of metal base

with fused porcelain to metal, giving tooth contour, shape, and cover.

- **veneer:** A **direct veneer** is placed and cured directly on the tooth surface to build up the area or to replace a missing tooth structure. For an **indirect veneer**, tooth material is prepared in the lab and later cemented onto the tooth structure. Figure 12-1B shows a before-and-after view of veneers of the anterior teeth.

Crown replacement and restorations may stand alone or may also be part of fixed bridgework. A **bridge** is a prosthesis used to replace one or more teeth. Dental bridgework may be of a fixed or removable nature. Figure 12-2 gives illustrated examples of bridges.

- **fixed bridge:** cemented into the oral cavity and not removed by the patient; the number of teeth involved in the appliance determines the amount or number of units (Figure 12-2A).

Figure 12-2 Illustrated examples of bridges

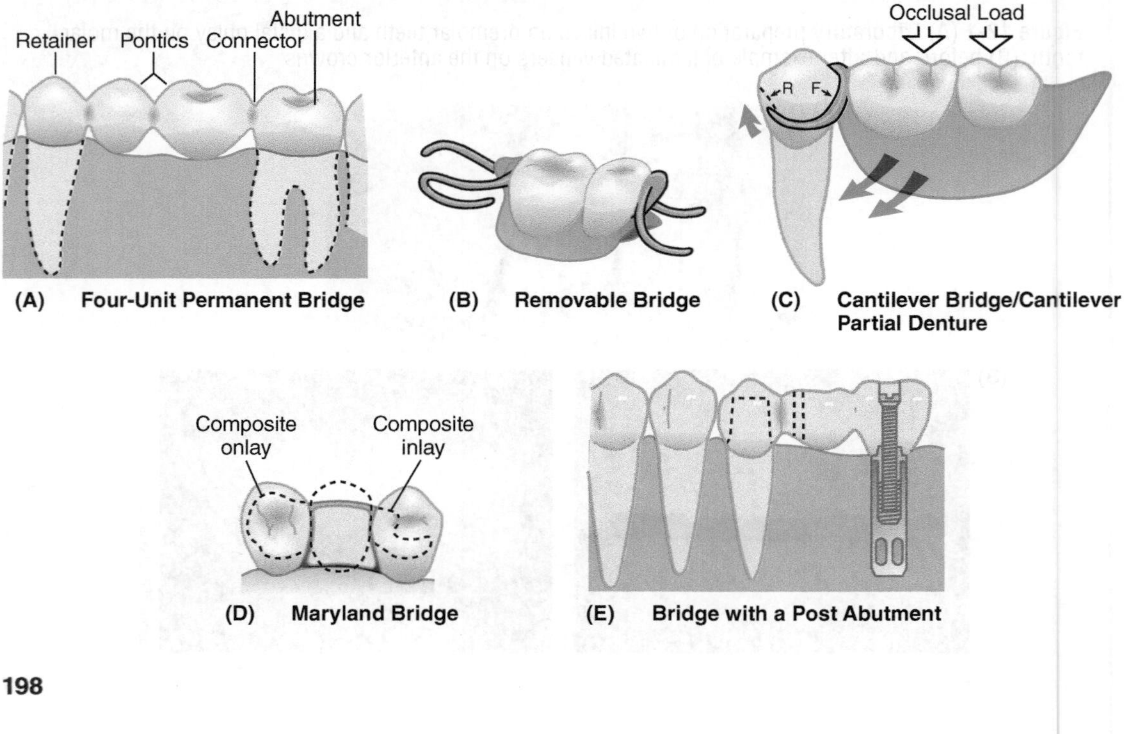

(A) **Four-Unit Permanent Bridge**

(B) **Removable Bridge**

(C) **Cantilever Bridge/Cantilever Partial Denture**

(D) **Maryland Bridge**

(E) **Bridge with a Post Abutment**

- **cantilever bridge** (**KAN**-tih-**lee**-ver): bridge with unsupported end, usually saddled (Figure 12-2C).
- **Maryland bridge:** replaces anterior or posterior tooth and is cemented directly to the adjacent or abutting teeth; also may be called a California bridge or resin-bonded bridge (Figure 12-2D).

A bridge has three components or structural parts:

1. **pontic** (**PON**-tick): artificial tooth part of the bridge that replaces the missing tooth and restores function to the bite.
2. **abutment** (ah-**BUT**-ment): natural tooth (or teeth) prepared to hold or support the retaining part of the bridgework in position.
3. **adjacent** (ah-**JAY**-cent = *nearby or adjoining*) **teeth:** may be included in units if they are involved in the bridge area.

REMOVABLE DENTAL PROSTHESES

Prostheses that the patient can take in and out at will are called removable prostheses. These devices include full mouth dentures as well as a replacement for single teeth. Terminology includes the following:

- **complete denture** (**DENT**-chur = *removable appliance composed of artificial teeth set in an acrylic base*): full denture designed to replace the entire dentition of an upper or lower arch.
- **partial denture:** removable appliance, usually composed of framework, artificial teeth, and acrylic material; replaces one or more teeth in an arch.
- **immediate denture:** denture prosthesis that is placed into the mouth at the time the natural teeth are surgically removed.
- **overdenture:** prosthetic denture that is prepared to fit and be secured on implant posts or on prepared retained roots.

Although all removable appliances are constructed to fit in a designated area and to return the mouth to a proper function, not all are fabricated in the same manner or using the same materials or components, such as:

- **framework:** metal skeleton or spine onto which a removable prosthesis is constructed.
- **saddle:** the part of the removable prosthesis that strides or straddles the gingival crest; used to balance the prosthesis. It serves as a base for the placement of artificial teeth.
- **rests:** small extensions of the removable prosthesis made to fit or sit atop the adjoining teeth. They provide balance and stability for the partial denture appliance. Rests are named for the area that is in contact with the tooth surface—occlusal, lingual, incisal, and so on.
- **clasp:** extension of partial framework that grasps the adjoining teeth to provide support and retention of the prosthesis.
- **retainer:** in fixed prosthesis, the part of the appliance that joins with the abutting, natural tooth to support the appliance, like the pillar holding the span of a bridge over the water. Some retainers are thin bars extending from quadrant to quadrant, called lingual bars, or some may be palatal bars.
- **connector** (*device used to unite or attach two or more parts* together): used to connect quadrants of a partial denture or connect and support an overdenture.
- **stress breaker:** a connector applied in stress-bearing areas to provide a safe area for stress relief and possible breakage.
- **artificial teeth:** anatomical substitutes for natural teeth; made of porcelain or acrylic material in various shades and shapes, called molds.
- **denture base:** acrylic part of the denture prosthesis that substitutes for the gingival tissue.
- **flange** (flanj): projecting rim or lower edge of prosthesis.
- **post dam:** posterior edge of the maxillary denture; helps to maintain the denture and suction.

Figure 12-3 Removable partial denture with structural components noted

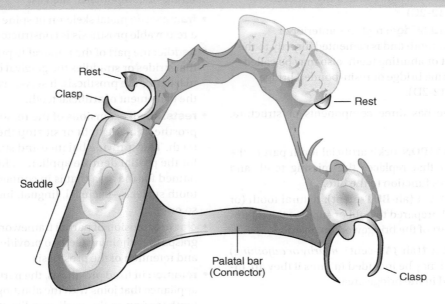

The structural components of dental appliances used in removable prostheses described in this section are illustrated in Figure 12-3.

PROCEDURES AND METHODS USED IN THE PROSTHODONTIC PRACTICE

Many of the operative procedures for fixed and removable prosthodontic appliances are similar in nature, with a few variations or step changes. Table 12-1 compares the operative steps for fixed and removable prostheses. The discussion of prosthesis fabrication is concluded in Chapter 19, Dental Laboratory Procedures.

Impression Procedure

Throughout the prosthodontic appointment, various impressions of the teeth and tooth preparations are taken. The choice of material to be used and the necessary items required for the procedure depend on the reason for the treatment and the condition or physical properties of the item to receive the impression. Impression materials must be **elastomeric** (**ee**-las-toh-**MARE**-ick = *having properties similar to rubber*), to be pliable during the impression process. Elastic impression items include hydrocolloids, rubber bases, and compounds. All materials must be carried and applied in the mouth by use of specially designed trays.

Hydrocolloids

An impression material that is both reversible and irreversible is **hydrocolloid** (**high**-droh-**KOHL**-oyd; *hydro = water, colloid = suspension of material*), an agar-like material that can change from one form to another. The types of hydrocolloid are:

- **reversible hydrocolloid:** impression material that can change from solid or gel state, to a liquid form, and back again, depending on temperature changes. This material is used in a water-cooled tray.
- **thermoplastic** (**therm**-oh-**PLAS**-tick; *thermo = heat, plastic = moldable*): quality of a material that changes from a rigid to plastic or movable form as a result of application of heat.

Table 12-1 Comparison of Operative Steps for Dental Prostheses*

Fixed Prosthodontics	Removable Prosthodontics
Exam, shade, mold selection, impression	Same procedure
Preparation of tooth and/or site	Mouth preparation, surgical adjustment
Impression of prepared tooth/site	Multiple impressions—custom trays
Try-in, unit adjustment	Try-in, wax adjustment
Adjustment, seating, and cementing	Adjustment and delivery

*Prosthesis fabrication is completed and discussed in the Chapter 19.

- **irreversible hydrocolloid:** once chemically set or in gel form, this material cannot be reversed or used again. An example of an irreversible hydrocolloid is **alginate** (**AL**-jih-nate) powder that is supplied in bulk containers or individual envelopes in regular or fast-set times. Alginate is stored in a dry, cool place until mixed with a premeasured water dose. Humidity can affect the water balance and stability of an irreversible hydrocolloid. Swelling from absorption of water is called **imbibition** (**im**-bih-**BISH**-un = *fluid absorption*), and evaporation or fluid loss causes shrinkage.

Rubber Bases

Rubber bases are common impression materials. They exhibit rubberized characteristics and are supplied in tubes, wash, and putty consistency or in a twin-cartridge (base and accelerator/activator), calibrated mixing dispenser called an **extruder** (ecks-**TRUE**-dur) **gun**. The base mixture requires an activator or **catalyst** (**CAT**-ah-list = *substance that speeds up a chemical reaction*) to instigate mixing together into a homogeneous mass and chemical set. The basic types of rubber bases are **silicone** (**SILL**-aih-kone), **polyether** (**pohl**-ee-**EE**-thur), **polysulfide** (**pohl**-ee-**SUL**-fide), and **polyvinyl siloxane** (**pohl**-ee-**VINE**-uhl-sil-**OX**-ain).

Compound

Another thermoplastic impression material is a **compound** (**CAHM**-pound), a nonelastic impression material that may be used in edentulous impressions. Compound is supplied in cakes or blocks and is heated to a soft, pliable mass; placed in an impression tray; and put into the mouth. After cooling in the mouth, it is removed, further cooled, and used as a customized impression tray for a future final wash with a zinc-oxide-eugenol paste or impression paste material.

Impression Trays

Dental impressions of the mouth are accomplished by placing the desired material into a carrying device and inserting it into the patient's oral cavity. The specific device used to transport the impression material depends on the site to be reproduced. Impressions can be of one tooth, a few teeth, or an entire **edentulous** (ee-**DENT**-you-luss = *without teeth*) arch. Some transport devices are copper tubes. Some are trays of *stock* metal or plastic purchased through dental suppliers. Trays may be custom constructed or purchased as full arch, quadrant, or sectional and anterior trays. Impression trays come in various sizes and shapes to accommodate specific areas of the mouth. Figure 12-4 shows a few examples. Impression materials are discussed further in Chapter 18, Dental Laboratory Materials.

Preparation of Teeth and Site

Site preparation must be accomplished before a prosthesis can be placed. The teeth and the area involved could receive one or a combination of a variety of preparations:

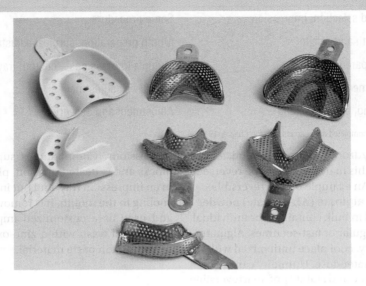

- **alveolectomy** (al-vee-oh-**LECK**-toe-mee): surgical removal of alveolar bone crests; may be required to provide smooth alveolar ridge for denture seating.
- **alveoplasty** (al-vee-oh-**PLASS**-tee): surgical reshaping or contouring of alveolar bone.
- **extraction** (ecks-**TRACK**-shun): surgical removal of teeth may be necessary. If completed before the insertion of an immediate denture, a clear **template** (**TEM**-plate = *guide or pattern*) may be used as a guide to prepare the alveolar surface.
- **coping** (**KOH**-ping = *coverings*): metal cover placed over the remaining natural tooth surfaces to provide attachments for overdentures.
- **reduction** (ree-**DUCT**-shun = *reducing or lessening in size*): removal of tooth decay and surfaces to receive the appliance. Various margin edges are prepared on the natural tooth to accommodate the thickness and material of the covering artificial crown, as illustrated in Figure 12-5.

- **chamfer** (**SHAM**-fur = *tapered margin at tooth cervix*): preparation for crown placement or full veneer covering.
- **shoulder** (**SHOL**-dur = *cut gingival margin edge*): preparation to provide junction of the crown and tooth; usually for metal on ceramic crown or porcelain jacket crown.
- **bevel** (**BEV**-el = *slanted edge*): tooth preparation for seating and holding of a crown.
- **core buildup:** use of synthetic material to enlarge tooth core area to provide support for an artificial crown and to protect the pulpal tissues. Small brass pins may be inserted into the material to aid retention and strength.
- **post placement:** addition of a metal retention post to teeth that have had pulp removal and root canal enlargement, to aid in stability and strength (see Figure 10-3 in Chapter 10, Tooth Restorations).
- **undercut:** removal of tooth structure near the gingival edge to provide a seat or placement for the extending edge of the appliance; same as tooth reduction.

Figure 12-5 Tooth margins for various types of preparations

Preparations at the gingival margin

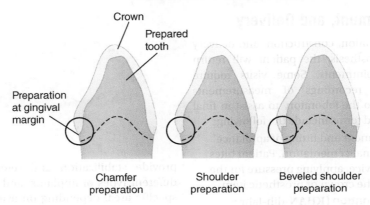

Crown

Prepared tooth

Preparation at gingival margin

Chamfer preparation

Shoulder preparation

Beveled shoulder preparation

- **retraction cord:** chemically treated cord placed in the gingival sulcus to obtain chemical or physical shrinking of the attached gingiva. These twisted or braided cords are plain or **impregnated** (im-**PREG**-nay-ted = *saturated*) with chemicals and packed into the gingival area to cause temporary shrinkage of the surrounding tissue and/or control bleeding (see Figure 12-6). Another method is to eject retraction paste into the sulcus prep for one to two minutes and then rinse away prior to impression taking.

Figure 12-6 Retraction cord placement on a model

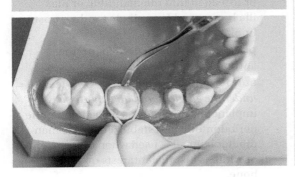

- **bite registration:** impression of the teeth while in occlusion. A bite registration is taken to assist with the fabrication of the prosthesis. The impression may be obtained from biting into a wax sheet, bite plates, or stock trays and prepared frames filled with impression material. Some dentists will eject impression material on the surfaces of the teeth to make a bite pattern for later use. Bite registrations may be classified in various ways:
  - **open bite:** patient bites into the impression material.
  - **closed bite:** the material is injected and expressed around the desired teeth while they are in occlusion.
  - **opposing arch:** impressions of the occlusal surfaces of both arches are taken in the same procedure.
- **work order:** written directions from the dentist to the laboratory completing the case; the impressions, bite registration, and orders are sent together.
- **temporary or provisional coverage:** temporary protection for the prepared tooth while laboratory work is being completed. Coverage may be in the form of an aluminum cap, acrylic custom cover, or preformed resin

crown form cemented onto the prepared teeth for protection until the final try-in and delivery.

Try-In, Adjustment, and Delivery

During the preparation, construction, and delivery of the dental prosthesis, the patient will return for various appointments. Some visits require adjustment and recordings of measurements that will be sent to the laboratory to assist in final fabrication. Related terms include the following:

- **seating:** placement and fitting of appliance for try-in and final cementation. Patient bites on a stick or device, applying pressure for the application of the crown or prosthetic item.
- **condylar inclination** (**KHAN**-dih-lahr = *pertaining to the condyle*) (**in**-klih-**NAY**-shun = *tendency, bending, bias*): observation of bite relationship and TMJ involvement. The following articulation movements involve the condyle:
  - **centric** (**SEN**-trick = *central, center*): occurring when the condyle rests in the temporal bone during biting, resting, and mouth movements.
  - **protrusion** (pro-**TRUE**-shun = *projecting or thrust forward*): measurement with the mandible thrust forward, with the lower jaw out.
  - **retrusion** (ree-**TRUE**-shun = *forcing backward*): measurement with the mandible drawn backward.
  - **lateral excursion** (**LAT**-er-al = *side,* ecks-**KERR**-shun = *movement*): measurement with side-to-side movement of the mandible.
  - **appearance indicators:** notations of the smile line and the length of the cuspid point.

USE OF IMPLANTS IN PROSTHODONTICS

When prosthodontic appliances do not fit properly or are difficult to retain in the mouth, the dentist may suggest titanium or zirconia implants to

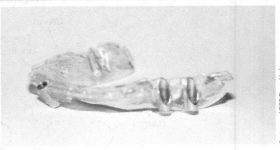

Figure 12-7 Example of surgical guide for implant placement

provide stabilization and retention. There are different types of implants, and each is used in a specific area, depending on available bone, type, and amount of stabilization needed. The related terms are:

- **implant** (**IM**-plant = *insertion of object*): surgical insertion of implant posts or prepared frame to provide stabilization for overdentures or appliance retention. Some implants may be a simple single insertion while others may be complicated and require study and preplanning such as CAD/CAM impression, cone beam radiograph measurements, and preconstruction of placement guides as shown in Figure 12-7. A surgical implant may be one or a combination of the following types:
  - **root form implant—endosseous** (en-**DOSS**-ee-us = *within the alveolar bone*): screw-type device that is cemented or threaded into the mandible or maxilla bone; used for a single tooth or post implant.
  - **plate form implant:** used for narrow jawbone; flat-plate style.
  - **subperiosteal** (**sub**-pear-ee-**OSS**-tee-ahl = *under the gingival and alveolar tissues*): implant plate or frame is placed under the periodontium and stabilized on the mandibular bone. It is used when bone height or width is insufficient; rests on top of the bone.

○ **transosteal** (trans-**OSS**-tee-ahl = *through the mandibular bone*): large plate is stabilized on the lower border of the mandibular bone with posts extending through the gingiva; used to anchor prostheses in difficult situations.

All transplant appliances must bond with the bone tissue to obtain stability. This process is called **osseointegration** (*osseo = bone, integrate = bonding*) and requires from three to six months to occur.

MISCELLANEOUS PROSTHODONTIC SERVICES

There are a variety of prosthodontic devices and treatments that can be rendered by the dentist or prosthodontist, depending on the operator's expertise. Figure 12-8 shows a few. Terms related to these services are:

• **maxillary obturator** (**ob**-two-**RAY**-tore = *body cavity obstruction*): palatal cover device worn

---

Figure 12-8 Assorted prosthetic devices: (A) bite adjuster/positioner, (B) anti-snore appliance, (C) Hawley orthodontic retainer, (D) removable orthodontic retainer, (E) habit suppressor

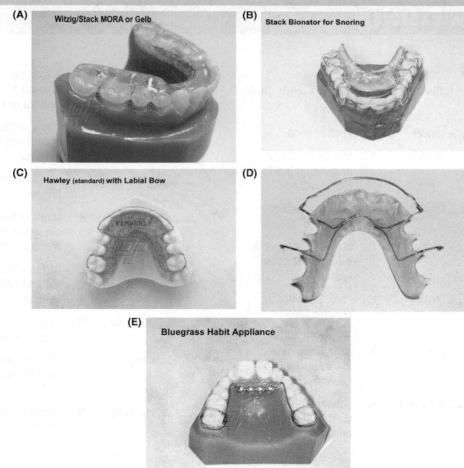

(A) Witzig/Stack MORA or Gelb

(B) Stack Bionator for Snoring

(C) Hawley (standard) with Labial Bow

(D)

(E) Bluegrass Habit Appliance

in the mouth to cover genetic openings into the nasal area, such as a cleft palate.

- **TMJ adjustors:** calibrated position splints for wear adjustment to maintain proper vertical dimension of occlusion.
- **sleep apnea and anti-snore forms** (*mandibular advancement splint*): custom-made dental-positioning device for tongue and mouth position during sleep period to avoid tongue drop and oxygen cutoff (see Figure 12-8A).
- **positioners:** individual patient devices to maintain mouth or tooth position or

to complete orthodontic positioning (see Figure 12-8B).

- **sport mouth guards:** custom-made semi-hard forms to be inserted in times of contact sports; may be space-adjusted for orthodontic brace wear (see Figure 12-8C).
- **repair and adjustment of devices:** broken dentures or those with teeth missing, lost treatment trays, adjusted movement devices, and various prosthodontic appliances may be repaired or reconstructed by the skilled prosthodontist or prosthodontic technician.

Review Exercises

Matching

Match the following word elements with their meanings.

1. _____ veneer
2. _____ acrylic
3. _____ abutment
4. _____ titanium
5. _____ retrusion
6. _____ pontic
7. _____ amalgam

8. _____ alginate
9. _____ obturator
10. _____ protrusion
11. _____ ductility
12. _____ clasp
13. _____ porcelain
14. _____ flange
15. _____ elasticity

A. implant metal
B. thin surface shell or layer applied to tooth surface
C. mandible drawn backward
D. claw-like framework extension to grasp teeth
E. hard, translucent ceramic shell or cover material
F. resin material used in denture gingiva fabrication
G. natural tooth used to support bridgework retainer

H. projecting rim or lower edge of denture or saddle
I. ability of material to stretch and return to shape
J. mandible projecting forward
K. ability to be drawn out into thin line without breaking
L. part of bridgework replacing missing tooth/teeth
M. body cavity obstruction
N. base metal or combination of metals
O. hydrocolloid that is irreversible

Definitions

Using the selection given for each sentence, choose the best term to complete the definition.

1. A full mouth maxillary denture is an example of what type of prosthesis?
   a. fixed
   b. removable
   c. immediate
   d. compound

2. A measurement taken with the mandible drawn back in occlusion is considered:
   a. centric
   b. protrusion
   c. retrusion
   d. lateral

3. An impression of the bite while the teeth are in occlusion is termed:
   a. centric bite
   b. protrusion bite
   c. closed bite
   d. open bite

4. A solid, cast restoration fabricated to fit into a prepared tooth is called a/an:
   a. inlay
   b. onlay
   c. crown
   d. composite

5. A thin-layered sheath to be placed over the surface of a tooth is a/an:
   a. taper
   b. bridge
   c. veneer
   d. jacket

6. An alloy of less than 25% of gold, palladium, and platinum is said to be:
   a. high noble alloy
   b. base noble alloy
   c. noble alloy
   d. semi-noble alloy

7. Aluminum caps, preformed crowns, and custom crowns used between appointments are:
   a. permanent coverage
   b. try-in applications
   c. temporary coverage
   d. restorations

8. A natural tooth used to support and become part of a fixed bridge is called a/an:
   a. restoration
   b. adjacent
   c. aperture
   d. abutment

9. Side-to-side movement of the mandible is which of the following movements?
   a. protrusion
   b. lateral
   c. retrusion
   d. centric

10. Retraction cord saturated with a chemical to resorb tissue is said to be:
    a. impregnated
    b. medicated
    c. resorptive
    d. regulated

11. A denture prosthesis placed in the mouth at the time of tooth removal is called a/an:
    a. overdenture
    b. partial denture
    c. immediate denture
    d. Maryland bridge

12. A hard, translucent, nonmetallic block material used in milling crowns and inlays at chairside is a/an:
    a. composite
    b. ceramic
    c. acrylic
    d. amalgam

13. The ability of a material to withstand penetration is an example of:
    a. hardness
    b. ductility
    c. tensile strength
    d. elasticity

14. The ability to be hammered or pressed into shape is an example of:
    a. elasticity
    b. elongation
    c. ductility
    d. malleability

15. The part of a partial denture that straddles the alveolar crest and gives support is a:
    a. saddle
    b. retainer
    c. clasp
    d. rest

16. The lower edge of a denture is called the:
    a. oblique ridge
    b. rest
    c. post dam
    d. flange

17. The posterior edge of the maxillary denture used to maintain position and suction is the:
    a. retainer
    b. denture base
    c. flange
    d. post dam

18. The term for a human dentition containing no teeth is:
    a. edentulous
    b. abutting
    c. undentated
    d. furnicated

19. A full gold crown with a porcelain facing is considered which type of prosthodontia?
    a. fixed
    b. removable
    c. immediate
    d. complete

20. A prosthesis constructed to fit over and attach to anchor post in the alveolar bone is a/an:
    a. immediate denture
    b. composite denture
    c. overdenture
    d. Maryland bridge

Building Skills

Locate and define the prefix, root/combining form, and suffix (if present) in the following words.

1. **hydrocolloid**
   prefix _____
   root/combining form _____
   suffix _____

2. **edentulous**
   prefix _____
   root/combining form _____
   suffix _____

3. **implantology**
   prefix _____
   root/combining form _____
   suffix _____

4. **alveolectomy**
   prefix _____
   root/combining form _____
   suffix _____

5. **subperiosteal**
   prefix _____
   root/combining form _____
   suffix _____

Fill-Ins

Write the correct word in the blank space to complete each statement.

1. A/an _____ is a prosthetic device used to replace the missing teeth of an entire arch.

2. A machine that holds two materials, unites them, and expresses one mixed material is a/an _____ syringe.

3. The acrylic crown cover placed on the prepared tooth between visits is called _____ coverage.

4. _____ is the taking on or absorption of moisture by alginate material.

5. To provide support and aid retention in a large prep of a nonvital tooth, a/an _____ may be placed and cemented into the enlarged nonfunctional root canal.

6. A/an _____ is a material or chemical that enables or quickens the chemical reaction.

7. A mouth without teeth present is said to be _____.

8. The process of gross removal of tooth structure during a crown prep is called _____.

9. A/an _____ is a slanted-edge prep of a tooth being prepared for a crown.

10. The prosthodontic closing of a cleft palate area is called a maxillary _____.

11. A _____ bridge is unsupported on the end and may be replaced with the saddle part of the appliance.

12. A registration of a bite while the lower jaw is relaxed is a/an _____ impression.

13. A prescription describing desired labor that is sent to the lab with the impressions is called a/an _____.

14. Another name for the metal skeleton of an appliance is the _____ of the device.

15. A tapered margin at the tooth cervix placed in preparation for a crown space is a/an _____ reduction.

16. An extension of bridge framework that sits on the occlusal surface to support and stabilize the bridge is called a/an _____.

17. A claw-like extension of a bridge that encircles a natural tooth and aids in retention of a crown is called a/an _____.

18. A full cover resembling the natural shape of the tooth that is placed over a large preparation is called a/an _____.

19. A _____ appliance is a prosthetic device cemented into the mouth.

20. A resin material that may be used in the core buildup of a tooth is _____.

Word Use

Read the following sentences and define the meaning of the word written in boldface letters.

1. The proportions for the base and **catalyst** must be accurately measured for a good mix.

   _____

2. To prevent shrinkage, the **alginate** impression should be poured up immediately.

   _____

3. The assistant placed the work order for the repair of the **prosthesis** into the laboratory box.

   _____

4. The condition of the **adjacent teeth** is important when preparing tooth replacement.

   _____

5. Always replace the lid of the alginate container to prevent **imbibition** to the material.

   _____

CHAPTER 13 | ENDODONTICS

✓ Learning Objectives

On completion of this chapter, you should be able to:

1. Identify the qualifications of an endodontist, and describe the practice of endodontia and the need for pulp treatment.

2. Identify and explain the diagnostic tests used to determine pulpal conditions.

3. Discuss the treatment steps required in pulpal and endodontic procedures.

4. List and identify the equipment and materials necessary for endodontic treatment.

5. Describe the surgical treatment plans employed in endodontic care.

6. Describe and discuss the treatment involved in the care of traumatized teeth.

7. List and identify the various methods and types of replantation procedures available in endodontic practice.

SCIENCE AND PRACTICE OF ENDODONTIC DENTISTRY

Endodontia (**en**-doh-**DAHN**-she-ah = *within the tooth*) is the branch of dentistry concerned with the diagnosis, treatment, and prevention of diseases of the dental pulp and its surrounding **periradicular** (pear-ee-rah-**DICK**-you-lar; peri = *around,* radi = *root*) tissues. The dental specialist who completes an additional two to three years of training and board testing becomes a Diplomate of Endodontics and limits his or her practice to this specialty as an **endodontist** (**en**-doh-**DON**-tist). Many

Vocabulary Related to Endodontics

This list contains selected new and important word parts and terms from this chapter. Take the time to learn these word parts and their meanings. You may use the list to review these terms and practice pronouncing them correctly. When you work with the audio for this chapter, listen to the word, repeat it, and then place a checkmark in the box. Proceed to the next boxed word, and repeat the process.

(hyphen before word means it's a suffix, hyphen after word means prefix, no hyphen means root word.)

Word Parts	Meaning	Word Parts	Meaning
apic/o	tapered tip of root	-ization	process/procedure
bi–	two	hyper–	above
bio–	life	mechan	machine
cuspid	elevation of enamel	sensi	capable of feeling
-ectomy	surgical removal of	-tivity	condition
-ical	pertaining to	trans–	through
illumina	light		

Key Terms

- ☐ **apicoectomy** (ay-pih-koh-**ECK**-toh-mee)
- ☐ **aseptic** (ay-**SEP**-tick)
- ☐ **autogenous** (aw-toh-**JEE**-nus)
- ☐ **avulsion** (ah-**VULL**-shun)
- ☐ **bicuspidization** (bye-cuss-pih-dih-**ZAY**-shun)
- ☐ **biomechanical** (bye-oh-meh-**KAN**-ih-kuhl)
- ☐ **cellulitis** (sell-you-**LIE**-tiss)
- ☐ **chelator** (**KEY**-lay-tor)
- ☐ **concussion** (kun-**CUSH**-un)
- ☐ **curettage** (**CURE**-eh-tahj)

Vocabulary Related to Endodontics *continued*

Key Terms *continued*

- ❑ cyst (SIST)
- ❑ debridement
  (deh-**BREED**-ment)
- ❑ desiccant (**DES**-ih-kant)
- ❑ endodontia
  (en-doh-**DAHN**-she-ah)
- ❑ extirpation
  (ecks-ter-**PAY**-shun)
- ❑ extruded (ecks-**TRUE**-ded)
- ❑ hemisection
  (**HEM**-ih-seck-shun)
- ❑ heterogenous
  (het-er-oh-**JEE**-nus)
- ❑ homogenous
  (hoh-**MAH**-jeh-nus)
- ❑ hyperextension
  (high-per-eck-**STEN**-shun)

- ❑ hypersensitivity
  (high-per-sen-sih-**TIV**-ih-tee)
- ❑ implantation
  (im-plan-**TAY**-shun)
- ❑ luxation (luck-**SAY**-shun)
- ❑ medicament
  (meh-**DICK**-ah-ment)
- ❑ mobility (moh-**BIL**-ih-tee)
- ❑ necrotic (neh-**KRAH**-tick)
- ❑ obturation
  (ahb-too-**RAY**-shun)
- ❑ osteomyelitis
  (oss-tee-oh-my-**LYE**-tiss)
- ❑ palpation (pal-**PAY**-shun)
- ❑ percussion (per-**KUSH**-un)
- ❑ pericementitis
  (pear-ih-seh-men-**TIE**-tiss)

- ❑ periradicular
  (pear-ee-rah-**DICK**-you-lar)
- ❑ pulpectomy
  (puhl-**PECK**-toh-mee)
- ❑ pulpotomy
  (puhl-**POT**-oh-mee)
- ❑ putrefaction
  (pyou-trih-**FACK**-shun)
- ❑ reamer (**REE**-mer)
- ❑ retrograde (**REH**-troh-grade)
- ❑ subluxation
  (sub-lucks-**AY**-shun)
- ❑ suppurative (**SUP**-you-rah-tiv)
- ❑ thermal (**THER**-mahl)
- ❑ transillumination
  (trans-ill-oo-mih-**NAY**-shun)
- ❑ traumatized (**TRAW**-mah-tized)

general dentists complete endodontic therapy in their practice but may refer difficult cases to the endodontic specialist.

Pulpitis (pul-**PIE**-tis) is an inflamed pulpal condition that usually needs endodontic treatment. The inflamed pulp tissue may be afflicted with a reversible treatable condition if the fibers are vital or alive and the pulp may recover. Diseased pulp tissue that cannot recover and repair itself is considered **necrotic** (neh-**KRAH**-tick = *dead or nonvital*), an irreversible condition. Diagnosis and future treatment is determined by endodontic diagnostic testing of the affected tooth and its surrounding tissues. Table 13-1 lists diagnostic conditions of pulpitis.

Table 13-1 Diagnostic Conditions of Pulpitis

Symptoms of Pulpitis	Reversible	Necrotic Pulp
Reacts to cold, sweet, heat	Yes	Yes, rapid onset
Pain after stimuli gone	No	Yes, lingers
Pain shifts to other tooth, areas	No	Possibly
Reacts to percussion	No	Possibly
Worse lying down or bending	No	Yes
Pulp test reaction	Yes	Not usual
Swelling	Not usual	Possibly
Spontaneous pain	Not usual	Possibly
X-ray reveals other involvement	Not usual	Possible abscess

DIAGNOSTIC PROCEDURES TO DETERMINE PULPAL CONDITIONS

Evaluation of the pulp's vitality consists of an assortment of tests, both subjective and objective. All evaluations begin with a review of the patient's dental history and questioning from the dentist to reveal the patient's complaints. Related terms are:

- **subjective symptoms:** conditions as described by the patient. An example of a subjective symptom may be a patient complaint of **hypersensitivity** (**high**-per-**sen**-sih-**TIV**-ih-tee; hyper = *over*, sensitivity = *abnormal reaction to stimulus*) or **pulpalgia** (puhl-**PAL**-jee-ah; pulp = *inner tooth tissue*, algia = *pain*); the type of pain, such as spontaneous or dull, throbbing. The endodontist will ask the patient particular questions regarding the patient's subjective pain to help determine pulpal life such as:

  ○ What causes the pain's onset?
  ○ What relieves the pain?
  ○ When does the pain occur?

- **objective signs:** conditions observed by someone other than the patient. Examples are a tooth **hyperextension** (hyper = *over*, extension = *movement*), a condition in which the tooth arises out of the socket, or a noticeable, unpleasant odor known as **putrefaction** (**pyou**-trih-**FACK**-shun = *decaying animal matter*). A dark-colored tooth may indicate internal bleeding from trauma or infection. Swelling of the face or gingival area may also be present.

Clinical Examinations

Clinical examinations used to diagnose the degree of pulpitis of an affected tooth may be any or all of the following:

- **palpation** (pal-**PAY**-shun): application of finger pressure to body tissues, including gingiva.
- **percussion** (per-**KU**-shun = *tapping of body tissue, tooth*): usually done by tapping a dental mirror handle on an affected tooth and comparing the sensation to tapping on a healthy or *control* tooth.

- **mobility** (moh-**BILL**-ih-tee = *capable of movement*): movement of a tooth in its socket during outside force or pressure application.
- **transillumination** (trans-ah-**lum**-mah-**NAY**-shun = *passage of light through object/tissue*): a light refraction test to reveal fractured tooth tissue.
- **thermal** (**THER**-mahl = *pertaining to temperature*): pulp sensitivity test with reaction to applications of heat and/or cold to tooth surface.
- **anesthesia:** numbing the questionable root or nerve ending to dissipate pain.
- **direct dentin stimulation:** scratching the exposed dentin with an explorer; the presence of pain indicates inflamed or irritated pulp tissue.
- **electric pulp testing:** applying an electrical current on the enamel surface of the tooth to register the tooth's pulpal sensitivity and presence of irritability (Figure 13-1).
- **digital radiograph:** X-ray examination with digital zoom and color contrasting ability permits a deeper insight to the pulp canal.
- **miscellaneous tests:** radiovisiography and magnetic resonance imaging (MRI) to demonstrate early changes of bone structure and periapical involvement of suspected tooth with an inflamed pulp; laser Doppler flowmetry (LDF) to determine blood flow of pulp tissue, and pulse oximetry to assess pulp vitality.

Periradicular Diagnosis

After the clinical testing has been completed, the dentist can determine the nature of the disease, or diagnosis, and develop a treatment plan. The principal diagnosis involving pulp tissues is to determine if the pulp is vital or nonvital. The periradicular tissue diagnosis may involve more pathologic conditions such as:

Figure 13-1 Examples of pulp vitality testers: (A) manual tester, (B) digital scanner

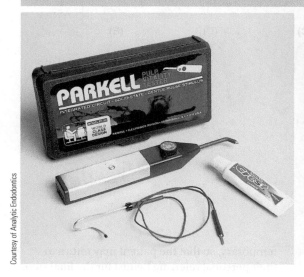

Courtesy of Analytic Endodontics

(A)   (B)

- **periodontitis** (**pear**-ee-oh-don-**TIE**-tiss; peri = *around,* dont = *tooth,* itis = *inflammation*): in acute apical periodontitis, a sharp, painful inflammation of tissues occurs around an affected tooth. Pain is lessened or eliminated by removal of the inflamed or necrotic pulp. A chronic apical periodontitis (CAP) requires management similar to the acute symptoms.
- **abscess** (**AB**-cess = *local pus infection*): an infection that may be an acute or chronic apical abscess; also called **suppurative** (**SUP**-you-rah-tiv = *producing or generating pus*).
- **pericementitis** (**pear**-ih-see-men-**TIE**-tiss; peri = *around,* cement = *cementuis,* itis = *inflammation*): inflammation and necrosis of the alveoli of the tooth.
- **cyst (SIST):** abnormal, closely walled fluid or exudates-filled sac in or around periapical tissues.
- **cellulitis** (sell-you-**LIE**-tiss): inflammation of cellular or connective tissue.

- **osteomyelitis** (oss-tee-oh-my-**LYE**-tiss): an inflammation of the bone and bone marrow, usually caused by bacterial infection.

ENDODONTIC TREATMENT PROCEDURES

After the diagnosis has been completed, a treatment plan is developed to provide dental care. An affected or irritated pulp may need one of several treatment procedures:

- **pulpotomy** (puhl-**POT**-oh-mee): partial excision of the dental pulp, usually reserved for children's teeth (see Chapter 17, Pediatric Dentistry).
- **pulpectomy** (puhl-**PECK**-toh-mee): surgical removal of pulp from the tooth, also known as root canal treatment (RCT) (see Figure 13-2 for steps in the procedure).
- **apicoectomy** (ay-pee-koh-**ECK**-toh-mee): surgical amputation of a root apex.
- **retreat:** endodontic retreatment of failed pulpal canal and core treatment with removal of existing filling material and re-obturation of the tooth.

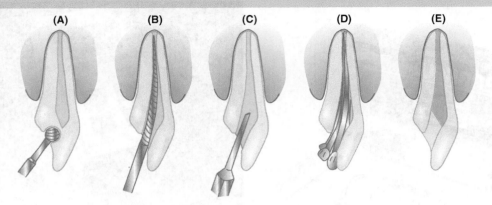

Figure 13-2 Pulpectomy procedure: (A) gaining canal access, (B) enlarging the canal, (C) cleansing the canal, (D) filling the canal, (E) finished RCT

(A)   (B)   (C)   (D)   (E)

ROOT CANAL TREATMENT

The standard treatment for a root canal has the following steps:

- **anesthesia:** local injection to relieve pain occurring during the procedure.
- **isolation of the operative area:** accomplished to provide safety and to assure an **aseptic** (ay-**SEP**-tick = *without disease*) site.
- **extirpation** (ecks-ter-**PAY**-shun = *to root out*): removing the pulpal tissue after the pulpal opening.
- **debridement** (deh-**BREED**-ment = *removal of foreign or decayed matter*): removing necrotic pulpal tissue and cleaning out the area.
- **irrigation and cleansing:** using chemicals and instruments to remove tissue dust and material matter from the pulp and pulp canals.
- **obturation** (ahb-too-**RAY**-shun = *to close or stop up*): filling and closing the canal area. This may consist of filling from the pulp to the apex or may be completed in a **retrograde** (**REH**-troh-grade = *backward step*) process of filling the canal beginning from the apex of the tooth to the pulp chamber, also called a retrofill endodontic restoration.
- **restoration:** returning the tooth to normal function and purpose, either permanent or temporary, so that the patient may return to their personal referring dentist for the final step.

ENDODONTIC TREATMENT EQUIPMENT AND MATERIALS

Specialized equipment is needed to perform endodontic treatment and procedures. Dental dam material is used to isolate the endodontic site.

Dental Dam

The purposes and procedures of the dental dam are discussed in Chapter 10, Tooth Restorations. The components of the dental dam (sometimes called *rubber dam*) isolation equipment are listed here and illustrated in Figure 13-3:

- **dental dam material:** thin layer of latex or nonlatex sheeting that varies in thickness, color, and size.
- **dental dam frame:** device used to hold material in place; may be metal or plastic, rigid or adjustable.
- **dental dam punch:** device used to place selected holes in the dam material for isolation of a tooth or teeth.
- **dental dam forceps:** hand device used to transport and place clamps or retainers around the selected tooth.

Figure 13-3 Dental dam equipment: (A) dam material, (B) dam frame, (C) dam punch, (D) dam forceps, (E) dam stamp and pad, (F) dam clamp assortment

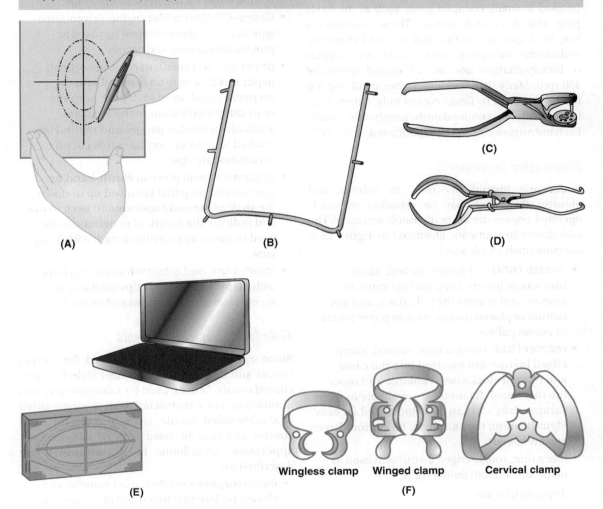

(A)   (B)   (C)   (D)

(E)   Wingless clamp Winged clamp Cervical clamp

(F)

- **rubber dam stamp and pad:** marking stamper and pad devices used to indicate alignment spots for puncturing the material with the punch.
- **dental dam clamp:** retaining device used to hold the material around the tooth; may be metal or resin and vary in size, shape, and style. A clear plastic "hat dam" may be closely fitted and trimmed to fit a damaged tooth crown and temporarily cemented onto the tooth crown with glass ionomer cement. The dental dam material fits under the device that is removed after treatment. Isolation may also be assisted by use of sealing materials that adhere the tooth structure or gingiva to dental dam material for a short time (approximately an hour).
- **dental dam ligature:** material used to hold and secure the dam material in the mouth; can be dental floss, latex stabilizing cord, or a small piece of dental dam.

RCT Instrumentation

Root canal instruments are specially designed to be used in small, cramped areas, such as the tooth pulp chambers and canals. These instruments may be engine-driven but must be used in special endodontic handpieces that usually are electric- or battery-charged and do not exceed speeds of 390 rpm. Many RCT instruments are small and are held and rotated by finger control only. Others have longer shafts to accommodate the length of the canals. Each instrument completes a specific task in the RCT.

Preparation Instruments

Endodontic instruments used to debride and obturate the canal may be classified as hand-operated, engine-driven, or ultrasonic and sonic. The endodontic instruments, illustrated in Figure 13-4, are quite small and delicate:

- **broach** (**BRO**-ch): a thin, barbed, wired instrument inserted into the root canal to ensnare and remove the pulp tissue and any natural or placed matter, such as paper points or cotton pellets.
- **reamer** (**REE**-mer): a thin, twisted, sharp-edged instrument inserted into the canal and rotated clockwise to enlarge and taper the root canal. Reamers are available in various sizes and can be color-coded for easy identification; they also may be engine-driven at slow speeds.
- **file:** a thin, rough-edged instrument used to plane and smooth pulpal walls.

  Types of files are:

  ○ **K-file:** has twisted edges and is used to enlarge as well as to smooth walls; color-coded to denote size.
  ○ **Hedstrom file (U-shaped and S-shaped):** cone-shaped, twisted-edged instrument used for enlargement and smoothing; nickel titanium alloy files provide more flexibility.
  ○ **flex file:** stainless steel or nickel titanium alloy file that is stronger and provides more flexibility; used in narrow, curved canals.

- **pesso** (**PESS**-oh) **reamers:** thicker, engine-driven reamer with larger and longer parallel cutting edges for use in canal openings.
- **Gates–Glidden drills:** engine-driven, latch-type burs with flame-shaped tip; used to provide an opening and access.
- **paper points:** small, narrow, absorbent, paper tips that may be inserted into the prepared canal; used to dry the prep site or to carry medication to the area; are available in various gauges and millimeter-marked lengths or may have tips cut off to accommodate size.
- **stopper:** a small piece of elastic band or commercial plug that is moved up or down the shaft of the endo instrument; used to mark and indicate the length of penetration; also used to measure insertion length with X-ray view.
- **rotary burs and stones:** friction grip burs with diamond or carbide tips used to gain access through restorations and crowns.

Endodontic Hand Instruments

Some endodontic instruments used for cutting tissues and filling canals are finger style for more curved canals. Others, used for micro-surgery and obturation, are constructed with a single-sided or double-sided handle, shaft, and nib for hand control and may be used with or without heat application. Endodontic hand instruments are described as:

- **microsurgery curettes:** used to incise and elevate periodontal tissue and fibers permitting easier and faster healing time.
- **root canal (endodontic) spreader:** longer shank with pointed nib; used to carry and insert cement or filling material.
- **root canal plugger:** longer shanked with a flat-tipped nib; used to condense and adapt the canal filling material.
- **root canal condenser:** handled, long-tip instrument that may be heated and used to condense gutta-percha to the canal walls.

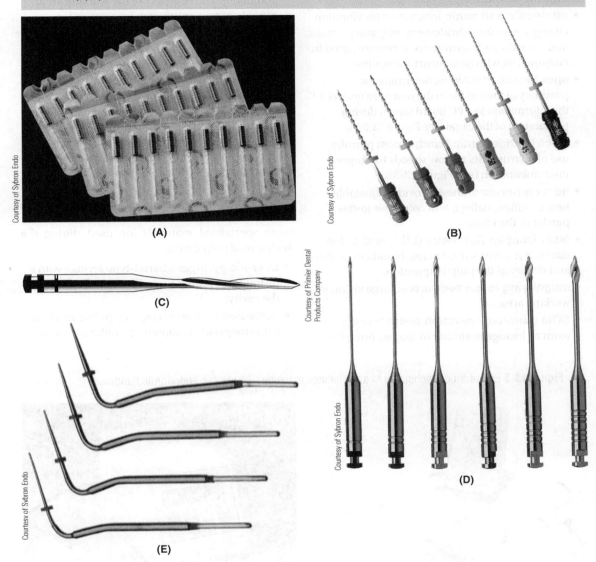

Figure 13-4 Endodontic instruments: (A) barbed broach, (B) reamers, (C) Pesso reamer, (D) Gates–Glidden drills, (E) spreaders

Courtesy of Sybron Endo

(A)

Courtesy of Sybron Endo

(B)

Courtesy of Primier Dental Products Company

(C)

Courtesy of Sybron Endo

(D)

Courtesy of Sybron Endo

(E)

- **Lentulo** (len-too-**LOW**) **spiral drill:** thin, twisted-wire, latch-type rotary instrument used to spread calcium hydroxide or cement into the canal. Materials may also be spread by small inserts from ultrasonic machines.

Assorted RCT Equipment

Not all root-canal equipment is small and manipulated by hand or instrumentation. Some special machines have been developed to assist the endodontist in the location, diagnosis, and treatment of the inflamed root tissue. Some of these include the following:

- **ultrasonic and sonic instruments:** vibration energy waves for debridement, irrigating canals, and spreading medicaments or cement; used in conjunction with hand instrumentation.
- **apex locator machines:** determine the proximity of the test file to the root apex and relate the information to a PC board screen during preparation of the canal (see Figure 13-5A).
- **electric endodontic handpieces:** permits use of instruments at slow speeds for finger instrumentation (see Figure 13-5B).
- **heat carrier machines:** provide adjustable heat to soften, deliver, and condense gutta-percha to the canal.
- **laser Doppler flowmetry (LDF) and pulse oximetry:** devices used to test blood circulation and vitality of the pulp in question.
- **magnifying loupe eyeware:** enlarge vision in working area.
- **SOM (surgical operation microscope):** worn as headgear, similar to loupes, but with

intense magnification possibilities (3–27 times) and improved halogen lighting. Enlarges vision and manipulative aspect of the working area; capable of transmitting image to monitor, camera, or possible assistant view.

- **assorted instruments:** include explorer, spoon excavator, and paddle-ended blades. These dental hand instruments have increased nib, blade, or neck length to accommodate extra depth to the working surfaces. Smaller instruments have been developed for working with SOM, and new techniques have been devised, but the procedure is the same: enter, debride, cleanse, fill, and restore.

Endodontic Materials

Some specialized materials are used during the treatment of pulpal tissue:

- **Luer-loc syringe:** a barrel-type syringe with a piston force plunger, used to inject fluids into the cavity.
- **gutta-percha points:** tapered points made of a thermoplastic compound; similar in size to

Figure 13-5 Endodontic machines: (A) apex locator machine, (B) electric endodontic handpiece

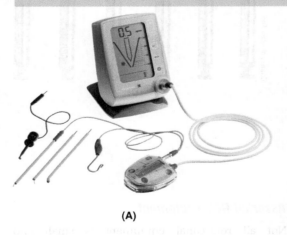

(A)

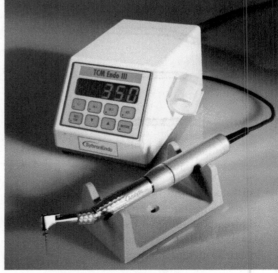

(B)

Courtesy of Sybron Endo

silver points or endodontic instruments, and used to fill the root canal; may be millimeter marked along length to help determine penetration insert length.

- **silver points:** tapered silver points comparable in size to files and reamers; used to fill canals.
- **cement pastes and fillers:** zinc oxide and eugenol mixes and commercial materials; used to cement points in canal.
- **chemicals:** chemical action used in conjunction with operator treatment to produce a result termed **biomechanical** (bye-oh-meh-**KAN**-ih-kuhl) action. Endodontic chemicals may be supplied in individual flexi-tip micro-tubes or placed in syringes to be used for cleaning and sterilizing (sodium hypochlorite, hydrogen peroxide), lubricating the canal (soap or glycerin), and softening dentin walls. **Chelators** (key-**LAY**-tor = *chemical ion softener*), citric acid and EDTA (ethylenediaminetetraacetic acid), are used to soften tissue.
- **desiccant** (**DIS**-ih-kant = *dry up, remove*): methanol or ethanol alcohol used to dry the area or clear away other chemical traces.
- **medicament** (meh-**DICK**-ah-ment = *medicine or remedy*): used for antimicrobial action, to prevent pain, and to neutralize the pulpal area. Major medicaments are phenols, aldehydes, halines, steroids, calcium hydroxides, and antibiotics.

SURGICAL ENDODONTIC TREATMENTS

Not all treatments of inflamed or necrotic pulps require RCT. Some endodontic procedures involve surgical treatment that may or may not be included in the endodontic RCT. Figure 13-6 depicts three of these treatments. Related terms are:

- **curettage** (**CURE**-eh-tahj = *scraping of a cavity*): scraping of the apical area; may be necessary to remove necrotic tissue.
- **apicoectomy** (ay-pih-koh-**ECK**-toh-mee): a procedure that may be necessary to remove the root apex, particularly where there is a radicular

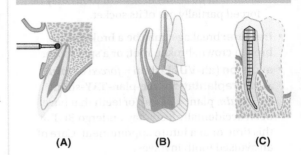

Figure 13-6 Illustrations of endodontic surgical treatments: (A) apicoectomy, (B) root amputation, (C) root hemisection

(A)   (B)   (C)

cyst involvement of the affected tooth; also called *root end resection* (see Figure 13-6A).

- **root amputation** (**am**-pew-**TAY**-shun = *surgical removal of body part, root*): separating and removing molar roots of affected tooth at the junction into the crown (see Figure 13-6B).
- **root hemisection** (**HEM**-ih-seck-shun = *cutting tissue or organ in half*): surgical division of multi-rooted tooth that may be performed in a lengthwise manner (see Figure 13-6C).
- **bicuspidization** (bye-cuss-pih-dih-**ZAY**-shun): surgical division of a tooth retaining both sides.

ENDODONTIC TREATMENT OF TRAUMATIZED TEETH

Besides treating the infected pulp, the endodontist performs varied procedures for **traumatized** (**TRAW**-mah-tized = *wounded*) teeth, with a variety of pulp injuries:

- **luxation** (luck-**SAY**-shun = *dislocation*): tooth movement that may be classified in one of the following ways:
  - **concussion** (kun-**CUSS**-un = *shaken violently*): tooth loosened as a result of a blow; usually recovers with minimal attention.
  - **subluxation** (**sub**-luck-**SAY**-shun; sub = *under*, luxation = *displacement*): tooth partially dislocated; evidence of bleeding but requires only minor attention.

- ○ **lateral luxation:** tooth may be partially displaced with the root apex tilted forward.
- ○ **extruded** (ecks-**TROO**-ded = *pushed out of normal position*) **luxation:** tooth may be forced partially out of its socket.
- **fracture:** breakage; may be a broken cusp, broken crown, broken root, or a split tooth.
- **avulsion** (ah-**VULL**-shun = *forced or torn away*) **replantation** (ree-plan-**TAY**-shun; re = *again,* plant = *place*): of teeth that have been accidentally lost; may undergo RCT at this time or at a future appointment. Care of an avulsed tooth involves:

1. Do not touch tooth root.
2. Rinse with tepid water.
3. Reinsert into the tooth socket, hold in place with finger; if unable, tuck under lip, or keep moist in milk or lightly salted water.
4. Seek immediate treatment—fast—because time is important.

TOOTH REPLANTATION PROCEDURES

Some additional endodontic procedures, although not common, are an essential part of pulpal therapy:

- **replantation:** replacing an avulsed tooth in its tooth socket. In some rare cases, if RCT cannot be completed in a conventional manner, the tooth may be extracted, undergo RCT, and then be reinserted and stabilized into the same alveolus.
- **transplantation** (**trans**-plan-**TAY**-shun; trans = *across,* planta = *plant*): transfer of a tooth from one alveolar socket to another; may be completed in one of the following manners:

- ○ **autogenous** (awe-toh-**JEE**-nus; auto = *self,* genous = *origin*): moving a tooth from one position in the oral cavity to another area in the same cavity.
- ○ **homogenous** (hoh-**MAH**-jen-us; homo = *same,* geneous = *origin*): transferring and inserting a tooth from one patient to another.
- ○ **heterogenous** (**het**-er-oh-**JEE**-nus; heter = *other,* geneous = *origin*): transfer from one species to another; not yet a feasible practice.

- **implantation** (**im**-plan-**TAY**-shun; in = *into,* planta = *place*): placing titanium metal extensions into the tooth root; may be performed endodontically to provide a longer crown-root ratio and stabilize the tooth.

Occasionally, traumatized teeth or other damaged and affected teeth may appear darker than adjacent teeth. Lightening of tooth color may be attempted by opening, debriding the canal, and placing an oxidizer chemical, such as sodium perborate inside. Heating or photo-oxidizing with ultraviolet rays may help to lighten the tooth color. This **intracanal bleaching** process is not to be confused with external or cosmetic bleaching.

Review Exercises

Matching

Match the following word elements with their meanings.

1. _____ abscess   **A.** inflammation of cellular or connective tissue

2. _____ hemisection   **B.** detachment, removal, or separation from others

3. _____ extruded   **C.** dislocation

4. _____ extirpation   **D.** medicine or remedy

5. _____ pulpitis

6. _____ isolation

7. _____ luxation

8. _____ apicoectomy

9. _____ necrotic

10. _____ curettage

11. _____ pulpotomy

12. _____ cellulitis

13. _____ desiccant

14. _____ medicament

15. _____ suppurative

E. chemical used to dry up or remove chemical traces

F. pushed out of place

G. producing or generating pus

H. cutting tissue or organ into half

I. local pus infection

J. scraping of a cavity

K. inflamed pulpal condition

L. removing the pulpal tissue from tooth interior

M. dead or nonvital

N. surgical removal of root apex

O. partial removal of pulp tissue

Definitions

Using the selection given for each sentence, choose the best term to complete the definition.

1. The removal of foreign or decayed matter is called:
   a. debridement
   b. necrosis
   c. apicoectomy
   d. isolation

2. Infection of the pulp tissue is called:
   a. pulpectomy
   b. pulpotomy
   c. pulpitis
   d. pulpalgia

3. The process of using chemical and operator treatment to produce a result is termed:
   a. obturation
   b. retrograde
   c. biomechanical
   d. supportive

4. The closing or stopping up of the root canal is a procedure called:
   a. amputation
   b. obturation
   c. transillumination
   d. curettage

5. A medicament used to dry up or clear away chemical traces inside the tooth is called a/an:
   a. desiccant
   b. chelator
   c. irrigant
   d. cleanser

6. A thin wire instrument with barbed edges that is used to remove pulpal tissue is a/an:
   a. broach
   b. reamer
   c. file
   d. gutta-percha

7. A synthetic material point used to fill the root canal is which of the following?
   a. broach
   b. reamer
   c. file
   d. gutta-percha

8. The process of placing or separating an object from others is called:
   a. amputation
   b. isolation
   c. pulpotomy
   d. pulpectomy

9. The surgical procedure of cutting an organ or tissue in half is called:
   a. amputation
   b. pulpectomy
   c. curettage
   d. hemisection

10. Of isolation, safety, visibility, and sterility, which are reasons for placing a dental dam before starting an RCT?
    a. all of them
    b. none of them
    c. isolation and safety

d. isolation, safety, and sterility
e. safety and sterility
f. visibility and isolation

11. The diagnostic application of finger or hand pressure on body parts is called:
    a. percussion
    b. healing hands
    c. handling
    d. palpation

12. Which of the four diagnostic tests requires heat and cold applications?
    a. thermal
    b. mobility
    c. transillumination
    d. anesthesia

13. An inflammation of the bone and bone marrow, usually caused by bacterial infection, is called:
    a. periodontitis
    b. pericementitis
    c. pulpitis
    d. osteomyelitis

14. An objective complaint by a patient is one that is:
    a. observed by the patient
    b. observed by someone other than the patient
    c. described by the patient
    d. described by someone other than the patient

15. Pulp tissue that is alive and healthy is considered to be:
    a. pulpitis
    b. necrotic
    c. regenerated
    d. vital

16. The removal of all of the pulpal tissue in a tooth is termed:
    a. pulpectomy
    b. pulpotomy
    c. alveolectomy
    d. amputation

17. Abnormal, closely walled fluid-filled or exudate-filled sac in or around periapical tissues is a/an:
    a. cyst
    b. cellulitis
    c. fistula
    d. osteomyelitis

18. Which of the following instruments does not need to be adapted for endodontic procedures?
    a. spreader
    b. files
    c. mirror
    d. plugger

19. The surgical removal of the apex of a root is called:
    a. apicoectomy
    b. pulpotomy
    c. pulpectomy
    d. amputation

20. A subjective complaint by a patient may be considered a/an:
    a. sign
    b. symptom
    c. observation
    d. registration

Building Skills

Locate and define the prefix, root/combining form, and suffix (if present) in the following words.

1. **apicoectomy**
   prefix _____
   root/combining form _____
   suffix _____

2. **hypersensitivity**
   prefix _____
   root/combining form _____
   suffix _____

3. **biomechanical**
   prefix _____
   root/combining form _____
   suffix _____

4. **transillumination**
   prefix _____
   root/combining form _____
   suffix _____

5. **bicuspidization**
   prefix _____
   root/combining form _____
   suffix _____

Fill-Ins

Write the correct word in the blank space to complete each statement.

1. The detachment or separation of an object or person from others is termed _____.
2. Passage of light through an object or tissue is called _____.
3. A diagnostic test using hot and cold applications to the tooth surface is called a/an _____ diagnostic test.
4. A _____ is a small marker placed on endo instruments to indicate the insertion depth of the instrument.
5. Bisecting a molar root in a lengthwise manner is considered a/an _____.
6. The closing up or filling of a prepared pulp canal is called _____.
7. The _____ is a small, thin, rough-edged instrument used to smooth and taper canal walls.
8. Scraping a cavity wall or enclosed area is called _____.
9. The instrument used to make holes in the dental dam material is the _____.
10. _____ is the act of removing foreign or decayed matter from the dental chamber and canal.
11. RCT is another term for _____.
12. The partial excision of dental pulp is termed _____.
13. A/an _____ transplantation of a tooth is when the tooth is moved from one position to another area in the same oral cavity.
14. An inflammation of the bone and bone marrow usually caused by bacteria is called _____.
15. Tapping of a mirror handle on the biting surface of a tooth is an example of the diagnostic testing called _____.

16. A diseased pulp tissue that cannot recover and repair itself is said to be _____.
17. _____ is the resetting of an avulsed tooth in its tooth socket.
18. _____ is a term for an inflamed, infected pulp.
19. A specialist limited to the treatment of tooth pulp and its surrounding tissues is called a/an _____.
20. _____ is a synthetic material used to fill the canal root in root canal treatment.

Word Use

Read the following sentences and define the meaning of the word written in boldface letters.

1. Hyperextension is an example of an **objective symptom** for a toothache.

   _____

2. **Percussion reaction** is tested on the affected tooth and a nearby control tooth.

   _____

3. After removing the pulp contents and cleansing the canal, the endodontist will **obturate** the prepared tooth.

   _____

4. Mrs. Baker brought her 14-year-old son to the office to receive treatment for an **avulsion** of his two central incisors.

   _____

5. During a root canal treatment, the **dental dam** will protect the patient from swallowing any small materials and will keep the tooth sanitary.

   _____

14 ORAL AND MAXILLOFACIAL SURGERY

✓ Learning Objectives

On completion of this chapter, you should be able to:

1. Describe the functions and roles of an oral/maxillofacial surgeon.

2. List and identify the instruments commonly used in the practice of oral surgery.

3. Discuss the various types of tooth extractions and the assorted types of tooth impactions.

4. Identify the common tissue surgeries, biopsy methods, and diseases encountered in oral/maxillofacial surgery.

5. Discuss the various minor bone surgeries performed with or without tooth extraction.

6. Identify and determine the differences between open and closed reduction of bone fractures.

7. List and describe the various types of complicated bone surgery, including arthrotomy and genioplasty alterations.

8. Discuss the classification of TMJ disorders, testing for diagnosis, and possible treatments.

9. Identify the various types of implants and their composition materials.

10. Discuss the practices of oral and maxillofacial surgery in cosmetic and esthetic completion of treatment and procedures.

Vocabulary Related to Oral Surgery

This list contains selected new and important word parts and terms from this chapter. Take the time to learn these word parts and their meanings. You may use the list to review these terms and practice pronouncing them correctly. When you work with the audio for this chapter, listen to the word, repeat it, and then place a checkmark in the box. Proceed to the next boxed word, and repeat the process.

(hyphen before word means it's a suffix, hyphen after word means prefix, no hyphen means root word.)

Word Parts	Meaning	Word Parts	Meaning
ankylo-	fused/growing together	endo-	within
-al	relating to	ex-	out
coron	crown	oste	bone
dont	tooth	peri-	around

Key Terms

❏ **allograft** (**AL**-oh-graft)

❏ **alveolectomy** (al-vee-oh-**LECK**-toh-me)

❏ **alveolitis** (al-vee-oh-**LIGH**-tiss)

❏ **ankyloglossia** (ang-kill-loh-**GLOSS**-ia)

❏ **arthrotomy** (ar-**THRAH**-toh-me)

❏ **asymmetrical** (ay-sim-**EH**-trih-kal)

❏ **benign** (bee-**NINE**)

❏ **blepharoplasty** (**BLEF**-er-oh-**plas**-tee)

❏ **crepitus** (**KREP**-ih-tus)

❏ **cyst** (SIST)

❏ **dentigerous** (den-**TIJ**-er-us)

❏ **diastema** (die-ah-**STEE**-mah)

❏ **endodontic** (en-doh-**DAHN**-tick)

❏ **endosteal** (en-**DOSS**-tee-ahl)

❏ **exfoliative** (ecks-**FOH**-lee-ah-tiv)

Key Terms *continued*

- ❏ **exodontia**
  (ecks-oh-**DAHN**-shah)
- ❏ **exolever** (**ECKS**-oh-lee-ver)
- ❏ **exostosis**
  (ecks-ahs-**TOH**-sis)
- ❏ **forceps** (**FOUR**-seps)
- ❏ **frenectomy**
  (freh-**NECK**-toh-me)
- ❏ **genioplasty**
  (**JEE**-nee-oh-plas-tee)
- ❏ **gingivectomy**
  (jin-jih-**VECK**-toh-me)
- ❏ **gingivoplastomy**
  (jin-jih-voh-**PLAS**-toh-me)
- ❏ **hemangioma**
  (heh-man-jee-**OH**-mah)
- ❏ **hemiarthroplasty**
  (**HEM**-ee-are-throw-**plas**-tee)
- ❏ **hemostat** (**HE**-moh-stat)

- ❏ **macrogenia**
  (mack-roh-**JEE**-nee-ah)
- ❏ **malady** (**MAL**-ah-dee)
- ❏ **malignant** (mah-**LIG**-nant)
- ❏ **mallet** (**MAL**-ett)
- ❏ **melanoma** (mel-ah-**NO**-mah)
- ❏ **microgenia**
  (my-kroh-**JEE**-nee-ah)
- ❏ **orthognathic**
  (ore-theg-**NATH**-ick)
- ❏ **osteoplasty**
  (**OSS**-tee-oh-plas-tee)
- ❏ **osteotomy**
  (oss-tee-**OT**-oh-me)
- ❏ **papilloma** (pap-ih-**LOH**-mah)
- ❏ **periosteal**
  (pear-ee-**OSS**-tee-al)
- ❏ **periosteotome**
  (pear-ee-**OSS**-tee-oh-tome)

- ❏ **pseudomacrogenia** (sue-doh-mack-roh-**JEE**-nee-ah)
- ❏ **ptosis** (**TOH**-sis)
- ❏ **radicular** (rah-**DICK**-you-lar)
- ❏ **ranula** (**RAN**-you-lah)
- ❏ **retractor** (ree-**TRACK**-tor)
- ❏ **rhinoplasty** (**RINE**-oh-plas-tee)
- ❏ **rhytidectomy**
  (rit-oh-**DECK**-toe-me)
- ❏ **rongeurs** (**RON**-jeers)
- ❏ **septoplasty**
  (**SEPT**-oh-**plas**-tee)
- ❏ **subperiosteal**
  (sub-pear-ee-**OSS**-tee-ahl)
- ❏ **suture** (**SOO**-chur)
- ❏ **torus** (**TORE**-us)
- ❏ **transosteal**
  (trans-**OSS**-tee-ahl)

DUTIES AND FUNCTIONS OF AN ORAL AND MAXILLOFACIAL SURGEON

A dentist who completes training and earns a state board certification in dentistry is able to perform extractions and some dental surgery. Prescription writing and hospital privileges are afforded to members of the dental profession, but in many cases, a dentist may not want to perform some surgical procedures. Certain procedures may be too complex, involve patients' with complex health conditions, or lack specific training. A general dentist may refer a patient to an oral and maxillofacial surgeon for treatment. An **oral maxillofacial surgeon** is a dentist who has completed additional oral surgical and anesthesia studies of two to three years, as well as a hospital internship and residency program. Studies may also be extended two to four years to receive a fellowship in a specific area or a double degree of DDS and MD.

The procedures performed by the specialist include **exodontia** (ecks-oh-**DAHN**-shah = *extraction of a tooth*); repair of a fractured maxilla and/or mandible; reconstruction of irregular facial bones and tissues; TMJ (temporomandibular joint) disorders; biopsies and surgical treatment of cysts, tumors, cancers, and other diseases of the oral cavity; placement of implant prostheses, cosmetic adjustments and corrections; and other miscellaneous surgery in the oral cavity.

Oral surgeons may work in private practice or hospital settings and perform solo or as a member of a reconstruction team with various specialists. They mainly work with referred patients who return to their family dentist after the surgical treatment is completed.

INSTRUMENTATION RELATED TO ORAL SURGERY

Each specialization requires instruments designed, adapted, or modified to complete certain desired effects. In addition to regular dental implements, there are numerous specialized oral surgical instruments. See Figure 14-1 for illustrations of common surgical instruments. Common instruments are:

- **forceps** (**FOUR**-seps = *pincers for seizing, holding, or extracting*): forceps are made for maxillary or mandibular use. Tooth forceps have a handle, a neck, and nib or beaks, which are angled and designed to grasp, hold, and provide leverage to a specific tooth for extraction. Many forceps come in right-sided and left-sided pairs and are numbered with an R or L, such as 88R or 88L molar forceps. Forceps that can be used on both the right and left sides are called *universal* (see Figure 14-1A).

- **scalpel:** a small surgical knife used to cut open or excise tissue from a surgical area. Made of metal or disposable plastic; may be one-piece style or composed of a detachable blade and handles of varying lengths. Blades are designed to work in a certain area and are numbered according to this design and shape. Much soft-tissue surgical work is completed using laser-machine tips that complete the tissue separation and cauterization of the area without the blood flow connected with surgery (see Figure 14-1B).

- **bone file:** heavier and thicker than the file used on tooth and restoration surfaces. Bone files may be single ended, but most are double ended with serrated file edges and different head sizes on opposite sides. They are used to smooth off irregular bone edges remaining from extracted teeth or bone restructure (see Figure 14-1C).

- **elevators:** devices used to raise the tooth; three types of elevators are used in oral surgery (see Figure 14-1J):

  ○ **periosteal** (**pear**-ee-**OSS**-tee-al = *concerning the periosteum*): used to loosen the periosteum tissue from bone, or detach the tissue around the cervix of the tooth and retract tissue in the surgical site, also called the **periosteotome** (**pear**-ee-**OSS**-tee-oh-tome = *cutting tissue around bone*).

  ○ **exolever** (**ECKS**-oh-lee-ver = *device to raise or elevate*): used to elevate or *luxate* a tooth from its natural socket; also called root elevators. Tips are designed to be used in the mesial or distal, and maxillary or mandibular area. Handles may be the grasp type or T-handed for extra leverage.

  ○ **apical** (**AY**-pih-kal = *pertaining to apex or tip*): used to elevate or pick out remains of a fractured root tip; also called root tip elevators/picks. These elevators have thinner handles and longer shanked tips than other tooth elevators.

- **hemostat** (**HE**-mow-stat = *device or drug used to arrest blood flow*): scissors-style device with a locking joint and serrated beaks; used to clamp off or hold onto and transfer. Hemostats come in various lengths and may have straight or curved beaks (see Figure 14-1G).

- **needle holder:** similar to a hemostat except that the nose of the instrument is rounded and blunted with serrated criss-crossed edges inside its beaks to assist with holding a needle. Suture needles are curved and triangular in shape to avoid tissue trauma during puncturing. Needles are numbered according to their sizes.

- **scissors:** various specialized scissors used in oral surgery (see Figure 14-1H).

- **tissue:** longer-handled scissors with a serrated blade edge that is used to grasp and hold the tissue during cutting.

- **suture:** smaller scissors with one curved, half-moon blade that is inserted under the suture thread during cutting.

- **bandage:** scissors used to cut materials and dressings during surgery; usually have one longer, blunted blade tip to insert under material.

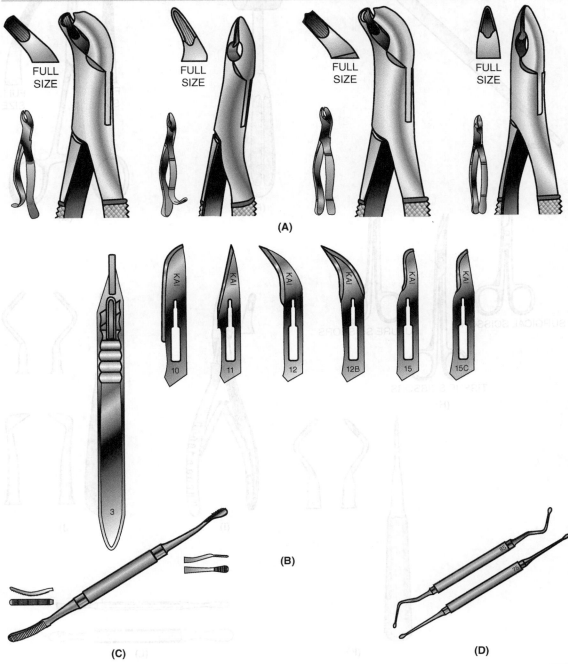

Figure 14-1 Assorted oral surgery instruments: (A) assorted dental forceps, (B) scalpel handle/surgical blades, (C) bone file, (D) double-ended curettes, (E) bone chisel, (F) surgical mallet, (G) hemostat, (H) surgical scissors, tissue scissors, suture scissors, (I) rongeur forceps, (J) root elevators, (K) root tip picks, (L) periosteal elevators

(A)

(B)

(C)

(D)

Figure 14-1 (Continued)

(E)

(F)

FULL
SIZE

FULL
SIZE

(G)

SURGICAL SCISSORS

SUTURE SCISSORS

TISSUE SCISSORS

(H)

(I)

(J)

79

80

78

(K)

(L)

- **rongeurs** (**RON**-jeers = *bone cutting*): grasp-handled instrument similar to forceps but with a spring in the handle to provide a "nipping" action. Beaks may be sharp cutting points (ends) or round sided (blades); used to snip off bony edges and rough areas (see Figure 14-1I).
- **aspirating tips:** disposable or metal suction tips with longer handles and narrower tip openings; used to aspirate sockets, deeper throat areas, and surgical sites.
- **chisel:** device that is longer, thicker, and heavier than tooth chisels. Available in small, medium, and large blade-width tips. Chisels are used to chip away bone and to apply force enough to break impacted molar teeth that will be removed in sections (see Figure 14-1E).
- **mallet** (**MAL**-ett = *surgical hammer*): hammer-like device used to apply pressure to chisels. A mallet may have a plain metal face or removable nylon-padded facing (see Figure 14-1F).
- **curette:** hand instrument with a spoon-shaped face that is inserted in the socket or surgical site to scrape out infection and debris. A surgical curette is larger than a dental operative curette. Curettes may be single ended or double ended (see Figure 14-1D).
- **retractor** (*draw back*): a hand device used to draw back cheeks and/or tissue to provide more access or light to the surgical area. Three types are used in surgery:
  - **tissue:** may be a hemostat-type device with notched tips to hold tissue. Assistants use these claw-like blades with holding tips to retract and hold tissue during surgical procedures.
  - **cheek retractor:** may be bent wire-shaped device or flat, curved handles used to scoop and hold cheek tissue; may be metal or plastic. After position is obtained, the retractor is hand stabilized against the bone to avoid cheeks and tissues from moving around. Excessive movement may be the cause of swelling and bruising after surgery.
  - **tongue retractor:** scissor type of instrument with longer shaft and padded or serrated edges; used to grasp and hold the tongue. Occasionally, the operator will use a sterile piece of gauze to grasp, hold, and extend the tongue for examination.
- **mouth prop:** small, medium, or large pieces of hard rubber; also called a bite block. Another style of prop, or gag, is a scissors-like instrument with padded ends instead of blades. The padded ends are placed into the tooth occlusion while in a "bite" and later used to spread the jaws apart while the patient is asleep during surgery.
- **suture** (**SOO**-chur = *closure*): used to close up a wound or incision. To remove the suture, suture thread of silk or nylon material is required. Resorbable suture material of gut or collagen substances does not require removal.
- **surgical bur:** similar to dental burs but larger in size; used to remove bone, to expose root tips, or to score and divide teeth in preparation for forced sectioning and removal.

SURGICAL PROCEDURES INVOLVED IN EXODONTIA

Tooth removal (exodontia) can be a simple or a complex procedure, depending on the tooth or teeth involved, the condition or disease of the site, and the patient's general health.

Single Extraction

A single extraction is a removal of one tooth during the procedure. The tooth may require a routine extraction, as in a single extraction of an impacted tooth. A single extraction may also entail additional surgical intervention, as when a tooth needs to be sectioned or severed in half.

Impacted Teeth

A soft tissue impacted tooth occurs when the tooth is covered with tissues of the periodontium. Consequently, an incision is required to expose the tooth for extraction. A bone- and tissue-impacted tooth is covered with tissue and bone. Bone-impacted teeth are typed and named for the tilt angle of the impaction. Examples of the impact classifications are given in Figure 14-2 and described here:

- **horizontal impaction:** the tooth is horizontally tilted (see Figure 14-2A). It may be leaning parallel to the floor at various angles; crown may be perpendicular to an adjacent tooth crown.
- **vertical impaction:** tooth is in upright position but in close proximity to or under the crown of a nearby tooth (see Figure 14-2B).
- **distoangular impaction:** crown of the tooth is slanted toward the distal surface and is covered by tissue and/or bone (see Figure 14-2C).
- **mesioangular impaction:** the crown of the tooth is mesially tilted and covered by tissue and/or bone (see Figure 14-2D).
- **transverse impaction:** tooth is situated sideways to the adjacent teeth and occlusal plane, and it is covered by tissue and/or bone.

Multiple Extraction

A multiple extraction involves the removal of two or more teeth during one procedure. When multiple teeth are extracted, the alveolar bone crests have to be removed and smoothed to prepare the ridges for denture or appliance wear. This reduction procedure is termed an **alveolectomy** (al-vee-oh-**LECK**-toh-me).

Full Mouth Extraction

In a full mouth extraction, all remaining teeth in the oral cavity are removed. Immediate dentures may be inserted over the sutured site at the time of surgery. A surgical **template** (**TEM**-plate = *pattern*) is used as a guide for the alveolectomy and resection of the area before the placement of the immediate denture. One potential complication resulting from extraction of teeth is **alveolitis** (al-**vee**-oh-**LIGH**-tiss = *infection or inflammation of the alveolar process*). This loss of the natural clotting is commonly called a **dry socket**.

Figure 14-2 Illustrated examples of impaction classifications

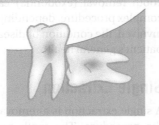

(A)   Horizontal Tooth Impaction

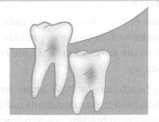

(B)   Vertical Tooth Impaction

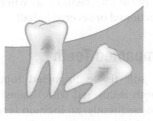

(C)   Distoangular Tooth Impaction

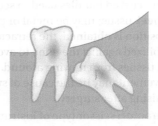

(D)   Mesioangular Tooth Impaction

PROCEDURES INVOLVED IN SOFT-TISSUE SURGERY

Many procedures performed by the oral surgeon are limited to, or involve, soft tissue of the oral cavity. Some of these soft-tissue surgeries are commonly completed by the general dentist and other specialists, particularly the periodontist, as well:

- **gingivectomy** (**jin**-jih-**VECK**-toh-me): surgical excision of unattached gingival tissue.
- **gingivoplasty** (**jin**-jih-voh-**PLAS**-tee): surgical recontour of the gingival tissues.
- **periodontal flap surgery** (*surgical excision and removal of pocket or tissue extensions*): laser or scalpel sectioning and tissue removal that may be necessary for extensive singular pocket involvement or when during tooth eruption, tissue flap coverage of incoming teeth, particularly third molars, obstructs or impacts food around the crown, causing gingival irritation and an infection termed **pericoronitis**.
- **frenectomy** (freh-**NECK**-toh-me = *surgical removal or resectioning of a frenum*): surgery that may be performed on the maxillary labial frenum to correct **diastema** (die-ah-**STEE**-mah = *a space between two teeth*), or on the mandibular lingual frenum to correct **ankyloglossia** (**ang**-kill-oh-**GLOSS**-ee-ah = *shortness of the tongue frenulum, tongue tied*).
- **incision and drainage (I&D):** procedure performed for a periodontal abscess. An incision is made into the affected area, and an opening is obtained to remove and drain infected matter. In some cases, a small piece of rubber dam, or Iodoform gauze, is inserted into the incision to maintain the opening for drainage.

Other tissue surgery may involve removal of the salivary glands, cysts, or any assorted **malady** (**MAL**-ah-dee = *disease or disorder*) of the mucous membranes and oral structures.

Tissue Biopsy

Another tissue surgical procedure performed by an oral surgeon is a **biopsy** (**BYE**-op-see = *small tissue incision*). The common types of dental biopsies are:

- **incisional biopsy:** removing a wedge-shaped section of affected tissue along with some normal adjacent tissue.
- **excision biopsy:** removal of the entire lesion of affected tissue with some underlying normal tissue.
- **exfoliative** (ecks-**FOH**-lee-ah-tiv) **biopsy:** scraping with glass slide or tongue depressor to collect tissue cells for microscopic study.
- **brush biopsy:** much like the exfoliative test, a pipe stem brush is drawn across the mouth tissues, scraped against a glass slide, fixed with a solution, and sent to the lab for a computer-assisted reading.

Tissue Diseases

The term applied to cancerous tumors is **malignant** (mah-**LIG**-nant = *harmful or growing worse*). By contrast, **benign** (bee-**NINE** = *nonmalignant*) tumors are not considered life-threatening or deadly. Some of the tissue diseases occurring in the oral cavity are:

- **leukoplakia** (**loo**-koh-**PLAY**-key-ah): formation of white patches on the mucous membrane of the oral cavity that cannot be scraped off and have the potential for malignancy (Figure 14-3).
- **fibroma:** benign, fibrous, encapsulated connective tissue tumor.

Figure 14-3 Leukoplakia of the tongue

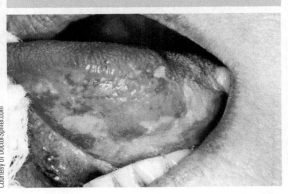

- **papilloma** (pap-ih-**LOH**-mah): benign, epithelial tumor of the skin or mucous membrane.
- **hemangioma** (he-**man**-jee-**OH**-mah): benign tumor of dilated blood vessels.
- **granuloma** (gran-you-**LOH**-mah): grandular tumor usually occurring with other diseases.
- **melanoma** (mel-ah-**NO**-mah): malignant, pigmented mole or tumor.
- **basal or squamous cell carcinoma:** malignant growth of epithelial cells.

PROCEDURES INVOLVED IN MINOR BONE SURGERY

Some tissue surgeries involve treatment of the alveolar bone (**osteoplasty** = **OSS**-tee-oh-**plas**-tee = *forming or recontouring bones*). Related terms are:

- **alveolectomy** (al-vee-oh-**LECK**-toe-mee): usually performed to remove alveolar bone crests remaining after tooth extraction in preparation for a smooth bone ridge for denture wear.
- **apicoectomy** (ay-pih-koh-**ECK**-toh-me): usually requires opening of the periodontium, including some alveolar bone, and exposure with removal of the root apex. Many times this

surgery is followed with a retrofill root canal treatment (RCT).

- **exostosis** (**ecks**-ahs-**TOH**-sis = *bony outgrowth*): removing overgrowths and smoothing off of bone edges in preparation for dentures.
- **torus** (**TORE**-us = *rounded elevation*): an excessive bone growth; a torus on the lingual side of the mandible is termed a *torus mandibularis* (man-dib-u-**LAIR**-iss = *concerning the mandible*). In the roof of the mouth, it is termed *torus palatinus* (**pal**-ah-**TEEN**-us = *in the palate*). See Figure 14-4 for an example of each.
- **cysts** (**SISTs** = *abnormal, closed-walled sac present in or around tissue*): usually X-ray detected and removed before they enlarge and destroy bone tissue. Some types are:
  - **dentigerous** (den-**TIJ**-er-us): cystic sac containing a tooth or tooth bud particle.
  - **radicular** (rah-**DICK**-you-lar): cyst located alongside or at the apex of a tooth root; also called periapical cyst.
  - **ranula** (**RAN**-you-lah): cystic tumor found on the underside of the tongue or in the sublingual or submaxillary ducts; usually the result of a blocked duct.

Figure 14-4 (A) Torus mandibularis, (B) torus palatinus

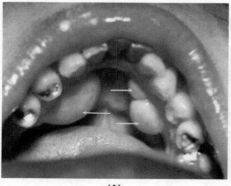

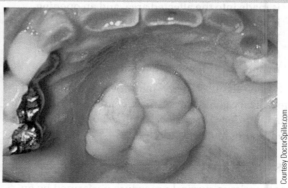

(A)   (B)

Courtesy DoctorSpiller.com

SURGICAL PROCEDURES INVOLVED IN FRACTURE REPAIR

Repair of fractured maxilla and mandible bones are reserved for treatment by an oral maxillofacial specialist. Fracture reduction can be completed in two fashions, closed or open reduction:

- **Closed fracture reduction:** repair with internal fixation, tooth wiring, or ligation methods in which the teeth are "wired together" in proper alignment while awaiting bone healing.

- **Open fracture reduction:** more complicated procedure involving osteotomy and rigid fixation, perhaps bone plate, mesh, pins, grafts, and other fixation devices. Open reduction requires not only alignment by fixation of the teeth but also repositioning and correction of fractures after surgical access through the periosteum.

PROCEDURES INVOLVED IN MAXILLOFACIAL SURGERY

More complicated or involved surgical intervention with tissue and bone elements is called maxillofacial reconstruction and beautification. Some procedures come as a result of congenital deformities, some from trauma occurrences, and others from disease damage. The oral maxillofacial surgeon may work alone or with other professionals in a team effort. Examples of reconstruction surgeries are:

- **genioplasty** (**JEE**-nee-oh-**plas**-tee): plastic surgery of the chin or cheek. Chin size is classified in one of six ways:

  ○ **macrogenia** (mack-roh-**JEE**-nee-ah): large or excessive chin.

  ○ **microgenia** (my-kroh-**JEE**-nee-ah): under-sized chin.

  ○ **lateral excessive/deficient:** excessive bone in one direction and deficient bone in another.

  ○ **asymmetrical** (ay-sim-**EH**-trih-kal): lack of balance of size and shape on opposite sides.

  ○ **pseudomicrogenia** (soo-doh-mack-roh-**JEE**-nee-ah): excess of soft tissue presenting a chin with the look of abnormal size.

  ○ **"witch's chin":** soft tissue **ptosis** (**TOH**-sis = *dropping or sagging of an organ*).

Chin size may be altered by chin augmentation, which could involve tissue liposuction or implanting bone cartilage, grafts, or alloplastic materials. **Osteotomy** (oss-tee-**AUGH**-toh-me = *bone incision*) is the surgical movement of bone, and **osteoplasty** (**OSS**-tee-oh-**plas**-tee = *to form bones*) is the removal of bone, usually completed with surgical burs.

- **chin augmentation:** may be termed *sliding genioplasty* because it is the option of moving the chin forward by making an incision inside the lower lip and inserting an artificial chin implant or moving the severed bone tip segment forward. In cases where the chin is too posterior, the cut segment may be advanced and secured to enlarge the chin.

- **ridge augmentation:** use of bone grafts to build or correct an underdeveloped or missing ridge possibly needed for tooth or denture implant or preparation for denture wear.

- **surgical correction:** in conjunction with the orthodontist and/or the prosthodontist, the oral surgeon may expose and band or peg erupting teeth to prepare the mouth for orthodontic treatment or may remove hidden or retained root tips, cysts, or foreign bodies before taking denture impressions.

Figure 14-5 An example of an alloplastic implant graft used in chin augmentation

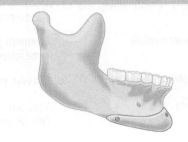

233

- **arthrotomy** (ar-**THRAH**-toh-me = *cutting into a joint*): reconstruction and alignment of the mandible for TMJ disorders. The mandible may be altered to obtain one of these three movements:
  - **retrusive** (ree-**TRUE**-sive): position with mandible backward.
  - **protrusive** (proh-**TRUE**-sive): position with mandible forward.
  - **lateral** (**LAT**-er-al): position to the side; mediolateral is toward the center of the face, and distolateral is toward the outside of the face.
- **cleft lip repair:** tissue fissure or incomplete juncture of maxillary lip tissues; congenital effect.
- **cleft palate repair:** congenital fissure in roof of mouth with an opening into the nasal cavity; may be unilateral (one-sided) or bilateral (two-sided); also may be complete or incomplete.
- **orthognathic** (ore-theg-**NATH**-ick) **surgery:** surgical manipulation of the facial skeleton to restore facial esthetics and proper function to a congenital, developmental, or traumatic-affected patient; performed in cooperation with orthodontic involvement in planning and treatment. Osteotomy and osteoplasty techniques are used on orthodontic prebraced teeth and jaws. This technique is further discussed in Chapter 15, Orthodontics.

ORAL SURGERY PROCEDURES INVOLVED WITH TMJ DYSFUNCTION

The temporomandibular joint (TMJ), composed of condyle of the mandible and the fossa eminence of the temporal bone, is responsible for vertical and lateral movement of the lower jaw. Any malposition or derangement of these parts of the TMJ may cause pain and dysfunction. Repair of a dysfunctional TMJ depends on the severity of the malady. One classification of internal derangement is listed in Table 14-1.

Medical tests used to determine malposition of the TMJ are:

- **computerized mandibular scan (CMS):** 3D tracking device to record functional movement of the jaw during opening, closing, chewing, and swallowing.
- **electromyography (EMG):** surface electrodes instrument to determine muscle activity during function; healthy muscles have low levels of electrical activity, and disarranged muscles register high activity.
- **electrosonograph (ESG):** recording of sounds during opening and closing of the jaw; also observed by use of a stethoscope.
- **CT (computed tomography, also known as CAT scan):** X-ray images are taken at different angles and computerized into a cross section of anatomical features. It is used for diagnosis

Table 14-1 Wilkes Classification of TMJ Internal Derangement

Stages	Symptoms	Motion Function
Stage I Early	Painless clicking	No restrictive motion
Stage II Early/Intermediate	Occasional painful clicking, headaches	Intermittent locking
Stage III Intermediate	Frequent pain, joint tenderness, headaches	Painful chewing, locking, restricted motion
Stage IV Intermediate/Late	Chronic pain, headaches	Restricted motion <35 mm
Stage V Late	Variable pain, joint **crepitus** (**KREP**-ah-tus): *grinding*	Painful function

Figure 14-6 An example of an i-CAT scan view involving the temporomandibular joint disorder (TMD)

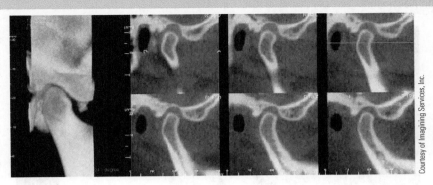

Courtesy of Imagining Services, Inc.

as well as for the preparation of Co-Cr-Mo (Cobalt-Chromium-Molybdenum) prostheses. See Figure 14-6 for an example of a CAT scan view involving the temporomandibular joint disorder (TMD).

Treatment of TMJ Dysfunction

Although some minor cases of TMJ dysfunction can be treated by selective grinding and aligning of tooth surfaces, night sleep guards, or temporary stabilization of the bite process, more severe cases of TMJ dysfunction require oral surgical services. Surgical intervention in TMJ treatment includes a variety of techniques, such as:

- **hemiarthroplasty** (**HEM**-we-are-throw-plas-tee)**:** surgical repair of a joint with a partial joint implant reconstruction. This may be completed by:

  ○ **autogenous reconstruction:** rebuilding of the joint using organic material supplied by the patient, such as toe or rib bone grafts.

  ○ **alloplastic reconstruction:** rebuilding of the joint using inert, synthetic man-made materials; can be manufactured to be resorbable or nonresorbable.

  ○ **allograft reconstruction:** graft material taken from human donors, which can be tested, sterilized, and accepted by the patient's body to rebuild the jawbone.

  ○ **xenograft:** harvested from animals, most commonly the cow; specially processed to become biocompatible.

- **total joint reconstruction:** surgical intervention and use of artificial prostheses for the condyle, disc, and fossa of the temporal bone.

- **revision surgery:** surgical correction of an area that has been operated on previously, occurring when further degeneration happens, when previous implants have failed, or when going from a partial joint implant to a total implant.

SURGICAL PROCEDURES INVOLVED IN IMPLANTOLOGY

The oral maxillofacial surgeon may work in association with a prosthodontist or dentist in the construction and completion of a dental appliance involving a single implant or multiple dental bone implants. After extensive X-ray, CT scans, measurements, examinations, and planning (Figure 14-7), the surgeon may perform one of the following types of dental implants:

- **endosteal** (en-**DOSS**-tee-ahl = *placement within the bone*)**:** also known as **osseointegrated** implants; can be used as an anchor for a single tooth or multiple areas, depending on the style of implant.

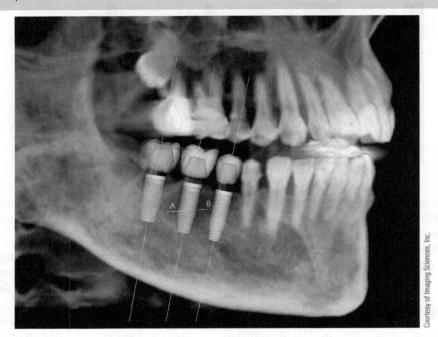

Courtesy of Imaging Sciences, Inc.

- **subperiosteal** (sub-pear-ee-**OSS**-tee-ahl = *beneath the periosteum and placed onto the bone*): usually a cast framework implant with protruding pegs that is placed over the bone and covered by the periosteum; used to hold a base plate for tooth-replacing device, similar to a denture base.
- **transosteal** (trans-**OSS**-tee-ahl = *through the mandibular bone*): anchor implants that are placed all the way through the mandible. These are also called staple implants.
- **endodontic** (**en**-doh-**DON**-tick = *within the tooth*): titanium post placed in the apex of endodontically treated tooth to improve the crown–root length ratio (Figure 14-8).
- **intramucosal insert:** indentations in the palate used to provide anchorage for special mushroom-shaped pads built into the gum side of a removable denture.

When the jawbone is too thin or insufficient to accommodate an implant device, a bone graft or ridge augmentation may be completed beforehand. With the use of bone-grafting materials and methods mentioned previously in the paragraph on TMJ arthroplasty, the jawbone may be repaired and later used for dental implants. Maxillary sinus openings may cause a lack of bone structure for implant placement. The sinus may be elevated, and bone-grafting materials may be placed to encourage bone growth thick enough for implant devices.

Implant Material

Implant pins or frameworks may be fabricated using any of several materials:

- **titanium:** biocompatible with high strength; oxidizes readily on contact with tissue fluid and has a minimum amount of corrosion.
- **zirconia (zircon oxide ceramic):** biocompatible, light colored; may be used in soft-tissue areas; for patients with allergies to

Figure 14-8 Illustrations of dental implants: (A) endosteal implant, (B) subperiosteal implant, (C) transosteal implant, (D) endodontic implant

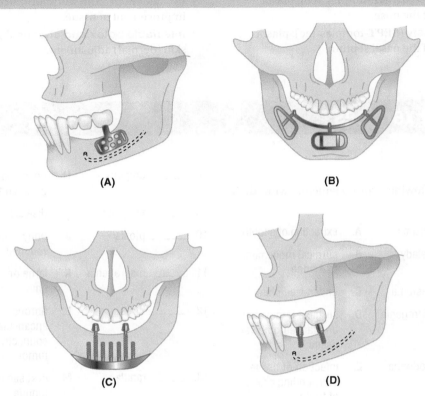

(A)

(B)

(C)

(D)

other materials and patients who do not want metal framework in the mouth.

- **polymers and composites:** in the research stage; may be used as abutments in partially edentulous mouths.
- **stainless steel and cobalt-chromium alloys:** older but less used metal materials.
- **cobalt-chromium-molybdenum:** implant material used in prosthesis construction for TMJ replacement.

ORAL SURGERY ROLE IN ESTHETIC DENTISTRY

As part of a combined project consisting of maxillofacial surgeons, prosthodontists, orthodontists, dentists, speech therapists, and others, the following procedures may be performed to alter, repair, give proper function, and present an improved cosmetic appearance:

- **cleft tongue repair:** bifid or split tongue; usually split at the tip.
- **cleft palate repair:** closing of lip and palatine tissues combined with orthodontic treatment.
- **cleft lip repair:** tissue closing and repair of opening tissue gap.
- **cosmetic alterations:** some cosmetic repair or improvement work is necessary with extensive bone and tissue replacement or movement. Examples that may be performed are:
  - **rhytidectomy (rit-ah-DECK-toe-mee):** excision of wrinkles by plastic surgery.

- **blepharoplasty** (**BLEF**-er-oh-**plas**-tee): plastic surgery of the eyelid.
- **rhinoplasty** (**RINE**-no-plas-tee): plastic surgery of the nose.
- **septoplasty** (**SEPT**-toe-plas-tee): plastic surgery of the nasal septum.

- **neck liposuction:** suction of fat tissue of the neck.
- **lip, cheek, or chin augmentation:** improvement of tissue.
- **injectable botox and chemical peel:** skin (dermal) adjustment.

Review Exercises

Matching

Match the following word elements with their meanings.

1. _____ fibroma

A. extraction of a tooth

2. _____ malady

B. surgical movement of a bone

3. _____ diastema

C. undersized chin

4. _____ microgenia

D. surgical removal of unattached gingival tissue

5. _____ exodontia

E. infection of tissue surrounding crown of tooth

6. _____ gingivectomy

F. white, precancerous patch on mucous membrane

7. _____ osteotomy

G. witch's chin

8. _____ crepitus

H. open space between two teeth

9. _____ template

I. disease or disorder

10. _____ ptosis

J. bony overgrowth or rounded elevation

11. _____ macrogenia

K. large or excessive chin

12. _____ torus

L. fibrous, encapsulated connective tissue tumor

13. _____ ranula

M. cyst sac under the tongue

14. _____ leukoplakia

N. pattern for surgical adaptation

15. _____ pericoronitis

O. grinding

Definitions

Using the selection given for each sentence, choose the best term to complete the definition.

1. Which instrument is used to clamp off the blood supply in an artery or vein?
   a. needle holder
   b. curette
   c. retractor
   d. hemostat

2. Ankyloglossia is an immobility or fixation of which tissue?
   a. uvula
   b. tongue
   c. tooth
   d. cheek

3. Which instrument is used to nip or cut off bony tissue ridges?
   a. rongeurs
   b. scissors

c. forceps

d. hemostats

4. A biopsy technique taking some normal tissue and the entire removal of the lesion is:
   a. excision
   b. general
   c. incision
   d. exfoliative

5. The building up of an undeveloped or missing mandible area is a/an:
   a. excision graft
   b. ridge augmentation
   c. reduction
   d. osteotomy

6. A blepharoplasty is a surgical correction of which body part?
   a. lip
   b. eyelid
   c. chin
   d. brow

7. A surgical hammer is a/an:
   a. retractor
   b. mallet
   c. chisel
   d. periosteal

8. The surgical contouring of the gingival tissue is termed:
   a. gingivoplasty
   b. osteoplasty
   c. gingivectomy
   d. osteoectomy

9. A surgical correction of a previously operated area is termed a/an:
   a. excision
   b. osteoplasty
   c. revision
   d. exodontia

10. An impaction of a tilted third molar with crown perpendicular to an adjacent tooth is which type of impaction?
    a. transverse
    b. distoangular

11. The infection of a tooth socket following an extraction may result in the condition called:
    a. alveolectomy
    b. alveolitis
    c. apicoectomy
    d. apicalalgia

12. A surgical overlay pattern used to prepare for immediate dentures is called a/an:
    a. template
    b. implant
    c. mouth prop
    d. pattern

13. A torus of the mandibular bone may be termed:
    a. torus palatinus
    b. torus lingualis
    c. torus mandibularis
    d. ranula

14. In the Wilkes classification of TMJ internal derangement, variable pain, crepitus, and limited motion is considered which stage?
    a. Stage II
    b. State III
    c. Stage IV
    d. Stage V

15. When the mandible is situated in a drawn backward position, it is said to be:
    a. anterior
    b. prognostic
    c. retrusive
    d. posterior

16. A cystic sac containing a tooth or tooth bud is termed:
    a. radicular
    b. cystic
    c. fibromic
    d. dentigerous

17. The rebuilding of a joint using man-made materials is which type of reconstruction?
    a. autogenous
    b. homogenous
    c. alloplastic
    d. arthrogenous

18. An implant appliance that is placed within the bone is termed:
    a. ossiferous
    b. exosteal
    c. subperiosteal
    d. endosteal

19. The rebuilding of a joint using organic material, such as a rib, is which type of reconstruction?
    a. autogenous
    b. homogeneous
    c. alloplastic
    d. arthrogenous

20. A surgical forcep designed to remove a maxillary or mandibular tooth is called:
    a. multipurpose
    b. general
    c. omnipotent
    d. universal

Building Skills

Locate and define the prefix, root/combining form, and suffix (if present) in the following words.

1. **pericoronitis**
   prefix _____
   root/combining form _____
   suffix _____

2. **ankyloglossia**
   prefix _____
   root/combining form _____
   suffix _____

3. **endosteal**
   prefix _____
   root/combining form _____
   suffix _____

4. **apicoectomy**
   prefix _____
   root/combining form _____
   suffix _____

5. **exodontia**
   prefix _____
   root/combining form _____
   suffix _____

Fill-Ins

Write the correct word in the blank space to complete each statement.

1. Another word for a tongue that has an unusual split at the tip is a/an _____ tongue.

2. A surgical implant appliance that is placed beneath the periosteum and onto the bone is a/an _____ implant.

3. _____ is the term given to a malignant, pigmented mole.

4. A/an _____ is a cystic tumor found on the underside of the tongue or in a sublingual or submaxillary gland.

5. A _____ is an abnormal, closed-walled tissue sac.

6. A protrusive mandible is positioned in a _____ position during a bite registration.

7. Another term given to a disease or ill condition is a/an _____.

8. A cystic sac containing a tooth or tooth part is a/an _____ cyst.

9. _____ is the term for surgical contouring of gingival tissue.

10. Rhinoplasty is plastic surgery of the _____.

11. The loss of a clot shortly after extraction is commonly called a/an _____.

12. The removal of a wedge piece and some nearby tissue for study is termed a/an _____ biopsy.

13. The surgical removal or resectioning of a frenum is a/an _____.

14. A/an _____ is a tumor of dilated blood vessels.

15. A torus mandibularis elevation is found on the _____ bone.

16. A rongeurs instrument is used to _____ bony edges.

17. A cyst located adjacent to or at the side of a tooth is a _____ cyst.

18. An implant device that is placed within the mandible bone is a/an _____ implant.

19. I&D is the abbreviation for the _____ procedure.

20. Another word for a surgical hammer is a _____.

Word Use

Read the following sentences and define the meaning of the word written in boldface letters.

1. To avoid **pericoronitis**, the dental hygienist instructed the teenager to carefully maintain a clean area round the erupting third molar.

_____

2. The office manager is sure to list the correct insurance code for the **alveolectomy** procedure.

_____

3. The **needle holder** has a blunt-ended nose while the hemostat's nose tip is pointed and long.

_____

4. When setting up the surgical tray for a full mouth extraction and immediate denture insert, the assistant makes sure the **template** is included.

_____

5. The surgeon advised Mr. Towers that there must be a long waiting period between the implant appointments to allow for **osseointegration**.

_____

✔ Learning Objectives

On completion of this chapter, you should be able to:

1. Discuss the orthodontic practice and describe the classifications and causes of malocclusion.

2. Describe the primary methods of treatment for malocclusion and the different approaches that may be taken.

3. Identify the various diagnostic tests and records for planning orthodontic care.

4. Discuss the various types of orthodontic appliances and the malocclusions they may be used to correct.

5. Discuss the need, purposes, and uses of headgear/ traction devices and the alternate methods of treatment for recessive mandibles.

6. Identify the assortment of special appliances and retainers necessary for orthodontic treatment.

7. List and identify the specialized instruments used in the orthodontic practice.

PURPOSE OF ORTHODONTIC PRACTICE AND MALOCCLUSION CLASSIFICATIONS

Orthodontia (**ore**-thoh-**DAHN**-shah; ortho = *straight*, dont = *tooth*) is the study dealing with the prevention and correction of abnormally positioned or misaligned teeth. The dentist specializing in this practice, the **orthodontist**, is a graduate dental student who has completed an additional two to three years of study in orthodontics. This specialist

Vocabulary Related to Orthodontics

This list contains selected new and important word parts and terms from this chapter. Take the time to learn these word parts and their meanings. You may use the list to review these terms and practice pronouncing them correctly. When you work with the audio for this chapter, listen to the word, repeat it, and then place a checkmark in the box. Proceed to the next boxed word, and repeat the process.

(hyphen before word means it's a suffix, hyphen after word means prefix, no hyphen means root word.)

Word Parts	Meaning	Word Parts	Meaning
-ary	pertaining to	maxillo	maxillary bone
-al	relating to	numer	number
facial	are of the face	occlus	bite/come together
-ion	condition	ortho	straight
mal-	bad	super	above, over

Key Terms

❏ **bracket** (**BRACK**-et)
❏ **cephalometric** (sef-ah-low-**MEH**-trik)
❏ **cervical** (**SIR**-vih-cull)
❏ **congenital** (kahn-**JEN**-ih-tahl)
❏ **distoclusion** (dis-toh-**KLOO**-zhun)

❏ **ectopic** (eck-**TOP**-ic)
❏ **extrusion** (ecks-**TROO**-zhun)
❏ **intrusion** (in-**TROO**-zhun)
❏ **ligature** (**LIG**-ah-chur)
❏ **mesioclusion** (me-zee-oh-**KLOO**-zhun)

❏ **myotherapeutic** (my-oh-thare-ah-**PYOU**-tick)
❏ **neutroclusion** (new-troh-**KLOO**-zhun)
❏ **orthodontia** (ore-thoh-**DAHN**-shah)

Vocabulary Related to Orthodontics *continued*

Key Terms *continued*

- ❏ **orthognathic surgery**
  (or-thug-**NATH**-ic)
- ❏ **orthopedic** (or-thoh-**PEE**-dik)

- ❏ **osteopenia**
  (ah-stee-oh-**PEE**-nee-ah)
- ❏ **prognathia**
  (prog-**NATH**-ee-ah)

- ❏ **retrognathia**
  (ret-tro-**NATH**-ee-ah)
- ❏ **rotation** (roh-**TAY**-shun)
- ❏ **torque** (TORK)

is concerned with the causes and treatment of malocclusion. With additional specialized training in the control and modification of facial growth, the orthodontist can practice dentofacial orthopedics, usually in conjunction with a team of other specialists. Some of these procedures can be TMJ dysfunction, cleft palate, and facial and tooth reconstruction.

Classification of Malocclusion

Dr. Edward Angle divided malocclusion into three classifications while the teeth are set in **centric relationship**, the most retruded position of the

mandibular condyle into the glenoid fossa (biting on the back teeth), also known as the *terminal hinge position*. The three classifications are illustrated in Figure 15-1 and are described here:

- **neutroclusion** (**new**-troh-**KLOO**-zhun): Class I condition in which the anteroposterior occlusal positions of the teeth or the mesiodistal positions are normal, but other malocclusion or positioning of the individual teeth occurs, such as crowding, misalignment, and crossbites.
- **distoclusion** (**dis**-toh-**KLOO**-zhun): Class II condition in which the mesiobuccal cusp of the maxillary first molar is anterior to the buccal

Figure 15-1 Classifications of malocclusion

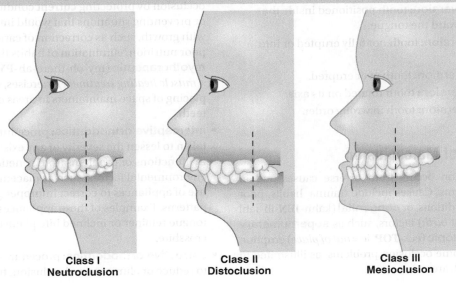

| Class I | Class II | Class III |
| Neutroclusion | Distoclusion | Mesioclusion |

groove of the mandibular first molar, resulting in an appearance of a retruded mandible. Class II is further separated into two divisions, according to the individual placement of the anterior teeth:

○ **Division 1:** maxillary incisors protruding with a V-shaped arch instead of a U-shaped arch; overjet present.

○ **Division 2:** maxillary incisors having a lingual incline with an excessive overbite and a wider than normal arch.

• **mesioclusion** (**me**-zee-oh-**KLOO**-zhun): Class III condition, in which the mesiobuccal cusp of the maxillary first molar occludes in the interdental space of the mandibular permanent first molar's distal cusp and the mesial cusp of the mandibular permanent second molar, resulting in an appearance of a protruded mandible.

An individual tooth position can also be classified as:

• **mesioversion:** tooth is positioned more mesial than normal.

• **distoversion:** tooth is positioned more distal than normal.

• **labioversion:** anterior tooth positioned outside the arch toward the lips.

• **buccoversion:** posterior tooth positioned toward the cheek.

• **linguoversion:** tooth positioned inside the arch toward the tongue.

• **infraversion:** tooth not fully erupted or into space.

• **supraversion:** tooth over erupted.

• **torsoversion:** tooth rotated on its axis.

• **transversion:** tooth in wrong order.

Causes of Malocclusion

Malocclusion occurs from diverse causes and in various forms. Causes include trauma, habits, poor mouth conditions, or **congenital** (kahn-**JEN**-ih-tahl = *present at birth*) factors, such as **supernumerary** teeth or **ectopic** (eck-**TOP**-ic = *out of place*) eruption of teeth. Some occlusion problems, as illustrated in Figure 15-2, are:

• **open bite:** anterior teeth do not contact with each other, or no contact exists between the maxillary and mandibular posterior teeth.

• **overjet:** also known as horizontal overbite, increased horizontal distance between the incisal edges of maxillary and the labial surfaces of the mandibular central incisors.

• **vertical overbite:** excessive amount of overlap of the maxillary and mandibular central incisors when they are in occlusion.

• **crossbite:** midsagittal alignment between central incisors not in agreement; posterior tooth crossbite can also occur when teeth do not meet correctly in the centric bite.

• **underjet:** maxillary incisors lingual to mandibular incisors.

• **end to end:** edges of maxillary and mandibular incisors meeting each other.

TYPES AND METHODS OF ORTHODONTIC TREATMENT

Malocclusion is treated with a variety of methods or treatment plans:

• **preventive orthodontics:** procedures taken to preserve the integrity of a normal developing occlusion by protecting current conditions or preventing situations that would interfere with growth, such as correction of caries, poor nutrition, elimination of habits through **myotherapeutic** (my-oh-there-ah-**PYOU**-tic = *muscle healing treatment*) exercises, or by the placing of space maintainers in areas of missing teeth.

• **interceptive orthodontics:** procedures taken to lessen the severity of any existing malfunctions or problems from genetic or environmental factors, such as placement or use of appliances to correct improper growth patterns. Examples of these appliances are a tongue retainer or inclined bite plane to move a crossbite.

• **corrective orthodontics:** procedures taken to reduce or eliminate malocclusion; treatment

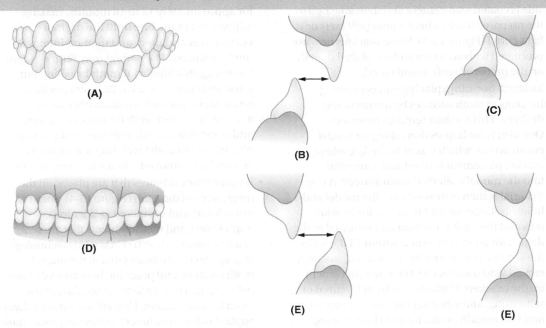

Figure 15-2 Assorted malocclusion conditions: (A) open bite: anterior teeth failing to meet and posterior teeth occluding; (B) overjet: increased horizontal distance between incisal edges of central incisors; (C) vertical overbite: vertical overlap that is not on incisal third of central incisor; (D) crossbite: midsagittal balance between maxillary and mandibular central incisors not in alignment; posteriors in improper occlusion; (E) underjet: maxillary incisors lingual to mandibular incisors; (F) end-to-end: edges of maxillary and mandibular incisors meeting each other

(A)

(B)

(C)

(D)

(E)

(E)

plans include the application of intraoral and extraoral appliances and auxiliary forces for tooth direction. Some movement forces are:

- **rotation** (roh-**TAY**-shun = *turn around on an axis*): altering the position of a tooth around its long axis.
- **translation:** bodily tooth movement; a change of teeth to alternate positions.
- **tipping:** change of a tooth position to a more upright direction.
- **intrusion** (in-**TROO**-zhun): movement of the tooth into the alveolus.
- **extrusion** (ecks-**TROO**-zhun): movement of the tooth out of the alveolus.
- **torque (TORK):** movement of the root without the movement of the crown.

Corrective orthodontic treatment is determined by many factors, including age, degree of malocclusion, cause of malocclusion, the patient's general health and attitude, and economics, as well as the orthodontist's expertise and training. Today's patient has many choices or methods of correction, including the following:

- **banding:** placing a metal band around the entire selective tooth or teeth. Brackets, tubes, hooks, springs, and other devices are placed on these bands and are used to attach push/pull pressure to the teeth movements and arch wire shaping.
- **direct bonding:** cementing brackets of stainless steel or gold-plated metal composite, ceramic with metal centers, or (monocrystalline sapphire) clear brackets on the surface of the tooth to

attach needed pressures and arch wire forms. Brackets may be plain hook style for attachments or a self-ligating system clip style that does away with elastics, requires fewer appointments, and is quicker in adjusting appointments. After the tooth is cleaned and etched, the bracket's back side is coated with cement and then attached to the prepared tooth, where it auto (self) sets or is light cured (Figure 15-3). Some brackets now are precoated with adhesive and are placed directly on the prepared surface and cured.

- **indirect bonding:** placing and cementing brackets to tooth surfaces by means of tray delivery. This method requires two visits. One visit is for impression taking for model construction, which is sent to the lab, where bracket placement is fitted and cemented into the model's selected tooth surface. A tray material is then expressed over the model and brackets. Upon set and removal, the bracket tabs and tray unit is cleaned and returned to the dentist for patient insertion within 14 days. On the second visit, the teeth are cleaned, isolated, etched, and then receive the tray with cement on the brackets. Cement may be light-cured or self-curing, and when set the tray is removed, the brackets remain on the tooth to have appropriate wires attached for continuing treatment.

- **Invisalign braces:** strong plastic (polyurethane) custom trays used in mild malocclusion cases. The specially trained orthodontist takes impressions, X-rays, and photos that are sent to the Align lab, which prepares a CT scan and a 3D model for the fabrication of trays. These trays are returned to the dentist who inserts and instructs the patient. Trays are changed every few weeks, for approximately 12 to 18 months, making adjustment in the bite until the desired occlusion is obtained, and then maintained until stabilized. The patient may remove them for eating, drinking, and tooth brushing but must wear them for 20 to 22 hours per day. Some tooth-colored attachments may be applied to rotated teeth for extra movement, and some molar teeth may have attachments placed to help assist with tray retention. These "knobs" are removed when treatment is done.

- **lingual braces:** braces that are placed on the tongue side of the teeth (Figure 15-4). Some orthodontists take required radiographs, impressions, and measurements that are sent to a laboratory to use 3D CAM/CAD technology to prepare custom braces that fit the lingual tooth surfaces, and precision bent wires that are delivered in a tray for indirect bonding to the tooth lingual surfaces. Lingual brackets are always applied using an indirect bonding tray procedure.

- **accelerated osteogenic orthodontic treatment:** surgical orthodontic "team" approach that involves placement of a regular orthodontic apparatus on the teeth and a periodontist or oral surgeon

Figure 15-3 Example of direct bonded brackets and arch wires

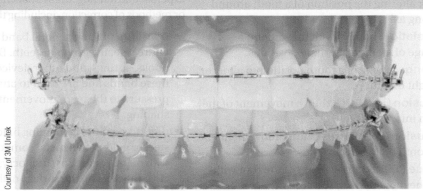

Courtesy of 3M Unitek

Figure 15-4 An example of the Incognito lingual brace system

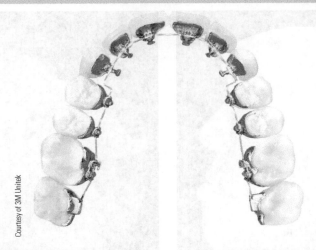

Courtesy of 3M Unitek

to incise the gingiva and expose the alveolar bone. Then, a surgical drill is used to remove some alveolar plate and score the mandible bone surrounding the teeth, which causes **osteopenia** (ah-stee-oh-**PEE**-nee-ah; *osteo* = bone, *penia* = lack of). An antibiotic bone graft mixture is placed in the site, and the area is closed. While the bone is in a weakened condition, the teeth move quickly into position (three to eight months) and are retained there while the bone remineralizes and strengthens. This procedure is also termed *Wilckodontics*. (See Chapter 11, Cosmetic Dentistry.)

- **adjunctive orthodontics:** Along with selective biomechanical movement, other procedures are taken to facilitate a proper outcome. Selective **enameloplasty** (removal of enamel surface) of adjacent teeth to allow increased space for movement is one. Occasionally, an existing tooth (a premolar on each side) is removed to provide ample space for movement of other teeth.

Orthognathic Surgery as a Team Effort

Other orthodontic procedures that are necessary to correct or restore function include cleft palate surgery, TMJ dysfunction, periodontal damage, pulp changes, closing of diastemas, jaw reduction, or other cranio-maxillofacial problems. This type of treatment called **orthognathic** (or-thug-**NATH**-ic) **surgery** combines the skills of several specialists. Usually the orthodontist's alignment of the teeth is completed along with services of an oral maxillofacial surgeon to reposition jawbones, the prosthodontist to provide prosthetic devices, and the family dentist for dental care of the patient. Other dental and medical specialists may also be involved in this type of surgery. The most common orthognathic surgical procedures involving tooth and jaw irregularities are:

- **open bite:** space between the upper and lower teeth when the mouth is closed.
- **retrognathia:** receding lower jaw or "weak chin."
- **prognathia:** protruding lower jaw, extending jaw.
- **temporomandibular joint dysfunction (TMD):** improper TMJ movement.

After extensive testing, examination (medical, clinical, CT, and 3D i-CAT radiology) photos, and planning, the teeth are orthodontically prepared and stabilized. Oral surgery for bone movement and jaw alignment will follow. The mouth may be temporarily "fixed" or held in place for a short time. Healing and after care will require appointments with all specialists and readjustment of stabilizers as progression occurs. Time involvement is from several months to two or more years; see Figure 15-5.

Figure 15-5 Postoperative 3D i-CAT scan report of jaw augmentation

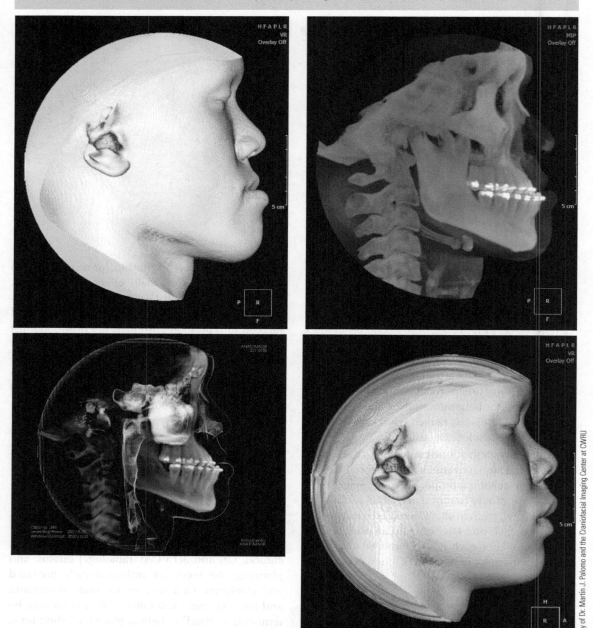

Courtesy of Dr. Martin J. Palomo and the Craniofacial Imaging Center at CWRU

REQUIREMENTS FOR DIAGNOSIS AND TREATMENT PLANNING FOR MALOCCLUSION

Diagnosing the type of malocclusion to enable the identification of subsequent treatment depends on a thorough workup exam that includes the following:

- **patient medical and dental history:** summary of health problems, dental hygiene habits, patient's desire to follow treatment instructions, and care plan for a long time period.
- **clinical examination:** inspection and charting of teeth, soft-tissue condition, and biting ability.
- **photographs (extraoral and intraoral):** photographic record of current condition; used to plan treatment and effective for before and after treatment status. Intraoral views are used for teeth and soft tissue while extraoral views are used to determine skeletal and tissue profile.

- **impression taking:** impressions of both arches and a bite registration are taken for the construction of a study model to be placed on an articulator and used for study and measurements.
- **radiographs:** full mouth series to view tooth conditions, panoramic X-ray exposure for growth projection, **cephalometric (sef**-ah-low-**MEH**-trik = *measurement of the head*) films for skeletal pattern, and possibly 3D i-CAT cone beam computerized tomography for bone depth and condition (see Figure 15-6).

After the workup appointment, the patient returns for a discussion about possible solutions, therapy, time, financial cost/payment, and participation matters. Both parents (if possible) are usually present for a child patient at this time. If any preliminary work such as dental restorations, removal of impacted third molars, or gingival therapy is needed, appointments are made with the appropriate dental provider before beginning orthodontic treatment.

Figure 15-6 Example of cephalometric X-ray used to determine growth measurements

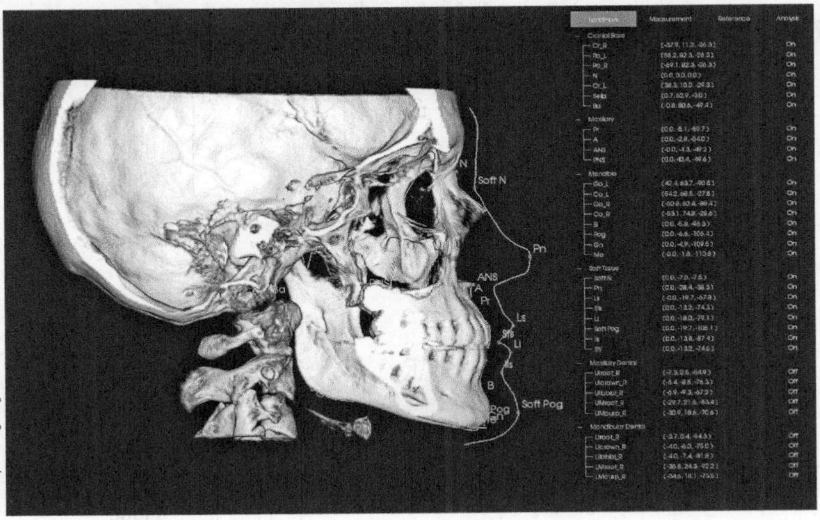

Courtesy of Imagining Sciences, Inc.

INTRAORAL APPLIANCES AND AUXILIARIES USED IN ORTHODONTICS

Treatment of malocclusion is accomplished by applying forces through an intraoral or an extraoral source, or a combination of both. They may be fixed or removable. Retainers, positioners, and habit avoidance devices are examples of removable items. The most common fixed orthodontic appliances, known as "braces," are fixed bands or brackets to which auxiliary devices are applied. Figure 15-7 shows a variety of fixed orthodontic appliances. Some intraoral items used are:

- **bands:** stainless steel circles or rings that are sized and cemented around a tooth. Bands are supplied as maxillary or mandibular in varying sizes, and they may be supplied with or without brackets or tubes attached.
- **bracket** (**BRACK**-et = *support*): a metal, ceramic, composite, or clear resin holding device used to support and stabilize the arch wire in the mouth. To hold the arch wire to the teeth, some brackets require ligatures (thin wires) to be tied around the bracket and the thicker arch wire. The newer brackets are self-ligating and require no ligatures. The arch wire clips into the bracket thus keeping the mouth cleaner and the braces less obvious to viewers. A bracket may be either **soldered** (**SOD**-erd = *joining of two metals*) or spot welded onto an orthodontic band. Other brackets may be cemented directly onto the facial surface of an anterior or posterior tooth and are called **DB** (direct bonded) brackets when cemented onto the pre-etched tooth surface. When more than four teeth are to receive brackets at the same seating, the tray delivery system called indirect bonding may be used.
- **arch wire:** horseshoe-shaped stainless steel or nickel titanium wire that may be round, rectangular, or square and removable or fixed. For the first year, round wires are normally used to move the tooth crown; during the second year, square or rectangular wires are used to move the root of the tooth. The arch wire is attached and held by ligatures to the brackets and tubes, and it maintains a pattern for development.

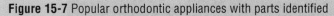

Figure 15-7 Popular orthodontic appliances with parts identified

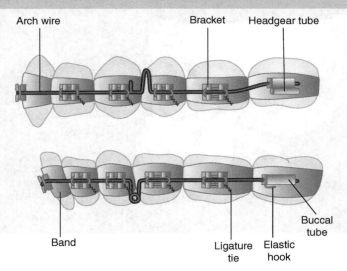

Arch wire   Bracket   Headgear tube

Band   Ligature tie   Elastic hook   Buccal tube

- **buccal tubes:** support devices soldered on bands into which headgear and arch wires are inserted. They also may serve as stabilization for elastics or power devices. Buccal tubes may also be used on molar brackets (pre-cemented or plain). Molar brackets can serve as retainers for arch wires or as stabilizers for spring and rod attachments.
- **button, cleats hooks, eyelets:** devices used for support and holding power devices, elastics, and wires.
- **ligature** (**LIG**-ah-chur = *binder or tie off*): thin, stainless steel wires used to tie on or attach arch wires and any necessary attachments. Ligatures are not needed for self-ligating brackets.
- **elastics:** sized latex circles providing various pull forces or elastomeric ties for holding.
- **auxiliary springs:** noble metal or stainless steel attachment to apply directional force.
- **separators** (**SEP**-ah-ray-tors = *device to set aside*): brass wire, steel springs, or elastomeric materials that are placed between the teeth to obtain space before placing the bands.

TYPES AND PURPOSES OF HEADGEAR AND TRACTION DEVICES

Many cases of corrective orthodontics require the application of external forces to obtain proper movement and alignment. The application of force stimulates the osteoclast cells to resorb the alveolar bone. After the misaligned tooth has moved into the proper place and is retained in that position, the osteoblast cells deposit mineral salts necessary to strengthen the alveolar bone, making the movement permanent. A combination of fixed intraoral appliances and removable extraoral devices is used to apply the proper amount of force. Related terms are:

- **headgear:** device composed of facebow and traction. It is used to apply external force.

- **facebow:** stainless steel external archbow device that is inserted into the fixed molar tubes on the maxillary first molars; the open wing ends extending from the oral cavity are connected with the prepared elastic traction strap devices. The facebow is used to move the molars distal for more anterior space.
- **traction device:** fitted, expandable device to be hooked onto a facebow after placement on the head. The traction device is custom made and placed to achieve desired movement of teeth. Figure 15-8 gives examples of these orthodontic traction devices:

  ○ **cervical device:** circles the patient's neck and attaches to the facebow to pull in a parallel position to retract teeth (see Figure 15-8A).
  ○ **high-pull device:** fits on top of the patient's head and hooks in downward position, perpendicular to occlusion, to retract anterior teeth and control maxillary growth (see Figure 15-8B).
  ○ **combination high-pull and cervical device:** traction combining both forces (see Figure 15-8C).
  ○ **chin device:** placed on the chin; incorporates high-pull and cervical forces and is used to control mandible growth.

In recent years, the popularity of the headgear apparatus has declined, partly because of the patient reluctance for wearing but mostly because of the use of temporary fixed anchoring and *Forsus* Class II correction devices, as described here:

- **temporary anchoring device (TAD):** titanium alloy miniscrew microplant device inserted into the interproximal bone to supply anchorage and a traction hold point; used to upright tilted teeth, open bites, and jaw movements.
- **Class II correction devices:** spring bar that clasps onto the buccal bracket on one end and arch wire placement on the other (see Figure 15-9). The pressure generated on the mandible is constant and provides movement

Figure 15-8 Example of orthodontic traction devices: (A) cervical traction device; (B) high-pull traction device; (C) combination high-pull and cervical traction device

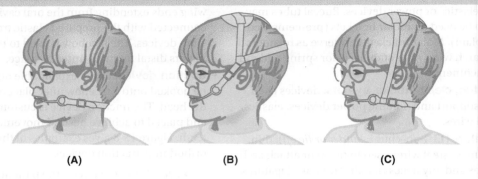

(A)   (B)   (C)

Figure 15-9 A Class II correction device that may replace headgear or traction wear

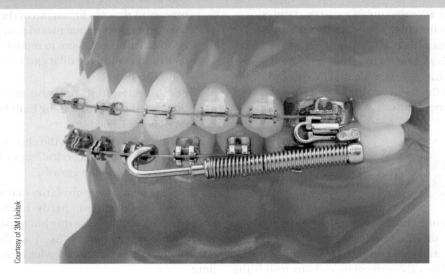

Courtesy of 3M Unitek

faster than with headgear/traction that is worn 20 or so hours a day and removed at times.

ASSORTED AND SPECIALIZED APPLIANCES AND RETAINERS

Each orthodontic treatment case is individualized for the patient. Devices and appliances are developed to accomplish a specific goal. Related terms are:

- **aligner:** an Invisalign system of computer-imaged and computer-generated clear plastic overlay trays used with milder cases of misaligned teeth. The patient wears this removable, personal aligner tray for a designated period of weeks and then progresses to the next tray until movement has been completed, and the teeth are in position.

- **activator:** appliance designed to guide, change, or alter facial and jaw functions for a more favorable occlusion position. Some popular activators such as Anderson and Quad Helix are constructed to conform to an acrylic plate on the inside of the mouth's palate area with bands and springs attached to the teeth.

- **Hawley appliance:** removable, customized, acrylic and wire appliance designed to maintain newly acquired tooth position that is worn at night and sometimes during the day. Newer retainers surround the teeth with clear wire (ASTICS), which are adjusted as need be.

- **Crozat appliance:** removable appliance made of precious alloy with body wires, lingual arms, and a high labial arch wire (maxillary); molar clasps hold the appliance in place.

- **lingual retainer:** mandibular lingual bar with cuspid-to-cuspid cemented unions to maintain lower incisors in position. When extended and attached to the mandibular molar-to-molar areas, it is known as a **lingual arch retainer**; also termed a fixed retainer.

- **orthodontic tooth positioner:** customized mouth tray device constructed of soft acrylic or rubberized material surrounding the crowns of all the teeth in both jaws; worn by the patient to maintain the newly acquired tooth placement until calcification and positioning are assured. They are not adjustable and differ from Invisalign trays that cause movement.

- **palatal expanders:** known as RPE (rapid palatal expanders), a fixed appliance cemented to the maxillary molar teeth with a spring insert in the palate area. The spring is activated by a key rotation to expand the appliance. This expansion applies force that rapidly expands the midpalatal suture and increases the size of the maxilla (see Figure 15-10).

- **fixed space maintainer:** custom-constructed appliance attached to the remaining teeth to hold a tooth pattern or to maintain space from the premature loss of a tooth.

- **nightguard:** removable plastic splint worn at night to lessen the harmful effects of patient's grinding of teeth (bruxism).

Figure 15-10 Rapid palate expander

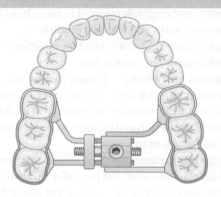

- **mouth guard:** removable custom-made plastic tooth covering piece worn as protection from trauma while engaged in sport activities.

- **oral shield:** device that fits into the vestibule space between the teeth and the lips; helps to train and maintain lip function by correcting habits, strengthening lip action, or correcting mouth-breathing faults.

- **dental appliances:** specialized mouth appliances for health disorders such as sleep apnea, thumb sucking, nail biting, and tongue thrusting.

INSTRUMENTATION FOR THE ORTHODONTIC PRACTICE

Each practice requires specialized tools and instruments to complete assigned tasks. Some of the most popular orthodontic instruments are listed here:

- **band remover pliers:** used to remove bands from teeth.
- **bird-beak pliers:** used to bend and shape appliance wires.
- **loop-forming pliers:** used to form and shape loops in wires.
- **Howe pliers:** used to make arch wire adjustment.
- **three-prong pliers:** used to close or adjust clasps.

- **contouring pliers:** used to contour bands for concave or convex tilt.
- **ligature-tying pliers:** used to tie or bind off ligature wires and to place elastics.
- **arch-forming pliers:** used for bending or holding dimensional wires.
- **stress and tension gauge:** narrow, handheld instrument with interior 1 oz. and 4 oz. smarked sliding scale; used to measure intraoral forces.
- **band seater:** rounded, serrated end is used to "seat" band onto a tooth.
- **ligature tucker:** straight-handled instrument with claw-like end that is used to guide ligatures and assist with the bending of cut wire edges.
- **bracket tweezers:** reverse-action, small-ended tweezers used to place direct bond brackets.
- **ligature cutter:** used to cut ligature wire, intraorally or extraorally.
- **pin and fine wire cutter:** used to cut or snip off ends of tied ligature wires.
- **Weingart utility pliers:** used for placing arch wires.
- **anterior band slitter:** used to shear upper and lower bands.

- **distal end cutter:** used to cut, hold arch wire that was inserted into the buccal tube.
- **band pusher:** used to push and seat bands onto the teeth.
- **ligature director:** used to direct and place ligature wires.
- **scaler:** hand instrument used to remove excess cement from bands, and to direct wires, bands, and elastics into placement.
- **direct bonding bracket holder:** used to hold DBs in position during placement.
- **edgewise pliers:** used to hold or adjust arch wires.
- **hemostat:** scissor-like clamps, straight and curved, which are used to carry or hold small objects.
- **Boone gauge:** measuring device used to establish the height of the orthodontic bands.
- **bite stick:** plastic- or metal-handled instrument with projecting serrated steel area that is used to help "seat" posterior bands.
- **protractor (orthodontic):** triangular premarked form used to make cephalometric tracing.

Review Exercises

Matching

Match the following word elements with their meanings.

1. _____ retainer
2. _____ supraversion
3. _____ centric relationship
4. _____ neutroclusion
5. _____ congenital
6. _____ open bite
7. _____ ligature
8. _____ crossbite

A. Class II malocclusion
B. study of malocclusion prevention and correction
C. midsagittal alignment not in agreement
D. custom device to maintain new tooth position
E. exceeding normal amount
F. tooth over erupted
G. horseshoe-shaped wire used as position pattern
H. Class I malocclusion

9. _____ temporary anchor device

    I. present at birth

10. _____ cephalometric X-ray

    J. tooth leaving arch toward the tongue

11. _____ arch wire

    K. biting on the back teeth

12. _____ orthodontia

    L. thin, stainless steel wire used to tie off or bind

13. _____ supernumerary

    M. anterior teeth do not contact with each other

14. _____ linguoversion

    N. inserted screw peg for traction and holding

15. _____ distoclusion

    O. radiograph for measurement of head

Definitions

Using the selection given for each sentence, choose the best term to complete the definition.

1. An intraoral device used to widen maxilla suture area is a:
   a. palate retainer
   b. Boone gauge
   c. Howe plier
   d. palatal expander

2. Selective removal of tooth tissue to provide interproximal space for tooth movement is:
   a. elongation
   b. osteoplasty
   c. enamelplasty
   d. reduction

3. The classification type of malocclusion that displays a projected mandible is:
   a. Class I
   b. Class II
   c. Class III
   d. Class IV

4. A large X-ray of the head area used to obtain bone measurement is a:
   a. panoramic X-ray
   b. cephalometric X-ray
   c. full mouth set
   d. tomography view

5. Which type of headgear traction device is placed around the patient's neck?
   a. high pull
   b. cervical
   c. combination
   d. facebow

6. Situation where the anterior teeth do not contact with each other or no contact exists between the maxillary and mandibular posterior teeth is:
   a. transversion
   b. closed bite
   c. open bite
   d. distoversion

7. An intraoral device used as a traction post instead of extraoral headgear is:
   a. temporary anchor (TAD)
   b. separator
   c. retainer
   d. Invisalign tray

8. To change a tooth position to a more "upright" direction is an example of:
   a. moving
   b. expanding
   c. rotating
   d. tipping

9. Correction of bad habits or carious conditions is an example of which type of orthodontics?
   a. preventive
   b. interceptive
   c. corrective
   d. base orthodontics

10. An increase of the horizontal distance between incisal edges of central incisors is called:
    a. crossbite
    b. overjet
    c. overbite
    d. open bite

11. Teeth affected by ectopic eruption are:
    a. missing
    b. malpositioned
    c. macrosized
    d. microsized

12. The class of malocclusion that is signified by a protrusive maxillary jaw is:
    a. Class I neuroclusion
    b. Class II distoclusion
    c. Class III mesioclusion

13. Congenital factors for malocclusion are:
    a. present at puberty
    b. a result of trauma
    c. present at birth
    d. a result of habit

14. A corrective treatment device cemented directly on the tooth surface is a/an:
    a. retainer
    b. arch wire
    c. separator
    d. bracket

15. Which of the following is not considered a "force" or power device?
    a. springs
    b. headgear
    c. elastics
    d. tubes

16. Which devices are placed between teeth to make space for placement of bands?
    a. separators
    b. pins
    c. buttons
    d. ligatures

17. A mandibular bar cemented from cuspid to cuspid on the tongue side of the teeth is a/an:
    a. arch wire
    b. activator
    c. lingual retainer
    d. positioner

18. Application of appliances and auxiliaries to improve occlusion is which form of orthodontics?
    a. interceptive
    b. preventive
    c. corrective
    d. base orthodontics

19. A bracket or a band is considered which type of orthodontic appliance?
    a. neutral
    b. extraoral

c. combination
d. intraoral

20. A removable plastic custom fit tray to be worn over the teeth during sports participation is:
    a. mouth guard
    b. space maintainer
    c. nightguard
    d. impression tray

21. A condition of normal jaw position but malpositioned teeth is termed:
    a. Class I neutroclusion
    b. Class II distoclusion
    c. Class III mesioclusion
    d. Class IV inclusion

Building Skills

Locate and define the prefix, root/combining form, and suffix (if present) in the following words.

1. **malocclusion**
   prefix _____
   root/combining form _____
   suffix _____

2. **maxillofacial**
   prefix _____
   root/combining form _____
   suffix _____

3. **mesioclusion**
   prefix _____
   root/combining form _____
   suffix _____

4. **orthodontist**
   prefix _____
   root/combining form _____
   suffix _____

5. **supernumerary**
   prefix _____
   root/combining form _____
   suffix _____

Fill-Ins

Write the correct word in the blank space to complete each statement.

1. A Boone gauge is used to measure the _____ of the bands.

2. Conditions occurring or evident at birth are said to be _____.
3. Classification of the occlusion is made when the teeth are placed in _____ relationship.
4. When maxillary incisors are lingual to mandibular incisors, a condition of _____ exists.
5. _____ orthodontics consists of procedures taken to reduce or eliminate malocclusion.
6. When anterior teeth do not contact with each other, the condition is called _____.
7. The movement of the tooth into the alveolus is termed _____.
8. _____ is the science that deals with the prevention and correction of abnormally positioned teeth and oral structures.
9. Classification of types of malocclusion is credited to Dr. _____.
10. Extra teeth present in the mouth are termed _____ teeth.
11. A tooth in a buccoversion position is moving to the _____ surface.
12. Teeth that have erupted in a malposition or in misalignment are said to result from _____ eruption.
13. Cephalometric radiographs are used to determine measurements of the _____.
14. Stainless steel rings/circles that are cemented onto teeth are orthodontic _____.
15. _____ are thin, stainless steel wires used to tie or bind off.
16. A misalignment between the central incisors of both arches result is a condition called _____.
17. The horseshoe-shaped wire tied onto brackets and tubes to align the teeth into position is called the _____.

18. When a bracket is cemented directly on the surface of the affected teeth, the procedure is termed _____.
19. Myotherapeutic therapy is the elimination of bad habits through _____ healing exercises and therapy.
20. Cleft palate repair is considered to be a type of _____ surgery.

Word Use

Read the following sentences and define the meaning of the word written in boldface letters.

1. The young girl did not like to expose her smile because her **crossbite** made her look unattractive.

   _____

2. **Indirect bonding** of brackets require less patient chair time when placing more than four brackets at a seating.

   _____

3. Some **orthognathic surgeons** donate free services for cleft palate clinics in many underdeveloped countries.

   _____

4. Many adults prefer the **Invisalign** orthodontic treatment because it is faster and less obvious.

   _____

5. The information from the **cephalometric radiograph** is used to measure the growth projection of the head during orthodontic treatment.

   _____

CHAPTER 16 | PERIODONTICS

✔ Learning Objectives

On completion of this chapter, you should be able to:

1. Identify and describe the major tissues comprising the periodontium.

2. Describe the cause of periodontal diseases and the symptoms involved.

3. List the various classes and types of gingivitis and periodontitis.

4. Describe the examination measures required to evaluate periodontal diseases.

5. Discuss the methods used to measure and record various periodontal conditions, and identify and explain the index ratings for tooth and periodontal conditions.

6. Identify the nonsurgical and surgical methods used to care for periodontal problems.

7. Identify the various types of bone implants and cosmetic procedures performed in periodontic dentistry.

8. Explain the use of instruments commonly used in periodontal treatment and care.

Vocabulary Related to Periodontics

This list contains selected new and important word parts and terms from this chapter. Take the time to learn these word parts and their meanings. You may use the list to review these terms and practice pronouncing them correctly. When you work with the audio for this chapter, listen to the word, repeat it, and then place a checkmark in the box. Proceed to the next boxed word, and repeat the process.

(hyphen before word means it's a suffix, hyphen after word means prefix, no hyphen means root word.)

Word Part	Meaning	Word Part	Meaning
gingiv	gum tissue	peri-	around
integra-	forming into one	sub-	under/below
-itis	inflammation	-tion	process/condition
-ology	study of	-trophy	nourishment
osse/oste	bone		

Key Terms

- ❏ allograft (**AL**-oh-graft)
- ❏ antimicrobial (an-tie-my-**KROH**-bee-al)
- ❏ augmentation (awg-men-**TAY**-shun)
- ❏ autograft (**AW**-toh-graft)
- ❏ cribriform (**KRIB**-rih-form)
- ❏ desquamative (des-**KWAM**-ah-tiv)
- ❏ endotoxins (en-doh-**TOCKS**-inz)
- ❏ exudate (**EX**-you-dayt)

- ❏ furcation (fur-**KAY**-shun)
- ❏ hyperplasia (high-per-**PLAY**-zee-ah)
- ❏ hypertrophy (high-per-**TROH**-fee)
- ❏ keratinized (**KARE**-ah-tin-ized)
- ❏ mucogingival (myou-koh-**JIN**-ih-vahl)
- ❏ osseointegration (oss-ee-oh-in-teh-**GRAY**-shun)
- ❏ pellicle (**PELL**-ih-kul)

- ❏ periodontology (pear-ee-oh-dahn-**TAH**-loh-jee)
- ❏ refractory (ree-**FRACK**-tore-ee)
- ❏ somatic (soh-**MAT**-ick)
- ❏ stippling (**STIP**-ling)
- ❏ suppurative (**SUP**-you-rah-tive)
- ❏ vestibuloplasty (ves-**TIB**-you-loh-**plas**-tee)

ANATOMY OF THE PERIODONTIUM

All dentists deal with the periodontal tissues in the course of their treatment, but complicated or complex cases can be referred to a periodontist—a dentist who has completed two to three years of additional education in the treatment of periodontal diseases. **Periodontology** (pear-ee-oh-dahn-**TAH**-loh-jee) is one of the ADA-recognized specialties and is the field of dentistry that deals with the treatment of diseases of the tissues around the teeth, commonly called the **periodontium**. The periodontium serves as an attachment apparatus and is composed of four major tissues (see Figure 16-1): gingival, periodontal ligaments, cementum, and alveolar process.

Gingival

The **gingival** tissues are fibrous, epithelial tissue surrounding a tooth. They may be divided into three types:

- **attached:** the portion that is firm, dense, stippled, and bound to the underlying periosteum, tooth, and bone. The **keratinized** (**KARE**-ah-tin-ized = *hard or horny*) tissue, also called *masticatory* mucosa, where the gingiva and mucous membrane unite, is indicated by the color changes from pink gingiva to red mucosa, and is called the **mucogingival** junction.

- **marginal:** the portion that is unattached to underlying tissues and helps to form the sides of the gingival crevice; also called the *free margin*

Figure 16-1 The tissues of the periodontium

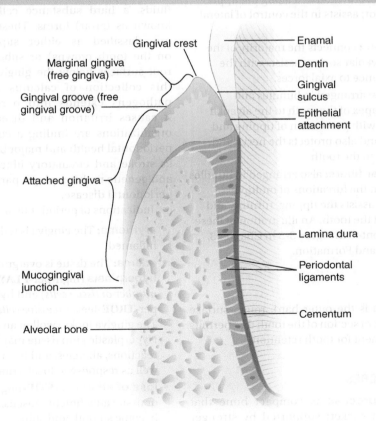

- Gingival crest
- Marginal gingiva (free gingiva)
- Gingival groove (free gingival groove)
- Attached gingiva
- Mucogingival junction
- Alveolar bone
- Enamal
- Dentin
- Gingival sulcus
- Epithelial attachment
- Lamina dura
- Periodontal ligaments
- Cementum

gingiva. It forms the gingival **sulcus** (**SUL**-kus = *groove*), approximately 1 to 3 mm in depth.

- **papillary:** the part of the marginal gingiva that occupies the interproximal spaces. Normally this tissue is triangular and fills the tooth embrasure area, and also is called the **interdental papilla.**

Periodontal Ligaments

The **periodontal ligaments** are bundles of fibers that support and retain the tooth in the alveolar socket. There are five principal types of periodontal membrane fibers:

- **alveolar crest fibers:** located at the cementoenamel junction; assists with the retention of the tooth in its socket and protects the deeper fibers.
- **horizontal fibers:** attached along the upper side of the root; assists in the control of lateral movement.
- **oblique fibers:** connects the majority of the root in the alveolar socket; assists with the tooth's resistance to axial forces.
- **apical fibers:** arranged in bundles and attaches the apex of the tooth to the alveolar bone; assists with prevention of tipping and dislocation, and also protects the nerve and blood supply to the tooth.
- **interradicular fibers:** also arranged in bundles and located in the furcations of multiple rooted teeth; assists the tipping, turning, and dislocation of the tooth. An illustration of these fibers is presented in Figure 3-5 in Chapter 3, Tooth Origin and Formation.

Cementum

The **cementum** is the outer hard, rough surface covering of the root section of the tooth that permits the fiber attachment for tooth retention.

Alveolar Process

The **alveolar process** is compact bone that forms the tooth socket; supported by stronger bone tissue of the mandible and maxilla and accepts periodontal fiber attachment. The alveolar process makes up the **cribriform** (**KRIB**-rih-form = *sieve-like*) plate to form and line the tooth socket. This outline is called **lamina dura** (**LAM**-ih-nah = *lining, thin layer*) and is easily viewed on radiographs.

ETIOLOGY AND SYMPTOMS OF PERIODONTAL DISEASES

In the etiology of problems affecting the periodontium, the major contributing factors are **plaque** (**PLACK** = *plate or buildup*) and **calculus** (**KAL**-kyou-lus). Teeth acquire an adhering biofilm or **pellicle** (**PELL**-ih-kul), which harbors an assortment of bacterial pathogens and enables plaque to build up. With the addition of calcium and phosphorus salts found in saliva and mouth fluids, a hard substance called calculus (also known as tartar) forms. These gingival irritants are classified as either supragingival (found on the tooth crowns) or subgingival (found on root surfaces below the gingival margin). When this collection of calculus and plaque with pathogens extends into periodontal pockets, it causes irritation and disease. Many health organizations are finding a correlation between periodontal health and major body diseases, such as stroke and circulatory illnesses. Tobacco use and genetic makeup play a part in the chances of periodontal disease.

Indications of periodontal disease are:

- **erythema:** The gingiva is red and appears inflamed.
- **edema:** The tissue is overgrown from **hyperplasia** (high-per-**PLAY**-zee-ah = *excessive number of tissue cells*) and **hypertrophy** (high-per-**TROE**-fee = *excessive cellular growth*). The gingiva looks swollen and irritated. Hyperplastic gum tissue may be caused by drug reactions, allergies, and hormonal changes, as well as response to local irritants and disease.
- **loss of stippling** (**STIP**-ling = *spotting*): Tone or tissue attachment loosens, and puffy gums become smooth and shiny.

- **pocket formation:** Gingiva is unattached, recession occurs, and the root may be observed.
- **alveolar bone loss with exudate** (**EX**-you-dayt = *passing out of pus*): A foul odor is present as supporting bone resorbs; retention is lessening.
- **mobility:** The tooth seems loose and moves under pressure because of loss of attachment. The tooth eventually is lost from lack of support or from extraction.

CLASSIFICATION OF PERIODONTAL DISEASES

Periodontal diseases can be divided into two main divisions:

1. Gingivitis, an inflammation of gingival tissue with no supporting tissue loss
2. Periodontitis, inflammation of gingival tissue with involvement of other tissues of the periodontium

Destruction of these tissues varies in degree, intensity, and overall action. To identify each stage and type of periodontal involvement, the American Academy of Periodotology (AAP) devised the following classification system for periodontal diseases.

Gingival Disease

- **Dental plaque involvement:** (most common) Tissues react to irritants.
- **Dental plaque with systemic factors:** These factors include pregnancy, hormone, medication, or malnutrition and may modify and intensify the disease course of action; sometimes called *induced gingivitis.*
- **Nondental plaque tensions:** These are of specific bacterial, viral, fungal, or genetic origin, such as gonorrhea, herpes, HIV, and candida infections.
- **Allergies:** The patient may be allergic to dental-restorative materials and have reactions to food, additives, and so forth.
- **Traumatic lesions, injury:** The patient may have been subjected to an external force or have been injured in some way.

Periodontal Disease

- **Chronic periodontitis:** Previously termed *adult periodontitis*, this is the most common type of slowly progressive periodontal disease. May be subdivided according to extent and severity into localized with less than 30% involvement and generalized with more than 30% involvement. Severity is measured based on the amount of clinical attachment loss (CAL) as slight, moderate, or severe.
- **Aggressive periodontitis:** Previously termed *early-onset periodontitis*, this is a rapidly progressive disease, with dramatic bone detachment affecting a specific area. It is subclassified into localized and generalized.
- **Refractory periodontitis:** The periodontitis progresses in spite of excellent patient compliance and provision of periodontal therapy. It may be applied to all types of periodontitis. Tissues that are painful, red, and sloughing are said to be **desquamative** (des-**KWAM**-ah-tiv = *shedding, or scaling off*).
- **Periodontitis as manifested of systemic disease:** Periodontal inflammatory reactions occur as a result of diseases and genetic disorders, such as leukemia, HIV, malnutrition, and hormones.
- **Necrotizing periodontal diseases:** Rapid gingival tissue destruction with bacterial invasion of connective tissue may be a manifestation of systemic disease, such as HIV infection. This category is subdivided into two divisions:
  - **Necrotizing ulcerative gingivitis (NUG):** This creates a foul odor and a loss of interdental papilla, sometimes called "trench mouth" (see Figure 16-2A).
  - **Necrotizing ulcerative periodontitis (NUP):** This presents with bone pain and rapid bone loss (see Figure 16-2B).

Figure 16-2 (A) Necrotizing ulcerative gingivitis, (B) X-ray evidence of significant bone loss around molar tooth.

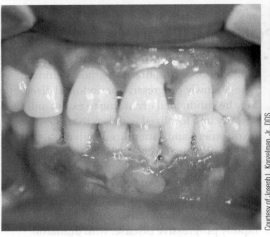

(A)

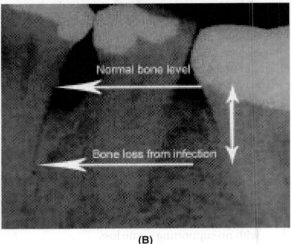

Normal bone level

Bone loss from infection

(B)

- **Abscesses of the periodontium:** Abscesses are classified according to location, such as gingival, periodontal, and pericoronal.
- **Periodontitis associated with endodontic lesions:** This simple classification was added to distinguish between periodontitis and periodontitis with endodontic inflammation involvement.
- **Developmental or acquired deformities and condition:** Deformities appear around teeth, edentulous ridges, and from trauma.

PERIODONTAL EXAMINATION AND EVALUATION

The patient must receive a thorough exam and evaluation before treatment can be established. This procedure involves:

- **medical history:** questions regarding diabetes, pregnancy, smoking, hypertension, dedication, substance abuse, and so forth.
- **dental history:** chief complaint, past dental records and radiographs, complete assessment of restoration condition, tooth position, mobility.

- **extraoral structure assessment:** exam of oral mucosa, muscles of mastication, lips, floor of mouth, tongue, palate, salivary glands, and the oropharynx area.
- **periodontal probing depth:** charting and recording findings of probe depths, assessing plaque and calculus presence, soft tissue, and implant conditions.
- **assessing intraoral findings:** exam for tori palatinus or tori mandibularis growths, abnormal frenum placement and size, and furcation involvement.

MEASUREMENT AND RECORDING OF PERIODONTAL CONDITIONS

The periodontal examination involves charting and recording tooth conditions and the status of the oral mucosa, particularly the periodontium. Prior to the perio exam, the teeth receive a **prophylaxis** (proh-fil-**LACK**-sis = *scaling, root planing, and polishing of teeth*). The professional cleaning of teeth involves the *scaling* or scraping off of calculus. This is usually accomplished by hand instruments and ultrasonic scaling tips that vibrate and remove the hard deposits from above the gingival crest (supragingival) and below the gingival crest (subgingival). Deposits in the periodontal pockets around the root area are planed by curettage or ultrasonic tips. The combination of the two processes is termed *scaling and root planing* (SRP) and is followed with a polishing by a slow handpiece with rubber cups or air polishers that spray a force of abrasive powder to cleanse the surfaces. Completion of this process leads to the periodontal survey.

Clinical examination requires obtaining and recording an **index** (**IN**-decks = *measurement of conditions to a standard*), which rates the status of a particular subject and provides a method to measure the progress of the tested item, such as bleeding or plaque.

To be effective, the index procedure must be followed for each patient, and the same method must be used from one dental source to another. Different indices apply to different conditions. The common indexes used in periodontics cover plaque, oral hygiene, calculus, debris, periodontal pocket depth, bleeding, grade mobility, root furcation, gingival margin, periodontal disease, and suppurative (pus) involvement, among others. Each practice will choose those measurements, which are considered most indicative, such as calculus, bleeding, and tissue attachment. To obtain measurements for indices, the dentist or hygienist will use a periodontal probe to insert into the gingival sulcus and record the findings.

The Periodontal Probe

The most common instrument used in measuring is the **periodontal probe**, a round- or flat-bladed hand instrument marked in millimeter increments. The probe tip is inserted into six specific areas with the deepest pocket marking measurement recorded for that spot. The six areas are facial (F), mesiofacial (MF), distofacial (DF), lingual (L), mesiolingual (ML), and distolingual (DL). Also available for measurement is an electronic probe such as the DiagnoPen with a perio probe that indicates the pocket condition after the teeth have been scaled and planed (Figure 16-3):

- <5 indicates clean gingival pockets.
- 4–40 indicates little calculus or residual calculus left.
- >40 indicates calculus in gingival pockets.

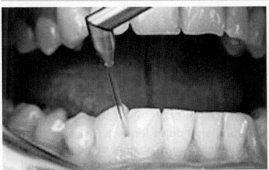

Figure 16-3 Perio point on DiagnoPen used to determine pocket condition after scaling and root planing

Courtesy of KaVo Dental

Measurements may be handwritten by the operator, dictated to a recording assistant, or spoken to a voice recorder that transmits the findings to a perio chart. When pocket markings are finished and recorded, the depths are connected by a continuous line giving a visual indication of the gingival crest, indicating the heights of the interdental papilla, and the depths of gingival pockets, including furcation involvement. Dental radiographs are examined to determine bone resorption and loss. The tooth is palpated and tested for mobility, and the patient's health history is reviewed and discussed.

PERIODONTAL TREATMENT METHODS

Treatments for periodontal conditions vary with the severity of the disease. Treatment may be of a nonsurgical nature, conducted in the dental office with a program of home care, or it may involve extensive surgical care.

Nonsurgical Treatment of the Periodontium

The nonsurgical treatment of periodontal irregularities and diseases involves a variety of procedures and therapies.

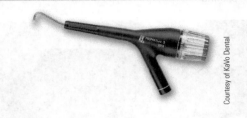

Courtesy of KaVo Dental

- **prophylaxis debridement:** removing supragingival and subgingival plaque, calculus, stain, and irritants through tooth-crown and root-surface scaling and root planing (SRP). This treatment usually involves ultrasonic tip scaling and hand instrumentation.

- **tooth and surface polishing:** polishing surfaces to remove accumulated **extrinsic** (ex-**TRIN**-sick = *outer*) stains on the tooth surface and **endotoxins** (**en**-doh-**TOCKS**-inz = *absorbed pathogens*) on the accessible surfaces. This treatment can be completed using air polishers, abrasive cleansing, and handpiece application of nonabrasive rubber cups and points with polishing paste or powder (see Figure 16-4).

- **selective polishing:** term applied to the polishing of chosen tooth sites or areas.

- **prophylaxis:** term applied to the combination of debridement and tooth polishing; used for purposes of insurance and scheduling. Tooth aids such as flossing and bridge cleaners, perio brushes, and the like are applied and used in necessary attention areas to complete a thorough cleansing.

- **patient education:** customized instruction in oral hygiene; the care of teeth and gingival tissue.

- **antimicrobial** (an-tie-my-**KROH**-bee-al = *against small life*) **therapy:** includes prescription mouthwashes (chlorhexidine digluconate); over-the-counter mouthwashes; systemic antibiotics such as tetracycline,

penicillin, clindamycin, erythromycin, and metronidazole medicines; and local delivery systems to the site using a gel pack, syringe insertion, or gelatin chip containing antimicrobial products. A new method called *Perio Protect* offers an antimicrobial medicated application in a custom-made patient tray for patient application.

- **occlusal adjustment:** selective grinding of occlusal cusps to eliminate premature contact.

- **tooth stabilization:** splinting, wire ligation, or bonding of teeth to lessen tooth mobility.

- **occlusal guards:** custom-formed acrylic night guard to protect from tooth grinding.

Periodontal Surgery Techniques

Various specialized surgical treatments are applied in cases of extensive disease of the periodontium. Surgery may involve periodontal knives, instruments, and scalpels. Lately, laser incision with controlled power levels and selected wavelengths to lessen bleeding, swelling, and discomfort is becoming more popular. Some procedures are:

- **mucogingival excision:** used to correct defects in shape, position, or amount of gingiva around the tooth; eliminates the pocket formation and **pericoronitis** typically found on erupting third molars.

- **gingivectomy:** excision of pocket tissue areas. One end of a pocket marker is inserted the entire depth of the pocket and squeezed until the opposite pointed tip penetrates the gingiva, thereby marking a setting for a surgical template pattern. Necrotic tissue is excised and removed.

- **gingivoplasty:** instrumental or laser surgical contour of gingival tissue to remove excessive tissue or pellicle edges.

- **periodontal flap surgery:** a loosened section of tissue is separated from the adjacent tissues to enable elimination of deposits and contouring of alveolar bone. The several types of flap surgery are:

- **envelope flap:** no vertical incision with the mucoperiosteal flap retracted from a horizontal incision line.
- **mucoperiosteal:** mucosal tissue flap, including the periosteum, reflected from the bone; also called full thickness flap.
- **partial thickness flap:** surgical flap, including mucosa and connective tissue but no periosteum.
- **pedicle flap:** tissue flap with lateral incisions.
- **positioned flap:** flap that is moved to a new position apically, laterally, or coronally.
- **repositioned flap:** surgical flap replaced into its original position.
- **sliding flap:** pedicle flap resituated to a new position.

- **osseous surgery:** tissue surgery with alteration in bony support of the teeth.
- **re-entry:** second-stage surgical procedure to enhance or improve conditions from a previous surgical procedure.
- **vestibuloplasty** (ves-**TIB**-you-loh-**plas**-tee): surgical alteration of the gingival mucous membrane in the vestibule of the mouth, including frenum reposition or frenectomy and change in muscle attachment.
- **ENAP (excisional new attachment procedure):** removal of chronically inflamed soft tissue to permit formation of new tissue attachment.
- **guided tissue regeneration:** placement of a semipermeable membrane (Gore-Tex) beneath the flap to prevent ingrowth of epithelium between the flap and the defect; encourages the growth of new periodontal attachment. See an example of tissue surgery in Figure 16-5.

Periodontal dressing packs are placed over the surgical site to assist with protection and healing. These packs are mixed, prepared, and

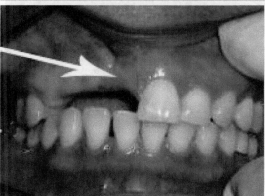

Figure 16-5 One type of periodontal surgery is restoration and adjustment of marginal ridge

Courtesy of Dr. Louis Poulos (www.drpoulosperio.com)

expressed on the surgical site. They are supplied in four ways:

1. Zinc oxide and eugenol powder and liquid are mixed to a paste, rolled, and pressed over the site.
2. Zinc oxide paste and a non-eugenol base paste are mixed together and applied to the area.
3. Syringe-dispensed periodontal paste is expressed on the site and light cured.
4. Gelatin packs dissolve and do not need to be removed.

Bone Grafting

Some periodontal surgical techniques require bone tissues. **Bone grafts** involve transplants to restore bone from periodontal disease (Figure 16-6). Related terms are:

- **allograft** (**AL**-oh-graft): human bone graft from someone other than the patient.
- **autograft** (**AW**-toh-graft): bone graft from another site in the same patient.
- **xenograft** (**ZEE**-no-graft): graft taken from another species, such as cow or pig bone (experimental).
- **allogenic** (al-loh-**JEN**-ick): addition of synthetic material to repair or build up bone.

Figure 16-6 Before-and-after examples of bone-grafting success

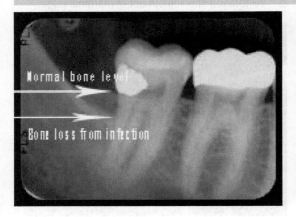
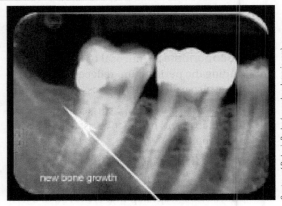

PERIODONTAL INVOLVEMENT WITH DENTAL IMPLANTS AND COSMETIC DENTISTRY

In addition to treatment of the gingiva and periodontium of the mouth, the periodontist performs a variety of tissue and bone augmentations or reductions needed for a functional or cosmetic improvement. Some of these procedures used to provide optimal dental care are listed in the following subsections.

Dental Implants

Dental implants are titanium or ceramic devices that are surgically placed into the alveolar bone to provide firm, fixed anchors for dental appliances or dentures. The bone and the implant complete a process of uniting called **osseointegration** (**oss**-ee-oh-in-teh-**GRAY**-shun = *union of bone and device*). Implants are explained and illustrated in Chapter 14, Oral and Maxillofacial Surgery, and terminology relevant to periodontics is defined here:

- **endosteal:** implants of various designs placed within the bone.
- **subperiosteal:** implant placement beneath the periosteum and onto the bone.
- **transosteal:** implant placement through the bone.

- **endodontic:** the implant is set within the apex of the root.

Periodontal cleaning and scaling procedures performed on implants must be completed with plastic, sonic instruments, or the newer titanium scalers to protect the implants from surface scratching.

Cosmetic Dentistry

Some treatments performed in a periodontist's practice are used for cosmetic purposes to complete the treatment plan or to improve the esthetic appearance of the patient. Some of these procedures are:

- **crown lengthening:** removal of excessive gingival covering tooth enamel in the sulcus area. May be done to gain access to areas of decay for restoration work or to remove a "gummy smile" appearance for esthetic reasons (see Figure 16-7).
- **soft tissue graft:** periodontal flap coverage of exposed root areas or repair of pocket damage.
- **pocket reduction:** eliminate collection area from pocket position; may include bone grafts.
- **ridge augmentation:** bone graft inserts to reshape to the natural contour of gingival and alveolar bone.

Figure 16-7 An example of a functional crown-lengthening treatment: (A) view of decayed tooth, (B) tooth prepared for crown with gingiva shortened, (C) completed crown placement on prepared tooth with crown lengthening

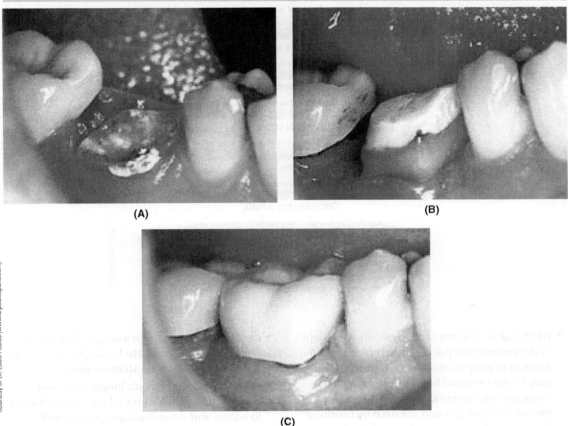

(A) (B)

(C)

Courtesy of Dr. Louis Poulos (www.drpoulossperio.com)

- **sinus augmentation:** raising the floor of the sinus cavity and building bone replacement may be necessary for placement of maxillary implants in cosmetic surgery.
- **combination procedures:** union of more than one procedure to achieve cosmetic effect.

INSTRUMENTATION FOR PERIODONTICS

Periodontal treatment requires specialized instruments, most of which are hand instruments, although ultrasonic, sonic, laser, and power-driven tools are also part of the necessary setup.

Periodontal Hand Instruments

Hand instruments employed in periodontal treatment, illustrated in Figure 16-8, are used in a push or pull method to accomplish a desired outcome. Push instruments use a push stroke direction with a blade-to-tooth angle of less than 45 degrees perpendicular to the instrument's shaft. An example is the chisel. Pull instruments use a pull stroke direction with a blade-to-tooth angle of between 45 and 90 degrees perpendicular to the instrument's shaft. The most effective pull angle is approximately 75 degrees. Examples include scalers, curettes, hoes, and files. Hand instruments are:

Figure 16-8 Assortment of periodontal hand instruments

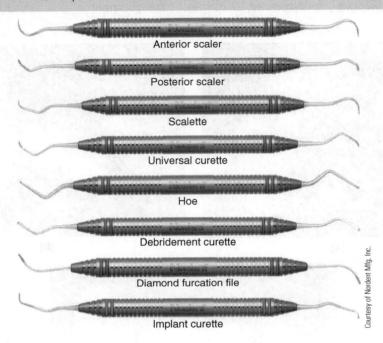

Anterior scaler

Posterior scaler

Scalette

Universal curette

Hoe

Debridement curette

Diamond furcation file

Implant curette

Courtesy of Nordent Mfg. Inc.

- **periodontal probe:** used to measure the depth of the periodontal pocket by determining the amount of gingival tissue attachment. A probe may be flat or round bladed and is marked in measured increments. Automatic periodontal probes are available and are used by inserting the probe wire into the sulcus area to determine and record the measurement on a computer.
- **explorer:** instrument with a longer, tapered, thin wire tip to determine calculus formation, restoration overhangs, and any root **furcation** involvement.
- **scaler:** instrument with a sharpened blade to remove supragingival calculus deposits and stains. Scalers are available in various shapes such as sickle for universal use, straight for anterior areas, and contra-angled for posterior areas.
- **hoe:** instrument with a long shank and a hoe-like tip; used to remove heavy or thick supragingival calculus in posterior areas.

- **chisel:** instrument with a longer shaft and a chisel-bladed tip; used to break off and remove heavy calculus in the anterior region.
- **curette:** instrument with longer shaft and working end with a rounded toe and back edge to access and remove subgingival deposits. A **universal** curette has a cutting edge on each side of the blade to enable use in all areas. Other curettes are designed for specific areas, such as the Gracey curettes with a cutting edge on one side of the blade.
- **file:** hand instrument with multiple cutting edges; used to smooth off rough and uneven tissues and remove stubborn calculus deposits.
- **ultrasonic and sonic instrument tip:** inserted into the ultrasonic handle; sonic forces move the tip in rapid, short (0.001 inch) waves at speed frequencies of 20,000 to 35,000 vibrations per second to break apart and dislodge deposits from the tooth surface. The tips or inserts are designed for specific areas and designated use.

Machine tips are cooled with a water spray to lessen friction heat. Some handpieces have light sources for better viewing.

Polishing Instruments

Instruments used to polish the tooth surfaces include straight handpieces, prophylaxis contra-angles, and rubber cups as well as polishing agents, such as pumice, cleaners, and chemically impregnated rubber points. Polishing and stain removal is completed by using an air-power-driven calcium carbonate powder spray unit or a slow handpiece rotary rubber cup with pumice.

Surgical Periodontal Instruments

The following are instruments used in surgery:

- **periodontal pocket marker:** set of instruments similar to tweezers with a sharp point on one tip for insertion into the depth of the pocket and then compressed to make puncture marks indicating pocket depth. There is one marker for each side of the pocket.
- **periodontal knives:** used to make incisions for removal of tissue or to obtain flap design. Blade shape may be round or pointed and long edged.
- **electrosurgery tips/unit:** apparatus using electrical current to incise tissue and coagulate blood at the same time; useful in periodontal flap, tissue grafting, crown lengthening, and other tissue surgeries.
- **laser tip/unit:** apparatus delivering energy in light form at different wavelengths; can be used in soft or hard tissue curettage surgery when regulated to the specific bacterial target.

Review Exercises

Matching

Match the following word elements with their meanings.

1. _____ papillary gingiva
2. _____ gingivectomy
3. _____ file
4. _____ allograft
5. _____ debridement
6. _____ transosteal implant
7. _____ sulcus
8. _____ endodontic implant
9. _____ furcation
10. _____ periodontal probe
11. _____ periodontal pocket marker
12. _____ prophylaxis
13. _____ etiology
14. _____ autograft
15. _____ keratinized gingiva

A. free marginal gingiva

B. used to measure depth of attached gingiva

C. professional cleaning of teeth

D. removal of subgingival and supragingival calculus

E. implant placed within apex of tooth root

F. hard gingival tissue called masticatory mucosa

G. hand instrument with rasp edges

H. bone graft from another site on the same patient

I. used to mark depth of tissue pocket for excision

J. marginal gingiva occupying interproximal space

K. branching or forking of tooth roots

L. implant placed through the mandibular bone

M. excision and removal of gingival tissue

N. bone graft from person other than patient

O. study of the cause of a disease

Definitions

Using the selection given for each sentence, choose the best term to complete the definition.

1. Transplanting bone to restore bone lost from periodontal disease is termed:
   a. osteoplasty
   b. bone graft
   c. bone therapy
   d. osseotectomy

2. Splinting, wire ligating, or bonding of teeth together are forms of tooth:
   a. stabilization
   b. mobility
   c. transplantation
   d. adjustment

3. Increase in the size of affected gingiva is termed:
   a. hypertrophy
   b. hypotrophy
   c. hypoextension
   d. hyperextension

4. Scraping or flaking off of any hard deposits or accumulated stain on tooth surfaces is:
   a. prophylaxis
   b. scaling
   c. root planing
   d. tooth polishing

5. Cleansing and shining of tooth surfaces and exposed tooth tissue is termed:
   a. prophylaxis
   b. scaling
   c. root planing
   d. tooth polishing

6. Which is not considered a periodontal pull hand instrument?
   a. periodontal probe
   b. scaler
   c. curette
   d. hoe

7. A bone graft insertion to provide a more natural ridge for dentures is termed:
   a. soft-tissue graft
   b. crown exposure

   c. ridge augmentation
   d. pocket reduction

8. A surgical flap replaced into its original position is what type of flap surgery?
   a. sliding
   b. pellicle
   c. partial
   d. repositioned flap

9. Which record is not considered an indexing recording of conditions?
   a. calculus
   b. bleeding
   c. radiograph
   d. stain

10. Another term for the common name "trench mouth" is:
    a. halitosis
    b. gingivitis
    c. ANUG
    d. periodontia

11. Hard substances formed from calcium and phosphorus salts and deposited on teeth are called:
    a. stains
    b. calculus
    c. plaque
    d. pellicle

12. Interradicular periodontal fibers may be found around which teeth?
    a. incisors
    b. cuspids
    c. bicuspids
    d. molars

13. Which is not considered a tissue of the periodontium?
    a. gingiva
    b. alveolar bone
    c. dentin
    d. cementum

14. Which of the following is not considered a periodontal index factor?
    a. bleeding
    b. color
    c. root furcation
    d. pocket depth

15. What is considered the proper amount of probe sites per tooth for pocket data?
    a. 1
    b. 2
    c. 4
    d. 6

16. Painful, red, sloughing gingival epithelium is called:
    a. irritated
    b. desquamative
    c. gingivitis
    d. refractory

17. Which of the following is not a symptom of gingivitis?
    a. redness
    b. mobility
    c. foul odor
    d. coral stippling

18. Calculus deposits found on the exposed coronal surfaces of the teeth are termed:
    a. coronal
    b. scaler
    c. subgingival
    d. supragingival

19. Selective grinding of occlusal edges of cuspids to eliminate premature contact is:
    a. occlusal guarding
    b. occlusal adjustment
    c. tooth stabilization
    d. cuspid alignment

20. The periodontium tissue that makes up the tooth socket is:
    a. alveolar bone
    b. gingiva
    c. periodontal fibers
    d. gums

Building Skills

Locate and define the prefix, root/combining form, and suffix (if present) in the following words.

1. **periodontology**
   prefix _____
   root/combining form _____
   suffix _____

2. **osseointegration**
   prefix _____
   root/combining form _____
   suffix _____

3. **subperiosteal**
   prefix _____
   root/combining form _____
   suffix _____

4. **hypertrophy**
   prefix _____
   root/combining form _____
   suffix _____

5. **gingivitis**
   prefix _____
   root/combining form _____
   suffix _____

Fill-Ins

Write the correct word in the blank space to complete each statement.

1. The _____ is a periodontal hand instrument with a longer shaft and neck to access subgingival areas.

2. The chisel is used to break off and remove heavy calculus deposits in the _____ region.

3. The major contributing factor to diseases of the periodontium is _____ formation.

4. Pus formation in a pocket area is called pocket _____.

5. An adhering tooth film that lacks the sticking quality of plaque is called _____ film.

6. Hard-tissue gingiva, also known as masticatory mucosa, is _____ gingiva.

7. The _____ is comprised of the tissue surrounding the teeth.

8. _____ gingiva is unattached to the underlying tissues and forms the gingival crevice.

9. Scalpels, lasers, and _____ are used to incise gingival tissue.

10. Periodontal instruments that vibrate rapidly using little strokes to break away deposits are called _____ instruments.

11. The uniting of the implant and bone tissue is a process called _____.

12. Using a bone graft taken from another species is termed a/an _____.

13. A/an _____ implant is placed under the periosteum and onto the bone.

14. A periodontal instrument used in a pushing motion should have less than a _____ degree angle on the blade.

15. The use of prescription mouthwashes and treated fibers to destroy microbes is termed _____ therapy.

16. The selective grinding of occlusal cusps to prevent premature contacts is _____.

17. Acrylic nightguards worn to protect from tooth grinding are called _____.

18. Polishing selected teeth during a prophylaxis is termed _____.

19. _____ refers to the procedure of contouring gingival tissue.

20. The measure of a condition to determine standards is called a/an _____.

Word Use

Read the following sentences, and define the meaning of the word written in boldface letters.

1. The dentist explained to Mrs. Bailey that her **induced gingivitis** is only temporary and will cease after the delivery of her baby.

   _____

2. Dr. Goldenberg's office called to arrange an appointment for a **gingivoplasty** procedure for her patient.

   _____

3. One of the treatment plan procedures for the ANUG patient involves **antimicrobial therapy**.

   _____

4. The dental hygienist uses a periodontal probe to establish the extent of the **marginal gingiva**.

   _____

5. The laboratory returned the study cast and the **occlusal guard** they have prepared for Mr. Mason.

   _____

CHAPTER 17 | PEDIATRIC DENTISTRY

✔ Learning Objectives

On completion of this chapter, you should be able to:

1. Discuss the practice and duties of a pedodontist and the types of teeth involved with children's dentistry.

2. List and identify the common concerns related to children's dental care.

3. Describe the preventive, operative, and home-care procedures provided to the deciduous teeth.

4. Discuss the restorative care given the primary dentition, and explain the various pulp-treatment procedures available.

5. Explain the need for control and/or sedation of the child patient and the methods employed to accomplish this state.

6. List and explain the classifications and treatment methods for fractured and traumatized teeth.

7. Discuss the various methods used to establish patient identification from the use of dental and personal records.

8. Identify the common childhood diseases that may affect the development and condition of the human dentition.

SCOPE OF PEDIATRIC DENTISTRY

Pediatric dentistry is one of the nine recognized specialties of the American Dental Association and is concerned with the care of the teeth and oral tissues of the child patient, from birth through adolescence. The dentist specializing in this practice is called a **pedodontist** and has completed dental school with an additional two years of concentrated training in the psychology,

Vocabulary Related to Pediatrics

This list contains selected new and important word parts and terms from this chapter. Take the time to learn these word parts and their meanings. You may use the list to review these terms and practice pronouncing them correctly. When you work with the audio for this chapter, listen to the word, repeat it, and then place a checkmark in the box. Proceed to the next boxed word, and repeat the process.

(hyphen before word means it's a suffix, hyphen after word means prefix, no hyphen means root word.)

Word Part	Meaning	Word Part	Meaning
gnath	jaw	nato	birth
intra-	within	neo-	new
implant	to insert	oma	tumor
micro-	small	re-	again
musc	muscle	-ular	relating to

Key Terms

- ❏ **amelogenesis imperfecta** (ah-**meal**-oh-**JEN**-ih-sis im-pur-**FECK**-tah)
- ❏ **ankylosed** (**ANG**-kihl-lowzd)
- ❏ **anodontia** (an-oh-**DON**-she-ah)
- ❏ **apexification** (ay-pecks-ih-fih-**KAY**-shun)
- ❏ **aplasia** (ah-**PLAY**-zee-ah)
- ❏ **candidiasis** (kan-dih-**DYE**-ah-sis)
- ❏ **cherubism** (**CHAIR**-you-bizm)

(Continued)

Vocabulary Related to Pediatrics *continued*

Key Terms *continued*

- ❑ **dentinogenesis** (den-tin-oh-**JEN**-eh-sis)
- ❑ **imperfecta** (im-per-**FECK**-tuh)
- ❑ **diastema** (dye-ah-**STEE**-mah)
- ❑ **enamoplasty** (ee-**NAM**-oh-**plas**-tee)
- ❑ **exfoliation** (ecks-foh-lee-**AY**-shun)
- ❑ **fissure** (**FISH**-er)
- ❑ **frenectomy** (freh-**NECK**-toh-me)
- ❑ **hyperdontia** (high-per-**DAHN**-she-ah)
- ❑ **hypodontia** (high-poh-**DAHN**-she-ah)

- ❑ **hypoplasia** (high-poh-**PLAY**-zee-ah)
- ❑ **infraorbital** (in-frah-**OR**-bih-tal)
- ❑ **intraligamentary** (in-trah-lig-ah-**MEN**-tah-ree)
- ❑ **intramuscular** (in-tra-**MUSS**-kyou-lahr)
- ❑ **intravenous** (in-trah-**VEE**-nus)
- ❑ **lymphangioma** (lim-fan-jee-**OH**-mah)
- ❑ **lymphoma** (lim-**FOH**-mah)
- ❑ **macrodontia** (mack-roh-**DAHN**-she-ah)
- ❑ **macroglossia** (mack-roh-**GLOSS**-ee-ah)

- ❑ **micrognathia** (my-kroh-**NAY**-thee-ah)
- ❑ **mucocele** (**MYOU**-koh-seal)
- ❑ **neurofibromatosis** (new-roh-fie-**broh**-mah-**TOH**-sis)
- ❑ **odontoma** (oh-dahn-**TOH**-mah)
- ❑ **scorbutic** (skor-**BYOU**-tick)
- ❑ **subcutaneous** (sub-kyou-**TAY**-nee-us)
- ❑ **submucosal** (sub-mew-**COH**-sul)
- ❑ **supraperiosteal** (soo-prah-pear-ee-**OSS**-tee-ahl)
- ❑ **verruca vulgaris** (ver-**OO**-kah vul-**GAIR**-iss)

management, growth development, health issues, and sedation of the child patient.

The first set of teeth to erupt is called the primary dentition. This combination consists of 20 **deciduous** teeth, which will be replaced by secondary or permanent teeth, plus 12 more adult teeth. The dental treatment and care given in pediatric dentistry is essentially the same as for adults, although instruments and some techniques may be modified.

DEVELOPMENT AND GROWTH CONCERNS OF THE PEDIATRIC DENTITION

Many of the dental problems of the child patient are the result of improper or irregular development of newly erupting teeth. Some congenital problems occur during the growth period in utero and are evident at birth or later when the teeth erupt, and others can happen when environment and habits affect the teeth.

Congenital or developmental problems may be:

- **ectopic arrangement:** a disturbance in the eruption pattern; tooth erupts out of place.
- **anodontia:** absence of teeth, usually of genetic origin.
- **macrodontia** (**mack**-roh-**DAHN**-she-ah): abnormally large teeth.
- **cleft palate or lip:** fissure of an organ; incomplete juncture.
- **hyperdontia** (high-per-**DAHN**-she-ah): excess number of supernumerary teeth.
- **hypodontia** (high-poh-**DAHN**-she-ah): congenital absence of teeth.
- **enamel hypoplasia:** underdevelopment of the enamel tissue.
- **dentinogenesis imperfecta:** incomplete or improper development of dentin tissue.
- **amelogenesis imperfecta** (ah-**meal**-oh-**JEN**-ih-sis, im-purr-**FECK**-tah): incomplete or improper development of the enamel tissue.
- **aplasia** (ah-**PLAY**-zee-ah): failure of an organ or body part to develop.

- **dens in dente:** tooth within a tooth.
- **germinated** (**JER**-mih-nay-ted = *sprout*): attempted division of a single tooth.
- **fusion of teeth:** union of two independently developing primary or secondary teeth.

Environmental or occurring problems can include the following:

- **caries:** dental decay; the number one disease of children.
- **epulis** (e-**PYU**-les): fibrous, sarcomatous tumor; also called *gum boil*.
- **abscess:** local collection of pus (see Figure 17-1).
- **cellulitis:** inflammation in the cellular or connective tissue.
- **early tooth exfoliation** (ecks-**foh**-lee-**AY**-shun = *shedding or falling off*): tooth loss resulting in the shifting of teeth and loss of tooth position.
- **ankylosis** (ang-key-**LOH**-sis): stiff joint, retention of deciduous tooth.
- **intrinsic** (in-**TRIN**-sick = *on the inside*): internal discoloration of teeth resulting from diet, medication, or excessive fluoride during tooth development.
- **baby bottle mouth:** mouth condition of badly decayed and rotted teeth with accompanying gum-tissue soreness that is caused from prolonged access to bottle feeding through sleep and eating. See Figure 17-2 for an example and the treatment received.

Figure 17-1 Decayed anteriors with abscess present in upper left area

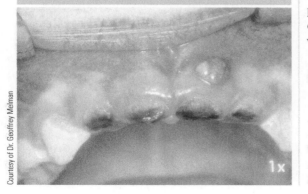

Courtesy of Dr. Geoffrey Melman

Figure 17-2 Nursing bottle mouth in upper view with crown treatment of affected teeth in bottom view

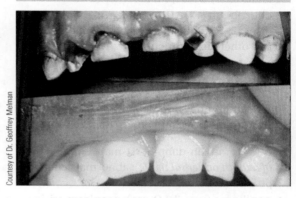

Courtesy of Dr. Geoffrey Melman

Some growth irregularities and mouth-affecting habits present future problems requiring interceptive or orthodontic care. Occasionally, a baby is born with a tooth present, called a *natal* tooth. Teeth erupting in the first month are termed *neonatal* teeth. Because of lack of stability, inability to nurse, or other reasons, these teeth may be removed. Other maladies include open bite, diastema (space gap), crossbites, tooth protrusions, oral habits such as thumb-sucking or lip sucking, and tooth crowding. Trauma and accidents, such as electric cord burn of lips and mouth tissues, require the attention of the pedodontist.

Developmental Tissue and Bone Problems

Not only are the developing teeth affected by growth problems, but sometimes the oral tissues and the child's bones may develop problems associated with dental care, such as the following:

- **macroglossia** (**mack**-roh-**GLOSS**-ee-ah; macro = *large*, glossia = *tongue*): enlarged tongue.
- **ankyloglossia** (**ang**-key loh-**GLOSS**-ee-ah): abnormally short lingual frenum causing limited tongue movement (tongue tied).
- **abnormal labial frenum:** enlarged or thick labial frenum that may cause **diastema**, an open area between the central incisors.

- **fissured (FISH**-ured) **tongue:** grooved division, cleft, or split of tongue.
- **micrognathia** (my-kroh-**NAY**-thee-ah): abnormally small jaw; undersized mandible.
- **cherubism (CHAIR**-you-bizm): a genetic disorder resulting in enlargement of the cheek and other facial structures.

Tumor and Cyst Growth

Some children develop neoplasms (new growths) of the oral soft tissue and bones. Related terms are:

- **odontoma** (oh-dahn-**TOH**-mah = *tumor of a tooth or dental tissue*): abnormal cell proliferation.
- **papilloma** (pap-il-**LO**-ma): neoplasm arising from epithelial cells; benign tumor.
- **verruca vulgaris** (ver-**OO**-kah, vul-**GAIR**-iss = *oral warts*): viral cause, possibly from finger sucking.
- **fibroma:** fibrous tumor, benign in nature.
- **granuloma:** grandular tumor usually of epithelioid or lymphoid cells.
- **neurofibromatosis** (**new**-roh-fie-**broh**-mah-**TOH**-sis): tumor on peripheral nerves.
- **hemangioma** (hem-an-**GI**-o-ma): vascular tumor, generally located in the neck/head area.
- **lymphangioma** (lim-**fan**-jee-**OH**-mah): tumor made up of lymphatic vessels.
- **lymphoma** (lim-**FOH**-mah): new tissue growth within the lymphatic system.
- **mucocele** (**MYOU**-koh-seal): mucous cyst.
- **ranula:** mucocele in the floor of the mouth in the sublingual duct.

MAINTENANCE AND PRESERVATION OF THE PEDIATRIC DENTITION

Maintenance and preservation of the primary dentition involves the same care and attention as that given to adult teeth. Visits to the dentist should begin around the child's first birthday and consist of the health and dental history, clinical and dental exam, prophylaxis, photos, and radiographs that have been modified in size for the smaller mouth. Parents may benefit from receiving instruction in nutrition and home care, including toothbrushing and other preventive measures at this time.

Prophylaxis treatment may include gingival care for simple, eruption, **scorbutic** (skor-**BYOU**-tick = *lacking vitamin C*), or acute gingivitis, as well as periodontitis and periodontosis, herpes simplex virus, aphthous ulcer, ANUG, or **candidiasis** (**kan**-dih-**DYE**-ah-sis = *fungus infection, thrush*; see Figure 17-3). Appliances may be constructed to correct bad habits, such as finger sucking or nail-biting. Other professional preventive care is discussed in the following sections.

Fluoride Application

The dentist may indicate a need for professional application of fluoride to the child's teeth. Fluoride care may be provided in the form of ingestion by drinking water with fluoride or taking prescribed fluoride supplements by topical application, placing upon the teeth, or a combination of both techniques. Topical application is supplied in the form of gel, varnish, liquid, spray, or other methods. The various types of dental fluoride, as recommended by the Division of Oral Health, National Center for Chronic Disease Prevention and Health Promotion, are given in Table 17-1.

Figure 17-3 Thrush in infant's mouth

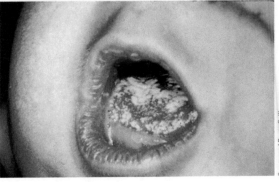

Table 17-1 Fluoride Supplementation

Fluoride Item	Form	Use	Availability	Recommendations
Fluoride toothpaste	Paste 1,000–1,500 ppm	Brush teeth 2× daily. Fl taken up by plaque and demineralized enamel, increases Fl in saliva.	OTC (over-the-counter)	Brush 2× daily, supervise children <6 small amounts, no swallowing; tots <2 by dentist advice.
Fl Mouth rinse	0.05% sodium fluoride OTC for daily use; 0.20% sodium fluoride (NaFl) for weekly school rinse program.	Used daily or weekly for prescribed time. Fl retained in saliva and plaque to help prevent tooth decay.	OTC for normal use; higher concentrations by Rx.	Not for use by children <6 unless Rx by DDS; danger of swallowing and causing fluorosis.
Fl supplements	Tablets, liquid, lozenges with (NaFl) sodium fluoride bases of 1.0, 0.5, or 0.25 mg Fl.	Useful for children without fluoride in water supply. Prefer sucking or chewing tablets for 1–2 minutes to maximize effects.	Rx by dentists.	Dentist to determine if child is high-risk without fluoride in water. Use proper dosage to avoid fluorosis.
Fl gel and foam	Gel = acidulated phosphate fluoride, gel, or foam of NaFl, or stannous fluoride.	Applied in dental office for 1–4 minutes; home use as prescribed.	Dental office = acidulated phosphate with 1.23% Fl concentration, 0.9% NaFl in office use, or 0.5% home use, or 0.15 stannous fluoride home use.	Applications at 3–12 month intervals; little risk of enamel fluorosis.
Fl varnish	Varnishes of 2.26% NaFl, or difluorsilane 0.1% fluoride amount.	Painted on teeth by dental professional; not intended to adhere permanently but holds Fl to teeth for hours.	Applied by dental professional in dental office.	Reapply at regular intervals, 2× year. No fluorosis risk from application.

ENAMOPLASTY

Enamoplasty (ee-**NAM**-oh-**plas**-tee) is the selective reduction of fissures and occlusal irregularities caused by grinding. Rather than filling deep pits or fissures with sealant material, the dentist may choose to perform some selective reducing or leveling of deep crevices to permit easier cleansing and home care of the teeth.

Pit and Fissure Sealant Application

At the age of six or seven years and thereafter as the permanent teeth erupt, the occlusal surfaces are covered with a sealant: a clear or tinted acrylic coating that is either **self-cured** (when mixed, base and catalyst are chemically polymerized) or **light cured** (polymerizes with the use of a curing light). Application to the enamel surface requires prophylaxis, isolation, and then acid **etching** of the tooth before placement of the topical sealant. When in place and hardened, the sealant will form an even, hard acrylic coating on the chewing surfaces, eliminating any deep pits or fissures.

Oral Surgery

Surgical intervention may be used to prevent future problems for developing teeth. Examples include extraction to remove **ankylosed** (**ANG**-kih-lowzd = *fixed, stiff*) teeth or a large labial frenum that requires a **frenectomy** (freh-**NECK**-toh-me = *incision and suturing of frenum to the periosteum*) to avoid a **diastema** (dyd-ah-**STEE**-mah) of the anterior central incisors or surgery of the lingual frenum to avoid a tongue-tied condition.

Space Maintenance

Professional care may involve placement of fixed or removable appliances to maintain or reclaim premature spacing in the arch until eruption of the secondary teeth. Some common space maintainers are the **band and loop** and the **distal shoe** appliances (see Figure 17-4). An acrylic **bite plane** appliance may be constructed to correct a simple crossbite, or the child may be fitted for a device to combat bad habits, such as thumb-sucking, nail-biting, or lip sucking.

RESTORATIVE DENTAL CARE FOR THE PRIMARY DENTITION

Restorative care of the deciduous teeth is basically the same as for the permanent dentition. Restorations are completed in the same manner, but some instruments can be modified in size, such as a T-band matrix in place of a larger adult matrix and retainer. A T-band matrix may be curved or straight. These bands are bent into a circle, and the T edges are folded over to hold the shape. The strips require no retainer and take less space in a smaller mouth.

Small cavities may be excised using a laser beam, small curette, or acid solution to eliminate impurities and then refilled with amalgam or a

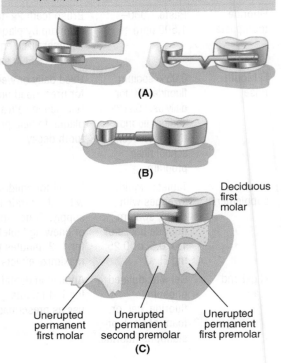

Figure 17-4 Space maintainers: (A) band and loop, (B) spring-activated, (C) distal shoe bar

(A)

(B)

Deciduous first molar

Unerupted permanent first molar

Unerupted permanent second premolar

Unerupted permanent first premolar

(C)

composite material. Larger decay areas are treated in the same manner as adults. Badly decayed or broken down teeth may need to receive a straight edge or contoured stainless steel crown. The crown is fitted, or **festooned** (fes-**TUNED** = *trimmed*), and cemented onto the tooth (see Figure 17-5). The child patient may receive composite resin bonding for tooth surfaces, ceramic and metal crowns, cores, fixed or removable partial or full dentures, implants, retainers, and protective mouth guards.

Pulpal Treatment

Because of the large opening in the **apex** of the erupting and developing tooth, pulpal treatment may be more aggressive in the child. There are two types of pulpal treatment:

- **apexogenesis** (ay-pecks-oh-**JEN**-ih-sis): treatment of a vital pulp to allow continued natural development.

Figure 17-5 Stainless steel crowns on deciduous teeth

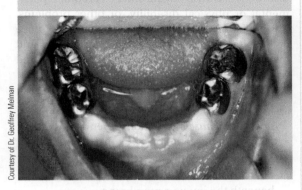

- **apexification** (ay-pecks-ih-fah-**KAY**-shun): treatment of a nonvital tooth to stimulate closure and the development of cementum.

The affected vital pulp of a primary tooth or a permanent tooth not fully calcified may receive any of a number of treatment procedures (Figure 17-6):

- **pulp capping:** placement of medication to sedate and treat inflamed pulp. **Indirect capping** is needed when the pulp has not yet been exposed. In **direct capping**, the medicament is placed directly upon the exposed, affected pulp (A).
- **pulpotomy:** partial or full removal of pulpal tissue located in the crown (B).
- **pulpectomy:** removal of pulpal tissue from the crown and root sections; may be endodontically filled immediately or followed later with endodontic treatment after apexification and closure of the apex of a young, secondary tooth (C).

Figure 17-6 Pulp treatment

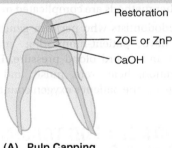

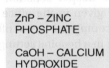

ZnP – ZINC PHOSPHATE

CaOH – CALCIUM HYDROXIDE

ZOE – ZINC OXIDE EUGENOL MIX

Restoration
ZOE or ZnP
CaOH

(A) Pulp Capping

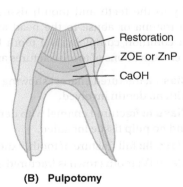

Restoration
ZOE or ZnP
CaOH

(B) Pulpotomy

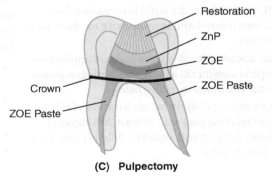

Restoration
ZnP
ZOE
ZOE Paste
Crown
ZOE Paste

(C) Pulpectomy

CONTROL AND SEDATION OF THE CHILD PATIENT

Pediatric dental care requires precise techniques completed rapidly and calmly. Control and sedation of the child patient is completed in various ways, such as:

- **Positive reinforcement:** compliments for good behavior, suggestions of positive actions.
- **Distraction:** change focus from dental work to school, friends, hobbies, sports.
- **Voice control:** friendly tone but firm, such as "we don't do that here" remarks.

Mechanical methods could include a dental (rubber) dam to provide control of the tongue and saliva, and maintain a sterile and open area; mouth props or gags; or a papoose board, which is a wrapping device used to restrain the patient for a difficult or precise treatment.

Some patients—anxious, with behavior problems, or medically compromised with diseases—may require deeper sedation. Various stages of sedation are given in the office practice while others may be completed in the office with monitoring controls or in a hospital setting.

Pediatric Sedation

Calming nervous anxiety without loss of consciousness is called conscious sedation. Loss of consciousness (sleep) is termed general anesthesia. There are various ways to achieve sedation:

- **oral medication:** the child is conscious but becomes relaxed and is responsive to touch and directions
- **local anesthetic:** after a preliminary application of topical anesthetic, a local anesthetic is injected into the work area to relieve pain.
- **inhalation sedation:** administration of nitrous oxide (relaxing gas) with at least 20% oxygen; reduces gagging and anxiety. Child is conscious but not anxious.

General anesthesia may be necessary for selected patients and perhaps those with seizure disorders, Down syndrome, cerebral palsy, mental or physical disability, or other problems. This sedation can be accomplished in the office or hospital but only after patient evaluation and informed consent. The patient must be monitored with emergency backup aid available.

Methods of administration are:

- **intramuscular** (in-tra-**MUSS**-kyou-lahr = *within the muscle*) sedation: parenterally administrated sedation.
- **submucosal** (sub-mew-**COH**-sul = *under the mucous membrane*): deposit of the drug beneath the mucous membrane.
- **subcutaneous** (sub-kyou-**TAY**-nee-us = *under the skin*): injection of the drug under the tissues.
- **intravenous** (in-trah-**VEE**-nus = *into the vein, vessel*): injection of the drug into the vein.
- **rectal insertion:** a possible method of drug administration, but usually not done unless other methods are complicated or unavailable.

Pedodontists who perform general anesthesia will have patient-monitoring machines that watch and record blood pressure, EKG readings, respiration, heart rate, pulse, and an oximeter measuring the patient's oxygen count.

TREATMENT FOR TRAUMA AND ABUSE

Injury to the teeth and mouth tissues can result from trauma or abuse to the head and face. The most common complaint is a tooth fracture. The four classifications of tooth fractures are:

- **Class I:** fractured enamel showing rough edges with no dentin involved.
- **Class II:** fractured enamel with dentin involved and no pulp tissue included.
- **Class III:** full fracture of tooth, exposing pulp.
- **Class IV:** tooth crown is fractured off.

Traumatized Tooth Difficulties

Traumatized primary and permanent teeth exhibit a variety of difficulties and effects:

- **pulpal hyperemia:** congestion of blood within the pulp chamber.
- **internal hemorrhage:** rupture of pulpal capillaries.
- **internal/external resorption:** destructive, dissolving process caused by odontoclastic action.
- **pulpal necrosis:** pulpal death.
- **ankylosis** (ang-kil-**LOH**-sis): fusion of cementum of the root with the cribriform plate of the alveolar bone with no intervening periodontal ligament.
- **intrusion:** tooth thrust into the alveolus with partial crown exposure.
- **extrusion:** tooth thrust away from the alveolus.
- **luxation:** tooth moved out of place.
- **avulsion:** tooth forced out of its socket.

Treatment of Traumatized Teeth

Treatment for injured primary teeth may include the following:

- Smoothing of rough edges
- Pulp capping
- Pulpotomy
- Pulpectomy with or without endodontic treatment
- Stainless steel banding, metal or resin crowns, placement of posts
- Replantation and stabilization (splinting) of replantation
- Partial denture tooth replacement (see Figure 17-7)

Other indications of abuse such as facial, neck, or hand bruises; bite marks; irregular walking gait; fear of adults; difficulty in sitting; eye contact avoidance; and unusual comments should be investigated and followed through proper channels.

Figure 17-7 Child wearing partial dental

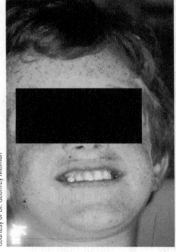
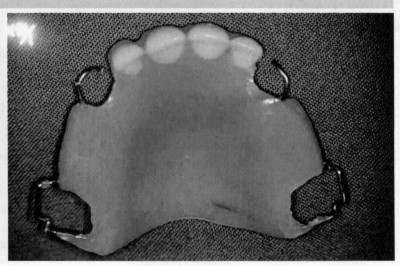

Courtesy of Dr. Geoffrey Melman

USE OF DENTAL RECORDS FOR PATIENT IDENTIFICATION

Dental records are being used extensively for identification in forensic and legal matters. The dental office offers many methods for recording and maintaining positive identification items for future reference. With particular attention to missing children, the pedodontist may supply information collected during routine visits.

- **Personal information data:** name, address, nicknames, ethnicity, hobbies, eyeglasses, tattoos, scars, birthmarks, and so forth.
- **Dental charting record:** current tooth development, dentition characteristics, and treatment data.
- **Radiographs:** current tooth placement, expected tooth development, and evidence of treatment received.
- **Photographs:** frontal and side views with profile and tooth growth. Digital photos have the advantage of providing immediate images that can be transmitted in missing child cases.

- **Saliva:** fluid collection containing the child's DNA and scent for use with tracking dogs in missing child cases.

MISCELLANEOUS CHILD HEALTH CONDITIONS

Dental care delivery depends on the child's total health condition. Children affected with systemic or genetic diseases may exhibit more dental distress and/or require more and specialized dental treatment. Some childhood diseases that may have additional dental concerns are:

AIDS	Down syndrome
asthma	fragile X syndrome
autism	hemophilia
blindness	juvenile diabetes
cerebral palsy	learning difficulties
congenital heart disease	leukemia
cystic fibrosis	rheumatic fever
deafness	viral hepatitis

Review Exercises

Matching

Match the following word elements with their meanings.

1.	_____ caries	A.	primary teeth
2.	_____ anodontia	B.	inside the tooth
3.	_____ ankyloglossia	C.	removal of pulp tissue in crown of tooth
4.	_____ cellulitis	D.	removal of enamel tissue
5.	_____ Class I fracture	E.	full tooth fracture, exposing pulp tissue
6.	_____ epulis	F.	inflammation in cellular tissue
7.	_____ permanent teeth	G.	under the mucous membrane
8.	_____ enamoplasty	H.	vascular tumor
9.	_____ Class III fracture	I.	tooth fracture of enamel, no other tissue included
10.	_____ deciduous	J.	torn or pulled away or out of
11.	_____ intrinsic	K.	dental decay
12.	_____ submucosal	L.	fibrous tumor, gum boil
13.	_____ avulsion	M.	secondary teeth
14.	_____ pulpotomy	N.	stiff or rigid tight tongue condition
15.	_____ hemangioma	O.	absence of teeth

Definitions

Using the selection given for each sentence, choose the best term to complete the definition.

1. Another term for a common gumboil is:
   a. oral wart
   b. gingival abscess
   c. inflamed uvula
   d. epulis

2. An abnormally short lingual frenum may cause a tongue-tied condition called:
   a. macroglossia
   b. microglossia
   c. papilloma
   d. ankyloglossia

3. An absence of teeth is a condition called:
   a. hypodontia
   b. anodontia
   c. hyperdontia
   d. osteodontia

4. Enamel hypoplasia is what type of condition of the tooth's enamel tissue?
   a. underdevelopment
   b. overdevelopment
   c. lack of tissue
   d. mottled enamel

5. Internal discoloration of the tooth surface is which type of stain?
   a. blanching
   b. exotrinsic
   c. intrinsic
   d. mesostain

6. Candidiasis is a fungus infection commonly referred to as:
   a. thrush
   b. ANUG
   c. gingivitis
   d. periodontitis

7. Scorbutic gingivitis is a result of which vitamin deficiency?
   a. vitamin A
   b. vitamin B
   c. vitamin C
   d. vitamin D

8. Sedation by swallowing medication involves which avenue of entrance?
   a. ingestion
   b. inhalation
   c. rectal placement
   d. intravenous

9. Trimming the gingival area of a stainless steel crown is called:
   a. alteration
   b. obturation
   c. crowning
   d. festooning

10. *Amelogenesis imperfecta* is the improper development of which tooth tissue?
    a. dentin
    b. enamel
    c. pulp
    d. cementum

11. Treatment of a vital pulp to allow continued natural development is termed:
    a. apexectomy
    b. apexotomy
    c. apexogenesis
    d. apexification

12. Intrinsic pigmentation is a coloring of which tooth surface?
    a. apical
    b. external
    c. gingival
    d. internal

13. The full or partial removal of pulp tissue from the crown portion of a tooth is a/an:
    a. apicoectomy
    b. pulpectomy
    c. pulpotomy
    d. pulp capping

14. Another word for the condition epulis is a/an:
    a. oral wart
    b. nosebleed
    c. gum boil
    d. cracked tooth

15. Dental caries is not a disease of which of the following mouth tissues:
    a. enamel
    b. dentin
    c. pulp
    d. mucous

16. Which pit and fissure sealant polymerizes without the use of the curing light?
    a. self-cure
    b. etched cure
    c. light cure
    d. polymer cure

17. The forced removal or knocking out of a tooth is known as:
    a. luxation
    b. avulsion
    c. intrusion
    d. extrusion

18. A fractured tooth showing evidence of dentin and enamel involvement is termed:
    a. Class I
    b. Class II
    c. Class III
    d. Class IV

19. Acid conditioning of a cavity preparation prior to the placement of a restorative material is called:
    a. etching
    b. sealant application
    c. composite auto curing
    d. composite self-curing

20. Which of the following is not a name for the teeth in a child's dentition?
    a. primary
    b. succedaneous
    c. baby teeth
    d. deciduous

Building Skills

Locate and define the prefix, root/combining form, and suffix (if present) in the following words.

1. **micrognathia**
   prefix _____

   root/combining form _____
   suffix _____

2. **odontoma**
   prefix _____
   root/combining form _____
   suffix _____

3. **intramuscular**
   prefix _____
   root/combining form _____
   suffix _____

4. **reimplantation**
   prefix _____
   root/combining form _____
   suffix _____

5. **neonatal**
   prefix _____
   root/combining form _____
   suffix _____

Fill-Ins

Write the correct word in the blank space to complete each statement.

1. A/an _____ arrangement occurs when there is a disturbance in the eruption placement, such as a tooth out of place.

2. Another term for a fissure of the palate or the lip is a _____.

3. A clear or lightly tinted acrylic substance painted on newly erupted teeth is called a _____.

4. Enlarged labial frenums may cause a space between teeth called a/an _____.

5. A tooth present in the baby's mouth at birth is called a _____ tooth.

6. Another word for pulpal necrosis is pulpal _____.

7. The failure of the development of an organ or body part is _____.

8. _____ is the treatment of the vital pulp to permit continued natural development.

9. A badly decayed deciduous molar may require a steel _____ restoration.

10. A _____ matrix may be used in the child patient during the placement of a restoration material.

11. Band and loop or distal shoe devices are types or methods for maintaining _____ after premature loss of a tooth.

12. A/an _____ is the congestion of pus at the apex of a tooth.

13. A tooth that is forced away from its socket is said to be _____.

14. A full fracture of the crown, involving all tissues, is a Class _____ fracture.

15. A toothprint is an ID dental record made of the child's _____.

16. An anesthesia of a gel, ointment, or liquid material that is used to obtain surface anesthesia prior to injection is called a/an _____ anesthetic.

17. Teeth erupting the first month of life are called _____ teeth.

18. Data about name, address, age, hobbies, nicknames, and so forth are considered to be _____ information.

19. Verruca vulgaris from a viral source such as finger sucking is another name for _____.

20. Pulpal treatment of children is usually successful because of the large opening of the tooth's _____, permitting more circulation.

Word Use

Read the following sentences, and define the meaning of the word written in boldface letters.

1. After completing the prophylaxis, the dental hygienist applied **sealants** to the newly erupted teeth.

   _____

2. The dentist advised the mother of the need of **conscious sedation** for the treatment of her son's steel crown appointment.

   _____

3. The baby girl exhibited a **natal** tooth in the lower mandibular incisal area.

   _____

4. Because of rapid growth patterns, it is the policy of this office to make a fresh **toothprint** at the child's yearly visit.

   _____

5. The dentist used **distraction techniques** with the child who was calling for his mother.

   _____

CHAPTER 18 | DENTAL LABORATORY MATERIALS

✓ Learning Objectives

On completion of this chapter, you should be able to:

1. Identify the various kinds of rigid and elastic impression materials, and give examples of each.

2. Discuss the assorted types of gypsum products used in dentistry, and give examples of their uses.

3. Identify the different kinds of dental waxes, and discuss a use for each type of wax.

4. Explain the process of polymerization and the factors that alter or modify the chemical reaction, as well as the uses for the polymer materials.

5. Describe the difference between precious and other metals, and state uses for the assorted types of gold.

6. Identify the common abrasives and polishing materials used in dentistry and the desired effect of each.

7. List the various types of dental cements, and state the uses for each type.

8. Discuss the different types of descriptive or manipulative characteristics of dental materials.

IMPRESSION MATERIALS

Dental laboratory procedures involve a variety of procedural steps or techniques and the use of many materials. These materials may be grouped into families according to composition or use. Each material exhibits its own particular characteristic, and

Vocabulary Related to Dental Laboratory Materials

This list contains selected new and important word parts and terms from this chapter. Take the time to learn these word parts and their meanings. You may use the list to review these terms and practice pronouncing them correctly. When you work with the audio for this chapter, listen to the word, repeat it, and then place a checkmark in the box. Proceed to the next boxed word, and repeat the process.

(hyphen before word means it's a suffix, hyphen after word means prefix, no hyphen means root word.)

Word Parts	Meaning	Word Parts	Meaning
electro	electric current	plated	thin layer
poly-	many	therm	heat
plastic	resin		

Key Terms

- ☐ **alloy** (AL-loy)
- ☐ **binary** (BYE-nar-ee)
- ☐ **calcination** (cal-suh-**NAY**-shun)
- ☐ **catalyst** (CAT-ah-list)
- ☐ **electroplated** (ee-**LECK**-troh-play-ted)
- ☐ **exothermic** (ecks-oh-**THER**-mick)
- ☐ **hydrophilic** (high-droh-**FIL**-ick)

- ☐ **hydrophobia** (high-droh-**FOH**-bee-ah)
- ☐ **hygroscopic** (high-groh-**SKAH**-pick)
- ☐ **imbibition** (im-bah-**BISH**-shun)
- ☐ **inhibitor** (in-**HIB**-ih-tore)
- ☐ **initiater** (ih-**NISH**-ee-ay-tore)
- ☐ **modifier** (MAH-dih-fye-er)
- ☐ **plasticizer** (PLAS-tih-sigh-zer)

- ☐ **polycarboxylate** (pahl-ee-kar-**BOX**-ih-late)
- ☐ **polymerization** (pahl-ee-mare-ih-**ZAY**-shun)
- ☐ **quaternary** (KWAH-ter-nare-ee)
- ☐ **quinary** (KWIN-ar-ee)
- ☐ **slurry** (SLUR-ee)
- ☐ **ternary** (TURN-ah-ree)

one substance may differ from another even within its own grouping or family. Knowledge of the general and specific use of a dental material is essential to successfully complete many laboratory procedures.

The assortment of materials needed to complete the various dental lab procedures is not limited to the lab area. They may be used alone, or they may be used in conjunction with the dental operatory/treatment room.

Types of Impression Materials

Impression materials are substances that are used to take and record the shape, size, or position of teeth, appliances, and oral anatomy. These materials may be rigid, plastic, or elastic.

Rigid Impression Materials

Rigid impression materials are used where no teeth are present, and material flexibility is unnecessary. The assorted types of rigid impression materials are:

- **impression plaster:** gypsum product, 60 cc of water to 100 grams of plaster.
- **metallic oxide paste:** two-paste system, zinc-oxide eugenol (ZOE) base with resin accelerator. This paste hardens through a chemical reaction.
- **impression compound:** supplied in cakes and sticks; color-coded for temperature flexibility; used to make a preliminary impression tray.

Plastic Impression Materials

Plastic impression materials are used with or without the presence of teeth. This movable material is employed where some material flexibility is needed for the impression. The three types of plastic impression material are:

- **thermoplastic:** material softens when heated and hardens when cooled.
- **compound:** supplied in sheets or stick form. The material is composed of a thermoplastic resin base with filers and plasticizers. It softens when heated and returns to a solid when cool; used in copper bands for independent crown preps.
- **wax:** used for registration of bites or for impression of a single tooth area.

Elastic Impression Materials

Elastic impression materials are used where teeth are present and material must be flexible for removal from the oral cavity or teeth. Elastic impression materials are either reversible or irreversible hydrocolloids:

- **reversible hydrocolloid:** impression material that can change repeatedly from gel to solid states depending on the thermal condition of the substance:
  - ○ **gel state:** material is soft and pliable.
  - ○ **solid state:** material has "set" or is rigid enough to hold the form.
- **irreversible hydrocolloid:** agar impression material that can be changed from gel to solid state as a result of a chemical reaction, and remain in that condition after mixing and using. For example, alginate powder or premixed packages are supplied in regular or fast set, tinted, and flavored (see Figure 18-1A for an example of an alginate impression).

Elastomeric Impression Materials

Elastomeric impression materials are used to make impressions of preparations and for demanding or accurate reproductions. These substances are composed of a base and an accelerator, or **catalyst** (**CAT**-ah-list = *substance that speeds up the chemical reaction*) and can be measured, mixed, and placed in a tray or syringe for use in the mouth. The material may be hand mixed or placed in an **extruder gun**, which is a device that contains two independent materials to be forced mixed and dispensed into a common tip as one material, thus eliminating measuring, mixing, and cleanup time.

- **polysulfide:** impression substance available in light, regular, or heavy-bodied **viscosity** (viss-**KAHS**-ah-tee = *thickness or tendency to flow*). Also known as mercaptan, this material will harden or set by means of chemical action.
- **silicone:** first supplied as a base putty with liquid accelerator drops and termed condensation or conventional silicone type or later as a two-paste system known as addition silicone type.

287

Figure 18-1 (A) alginate impression, (B) elastometric impression, (C) laboratory reproduction result from a digital impression

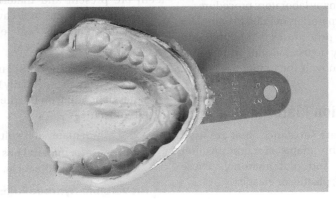

(A)

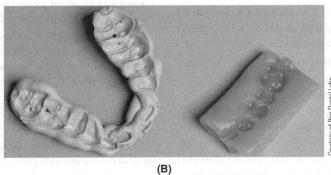

Courtesy of Roe Dental Labs

(B)

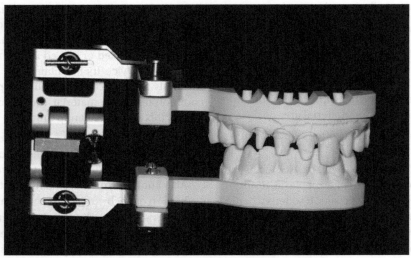

Courtesy of Roe Dental Labs

(C)

- **polyether:** supplied in regular viscosity, with a thinner **modifier** (**MAH**-dih-fye-er = *material to change conditions*) for reduced thickness.
- **vinyl polysiloxane:** impression material supplied in tubes, putty, paste-to-paste system, and cartridge styles. The material may be heavy, medium, or wash viscosity; impressions may be poured more than once. The material is stable. Some have bubble gum flavoring. See Figure 18-1B for an example of an elastometric impression using a heavyweight and lightweight viscosity material.

Digital Impression Technique

Another method to take an impression of a prepared site to present to the dental laboratory scene is digital capture and file transfer. Without the use of trays, tubing, or impression material, an impression of a prepared procedure, either one or multiple preps, may be obtained by an optical scan of the area. Using a wand device, one or both dentitions may be scanned, reviewed by the dentist, and forwarded to the dental laboratory for polyureothane model construction. The prosthodontist or lab technician then constructs the prescribed prosthesis for that case. See Figure 18-1C for an example of the finished impression made from the digital reading of the preparation.

GYPSUM MATERIALS

Gypsum products generally are obtained from the same rock or ore source: calcium sulfate. It is the **calcination** process of preparing and handling the gypsum material that determines the final classification and purpose of a gypsum product. Gypsum products can be color-coded for types and speeds.

Types of Gypsum

There are five types of gypsum:

- **Type I plaster—impression:** used to take an impression but is not popular because of its weakness and replacement by better impression materials.

- **Type II—model:** also known as *plaster of paris*, used mostly for impression and study models. Prepared by dehydrating calcium sulfate at atmospheric pressure to beta-hemihydrate form.
- **Type III—dental stone:** white or buff colored, Class I stone, used for orthodontic, diagnostic, and working casts. Prepared by dehydrating gypsum under pressure for alpha-hemihydrate form.
- **Type IV—improved or die stone:** stronger Class II stone used for dental dies and casts. It is dehydrated in a solution of calcium chloride to obtain a modified alpha-hemihydrate form; also known as densite.
- **Type V—casting investment:** gypsum-bonded material that can withstand extreme heat; used for casts of a prosthesis.

Other casting substances include phosphate and silica-bonded investment materials.

Use of Gypsum Materials

Gypsum products have a variety of uses in the dental office and the laboratory setting in the construction and fabrication of dental prostheses. Related terms are:

- **model and cast:** used for a positive reproduction of the mouth and oral conditions. The gypsum model, called a diagnostic cast or study model, consists of an art portion (base) and an anatomical (tooth) portion. Study models can be used as patterns for construction, legal records, and examples of before-and-after treatment, as well as planning and preparation (Figure 18-2A). Study models may also be constructed by 3D digital methods. A wand scan is taken of the mouth, and the readings are sent to a laboratory for construction of a study model. Figure 18-2B shows an example of a digital study model set.
- **die:** reproduction of prepared tooth; usually Class II stone poured into an impression of the preparation. Dies can be **electroplated** (ee-**LECK**-troh-play-ted = *thin metal covering through electrolysis*) with copper, silver, amalgam, or low-fusing metals for a stronger surface and working area.

Figure 18-2 (A) Plaster study model, (B) digital study model

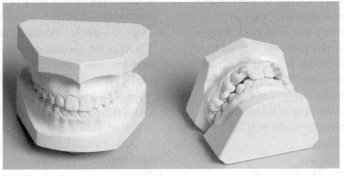

(A)

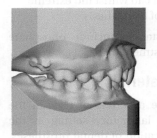 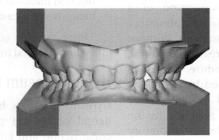 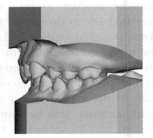

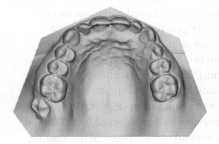 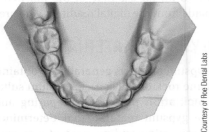

(B)

Courtesy of Roe Dental Labs

WAX MATERIALS

Wax is supplied in sheet, stick, round and square-shaped wire rope, and block forms for use in various dental procedures. Figure 18-3 gives examples of dental waxes. They include both synthetic and natural products from animal, mineral, and vegetable sources. The combination of material and the manufacturing process determines the ability of the wax to complete its designed purposes. Types of wax materials are:

- **inlay wax:** hard wax; blue, purple, green, or ivory colors; available in 3- to 4-inch sticks. Type I is for direct oral use; Type II is for laboratory or indirect use for inlay, crown, and casting patterns.

- **baseplate wax:** supplied in 3 × 6-inch sheets, pink in color and soft, medium, or hard; used

Figure 18-3 Examples of various waxes: (A) inlay wax, (B) occlusal bite rims, (C) boxing wax, (D) wax rope

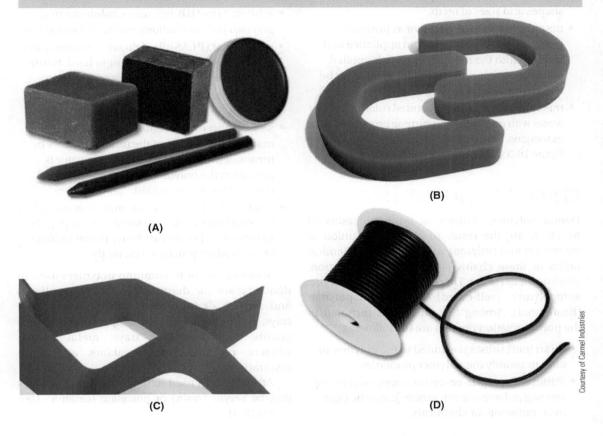

(A)

(B)

(C)

(D)

Courtesy of Carmel Industries

for denture construction, bite registration, and prosthesis construction.

- **casting wax:** available in square sheets of various thicknesses; colors denote its softening point; used for construction of patterns for cast partial dentures.
- **boxing wax:** supplied in 1½ × 12 × ⅛-inch strips; used to box or wrap around an impression prior to pouring. The strips hold the plaster or stone in place to form the art base of a study model.
- **occlusal bite blocks:** wax blocks in arch shape; used to set in teeth to be used for denture constructions. They are laboratory made by folding boxing wax and shaping, or they can be purchased premade, which saves time and is more consistent.

- **bite wafer wax:** used to check occlusion relationships; supplied in a preformed bite shape with a foil center to prevent bite through.
- **orthodontic wax:** soft, white stick wax used in orthodontics; used to line borders of impression trays.
- **wax round wire:** supplied on reels in various gauges; used to make lingual bars, sprues, and metal framework space.
- **utility wax:** soft, adhesive wax, supplied in stick or sheet; used to mount casts and to adapt or modify impression tray edges; also called rope wax.
- **sticky wax:** hard, brittle wax stick that is melted to hold dental units together.

- **preformed wax pontic shapes:** eliminates wax buildup process; supplied in various shapes and sizes of teeth.
- **disclosing wax:** also known as pressure indicator paste; painted on an appliance and inserted into the mouth. Pressure is applied to indicate high, sore, or tender areas; may be used to repair wax pattern voids.
- **miscellaneous waxes:** assorted color-coded waxes with particular fine-turning properties, such as margins, sculpturing, blocking out, and dipping. Figure 18-3 shows an assortment of dental waxes.

DENTAL POLYMER MATERIALS

Dental polymers, known as synthetic resins or **acrylics**, are the result of a chemical union of **monomer** and **polymer** substances. The chemical union of these chains is called **polymerization**, also known as *curing*. There are two types of acrylic: autopolymer (self-cured) and thermopolymer (heat-cured). Among the substances included in the polymerization process are the following:

- **filler:** inert substance added to the polymer to alter or modify the polymer properties.
- **initiator** (in-**NISH**-ee-ay-tor = *agent capable of starting polymerization process*): may be light, heat, radiation, or chemicals.

- **activator:** reacts with initiator to start polymerization.
- **inhibitor** (in-**HIB**-bih-tore = *substance that prevents polymerization*): maintains storage life.
- **plasticizer** (**PLAS**-tih-sigh-zer = *substance that causes a softening effect*): changes hard, brittle resin into a flexible, tough material.
- **composite:** polymer matrix bonded to glass particles; used for dental restorations.
- **self-curing resins:** autopolymerization materials that perform the uniting process by means of a chemical union; the activator is present in the polymer powder or base and does not have to be added.
- **heat-cured resins:** acrylic materials are united but need outside heat to set up; not as popular as self-cured but less likely to present bubbles or voids when processed correctly.

Some of the more common polymers used in dentistry are for denture bases, denture liners and repairs, denture teeth, custom impression trays, orthodontic and dental appliances, mouth guards, tooth-bleaching trays, metal casting veneers, pit and fissure sealants, and tooth restorations.

Artificial teeth used in dentures and appliances may be acrylic (resin) or porcelain (ceramic) (see Figure 18-4).

Figure 18-4 Examples of resin used with (A) partial framework or (B) complete denture

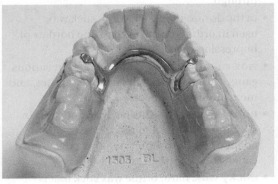

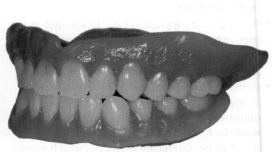

(A)

(B)

Table 18-1 Types of Gold Casting Alloy

Types	Consistency	Use
Type I (A)	Soft	Used for simple, nonstress surface, inlays
Type II (B)	Medium	Preferred in stress-bearing inlays or onlays
Type III (C)	Hard	Used in crowns and short-span bridgework
Type IV (D)	Extra-hard	Preferred for partial denture frames, saddles, and clasps

PRECIOUS AND BASE METALS

Metals are used in dental procedures. Some are used in their pure state, and others are used in combination with other metals. A combination of two or more metals is called an **alloy** (**AL**-loy). Combinations of two metals are **binary** (**BYE**-nar-ee); three metals are **ternary** (**TURN**-ah-ree); four metals are **quaternary** (**KWAH**-ter-nare-ee); and five different metals make up a **quinary** (**KWIN**-ar-ee) alloy.

Metals are classified as precious metals or base metals. Precious or "noble" metals—gold, platinum, palladium, and silver—are used for crowns, bridges, and dental appliances.

Gold Alloy

Pure gold (24 carat) may be used for gold foil restorations, and gold alloys formed with other precious metals, copper, or zinc may be supplied in sheet, wrought, or solder forms. Gold alloys can be **tempered** (hardened) or **annealed** (softened). They can also be whitened by adding silver, platinum, or palladium. Gold alloy solder is used to join parts of dental appliances or for repairs. Gold castings are classified into the four types shown in Table 18-1.

Type III is the most commonly used noble alloy. The basic combination for this alloy is:

- **75% gold:** resists tarnish/corrosion, nontoxic, hypoallergenic, docile, malleable, low melting point, and *burnishes* (smooths out) well.
- **10% silver:** lessens the red cast from copper and gold, increases ducility and malleability; gives strength to the alloy.
- **10% copper:** hardens in heat and high temperature; adds flowability.

- **3% palladium:** increases hardness, whitens gold, and prevents tarnish and corrosion.
- **2% zinc:** prevents porosity of surface areas, and provides smoothness.

Base Alloy

Base metal alloys contain less than 25% of noble metals and usually consist of chromium, nickel, and cobalt. They are used in partial denture frameworks or as substitutes for gold alloy. Other metals include stainless steel for crowns, orthodontic materials, nickel chromium, and cobalt-chromium for orthodontic wires.

ABRASIVE AND POLISHING MATERIALS

Finishing a dental prosthesis is a matter of smoothing and polishing. An abrasive material reduces or removes bumps, overhangs, and excesses but leaves behind scratches and surface cuts. A polishing agent reduces these scratches to an unnoticeable flat surface that reflects light. The technician begins the procedure with an abrasive material and then changes to a polishing agent to produce a shining surface. Abrasive and polishing materials may be supplied as powder to form a paste or **slurry** (**SLUR**-ee = *thin, watery mixture*), or luted to paper or cloth into sheets. Abrasives can be impregnated into wheels and points, or supplied in solid bricks that may be rubbed on rag or brush wheels for use with the dental lathe machine. Some common abrasive and polishing materials supplied in various grits on strips, discs, wheels, bricks, and powders are listed in Table 18-2.

Table 18-2 Common Abrasive and Polishing Agents

Material	Supplied As	Agent	Use
aluminum oxide	mounted stone, slurry	abrasive/polish	acrylic resin
carborundum	stones, points, disc	abrasive	metal, resin, tooth
chalk	soft powder	polishing	gold, resins
chromium oxide	powder	polishing	stainless steel
cuttle	powder of fish shell	abrasive	gold alloys
diamond	various size particles	abrasive	tooth structure
emery	particle or luted to cloth	abrasive	trim acrylic
garnet	stone, points	abrasive	resin, composite
pumice	powder, slurry	abrasive	metal, enamel, resin
quartz	grits, luted to paper, discs	abrasive	general use
rouge	powder, brick	polishing	gold, denture resin
tin oxide	powder, slurry	polishing	metals
tripoli	stone, brick	polishing	gold alloy
zirconium silicate	powder	polishing	enamel

CEMENT MATERIALS

Dental cements are used to temporarily or permanently lute dental castings, crowns, and bridges in place. These same cements, in thicker viscosities, can be used as bases or as restoratives in operative dentistry. The most common luting cements used with the dental laboratory products are zinc phosphate, ZOE, **polycarboxylate** (**pahl**-ee-kar-**BOX**-ih-late), and resin. The common cements used in dentistry are listed in Table 18-3.

Table 18-3 Dental Cements or Luting Agents

Material	Use
zinc phosphate	Permanent luting of casting, orthodontic appliances. Type II is used as a base.
ZOE	Temporary luting for castings, pulp capping, cavity liner, periodontal dressing, temporary restoration, insulating base, and wash.
ZOE and EBA (orthoethoxybenzoic acid)	Type II permanent cement for inlays, onlays, crowns, and bridges.
polycarboxylate	Luting for castings, stainless steel crowns, orthodontic cement.

Table 18-3 Dental Cements or Luting Agents *(Continued)*

Material	Use
silicophosphate	Luting for orthodontic appliances.
resin (light and self-cure), ESPE	Luting for castings, porcelain restorations, Maryland bridge.
glass ionomer	Type I cementation of metal castings, direct bond ortho bands, and core buildup. Type II is for anterior restorative.

CHARACTERISTICS OF DENTAL LABORATORY MATERIALS

When working with the various dental laboratory materials, you must be aware of and understand the descriptive or manipulative characteristics of strengths of each material. Related terms are:

- **bonding:** force of the union of one substance with another substance.
- **coefficient of thermal expansion:** amount of form change that takes place in a dental material and tooth during heat exposure in the oral cavity.
- **color:** has three components:
  - hue: color of object—red, green blue, and so on.
  - chroma: strength of specified hue.
  - value: darkness or brightness of specified hue.
- **creep:** tendency of amalgam to deform under constant applied pressure.
- **cure process:** hardening of the material through auto- (chemical) or light-activated response.
- **ductility:** ability of the material to withstand permanent deformation without fracturing under elongation stress.
- **elasticity:** ability of a material to return to its original form when stress is removed.
- **exothermic** (**ecks**-oh-**THER**-mick): chemical release of heat, as in zinc phosphate cement.
- **flow:** slow bending or movement of material under its own weight.

- **galvanization:** tendency of certain metals to produce an electrical charge when in contact with each other.
- **hardness:** maximum amount of resistance before penetration or scratching can occur.
- **hydrophilic** (high-droh-**FIL**-ick = *ability to attract and hold water*): absorption of water.
- **hydrophobia** (high-droh-**FOH**-bee-ah = *fear of water*): giving off or shedding of water.
- **hygroscopic** (high-groh-**SKAH**-pick) **expansion:** submersion into, or the addition of, water to a material prior to initial set.
- **initial set:** period of time when material assumes shape but remains pliable.
- **imbibition** (**im**-bah-**BISH**-shun = *absorption of fluid*): taking on of water.
- **malleability:** ability to withstand deformation without fracture while undergoing maximum compression stress.
- **setting time:** amount of time required for the material to become as hard as it will be.
- **tensile strength:** maximum amount of pulling stress required to rupture the material.
- **thermal conductivity:** capability of the material to transmit heat.
- **toughness:** ability of the material to resist fracture.
- **trituration:** mixing of mercury with other alloy material to form an amalgam.
- **working time:** period during which a material can be molded, shaped, or manipulated without any adverse effect on the material.
- **yield strength:** maximum amount of stress a material can withstand without deformation.

Review Exercises

Matching

Match the following word elements with their meanings.

1. _____ catalyst
2. _____ plasticizer
3. _____ study model
4. _____ filler
5. _____ imbibition
6. _____ boxing wax
7. _____ Type IV gypsum
8. _____ alloy
9. _____ sticky wax
10. _____ slurry
11. _____ reversible hydrocolloid
12. _____ acrylic
13. _____ inhibitor
14. _____ modifier
15. _____ die

A. inert substance added to alter properties

B. gypsum reproduction of a prepared tooth

C. substance that changes material's action

D. strip to encircle impression tray prior to pour-up

E. synthetic resin

F. hard, brittle wax used to hold objects together

G. taking on of water

H. substance to prevent polymerization; helps storage

I. runny, watery mix

J. elastic impression material

K. positive reproduction of the mouth

L. combination of two or more metals

M. improved stone

N. substance that causes softening effect

O. substance to speed up chemical reaction

Definitions

Using the selection given for each sentence, choose the best term to complete the definition.

1. Which of the following is not considered a precious or noble metal?
   a. amalgam
   b. gold
   c. platinum
   d. silver

2. A dark blue wax used to make wax patterns for cast restorations is:
   a. baseplate wax
   b. boxing wax
   c. inlay wax
   d. sticky wax

3. A hard, brittle stick wax that is melted to hold together dental items is:
   a. baseplate wax
   b. boxing wax
   c. inlay wax
   d. sticky wax

4. A pink sheet wax that is used for denture construction of the gingival area is:
   a. baseplate wax
   b. boxing wax
   c. inlay wax
   d. sticky wax

5. An inert substance added to the polymer to alter or modify the polymer's properties is:
   a. composite
   b. filler
   c. plasticizer
   d. inhibitor

6. Which type of gold alloy is preferred for use in crown and bridge work?
   a. Type I
   b. Type II
   c. Type III
   d. Type IV

7. Which of the following is not considered an impression material?
   a. gypsum
   b. amalgam
   c. compound
   d. metallic oxide

8. Gypsum products may be used for all of the following except:
   a. restorations
   b. impressions
   c. study models
   d. investment

9. Which wax is supplied in strips and placed around the impression tray prior to pouring?
   a. boxing
   b. casting
   c. inlay
   d. sticky

10. Which class of stone is classified as improved stone and used to make dies?
    a. Class I
    b. Class II
    c. Class III
    d. Class IV

11. The period of time when material assumes shape but remains pliable is called:
    a. working time
    b. initial set
    c. setting time
    d. form time

12. A material that softens when heated and hardens when cooled is said to be:
    a. exothermic
    b. intrusive
    c. rigid
    d. thermoplastic

13. A substance composed of two or more different substances is called a/an:
    a. union
    b. compound
    c. hygroscopic
    d. elastic

14. Which of the following metals is used in a Type III alloy to provide porosity to the alloy?
    a. zinc
    b. copper
    c. gold
    d. silver

15. In a comparison of two materials, the one with a heavier viscosity would be:
    a. thicker
    b. less stable
    c. same thickness
    d. thinner

16. A substance used to take and record the shape, size, or position of items is a/an:
    a. implant
    b. investment
    c. inlay
    d. impression

17. How many carats are in the precious metal pure gold?
    a. 10
    b. 12
    c. 20
    d. 24

18. Polysiloxane impression material is not supplied in which of these viscosities?
    a. slurry
    b. heavy
    c. wash
    d. medium

19. Which of the following finishing agents is considered an abrasive agent?
    a. chromium oxide
    b. chalk
    c. carborundum
    d. tin oxide

20. Trituration is another term for which process?
    a. heating
    b. polymerization
    c. amalgamation
    d. curing

Building Skills

Locate and define the prefix, root/combining form, and suffix (if present) in the following words.

1. **thermoplastic**
   prefix _____
   root/combining form _____
   suffix _____

2. **polycarboxylate**
   prefix _____
   root/combining form _____
   suffix _____

3. **exothermal**
   prefix _____
   root/combining form _____
   suffix _____

4. **polymerization**
   prefix _____
   root/combining form _____
   suffix _____

5. **electroplated**
   prefix _____
   root/combining form _____
   suffix _____

Fill-Ins

Write the correct word in the blank space to complete each statement.

1. The mixing of mercury with other metal alloys is a/an _____.

2. A thin, watery mixture of an abrasive material is a/an _____.

3. A mixture of five different metals is a/an _____ alloy.

4. A/an _____ is added to resin material to cause a softening effect.

5. A/an _____ is a reproduction of a prepared tooth for a crown or bridgework.

6. The time period when it is possible to mold, shape, or manipulate a material without an adverse effect upon the material is called _____ time.

7. A/an _____ is a substance that speeds up chemical reactions.

8. Model plaster is also known as _____ of _____.

9. A/an _____ process is used to coat a stone die with a thin metal sheeting cover.

10. An extruder gun is used to express _____ material to a preparation.

11. Slow bending or movement of a material under its own weight is termed _____.

12. Toughness is the ability of a material to resist _____.

13. Hue, chroma, and value are the three components of _____.

14. The forced union of one substance with another substance is _____.

15. Tin oxide, chalk, rouge, and tripoli are examples of a/an _____ agent.

16. _____ is used to unite two metals in a prosthesis.

17. _____ is a fear of water or shedding off of water.

18. The polishing agent—rouge—would be used to obtain a shine on denture resin or _____.

19. _____ wax may be used for construction of patterns for partial dentures.

20. The maximum amount of stress at which metal will return to the original form when stress is removed is termed _____.

Word Use

Read the following sentences, and define the meaning of the word written in boldface letters.

1. The dental technician warned the trainee to be careful of the **exothermic** chemical reaction that occurs when mixing the cement material.

_____

2. When following the fabrication prescription order for the prosthesis, the technician works with the **alloy** the dentist prefers.

_____

3. The dental assistant noted that the **setting time** of the new cement was different from the former brand of cement used in the office.

_____

4. The dentist asked the assistant to pour up the **die** impression with Class II improved stone.

_____

5. The technician noted that using some plaster **slurry** in the mix hastens the setting time.

_____

CHAPTER 19 | DENTAL LABORATORY PROCEDURES

✓ Learning Objectives

On completion of this chapter, you should be able to:

1. Identify the professional personnel related to the construction of dental prostheses or appliances made in the lab setting.

2. List and identify the assorted machinery and equipment articles necessary for laboratory procedures.

3. Describe the divisions of prosthodontia into fixed or removable sections and the major differences between these areas.

4. List and describe the assorted appliances that may be included in the partial reconstruction of the oral cavity and dental care.

5. List and describe the major fixed prosthodontic items and the variety of crowns and bridgework available.

6. Discuss the miscellaneous assortment of dental appliances and items used to protect, maintain, or correct dental care.

7. Explain how computer-assisted systems assist with dental laboratory procedures, and discuss the available units.

RANGE AND SCOPE OF THE DENTAL LABORATORY

A dental laboratory is the area where laboratory procedures necessary to complete dental health care are accomplished. The laboratory can be located in an independent building or in a specified area of a dental office facility. The dentist or prosthodontist may perform the dental laboratory work, or it may be assigned to others. A **dental laboratory technician** is trained in this

---

Vocabulary Related to Dental Laboratory Procedures

This list contains selected new and important word parts and terms from this chapter. Take the time to learn these word parts and their meanings. You may use the list to review these terms and practice pronouncing them correctly. When you work with the audio for this chapter, listen to the word, repeat it, and then place a checkmark in the box. Proceed to the next boxed word, and repeat the process.

(hyphen before word means it's a suffix, hyphen after word means prefix, no hyphen means root word.)

Word Part	Meaning	Word Part	Meaning
inter-	between	techne	art, skill, craft
later/latus	side	uni-	one
proxi	joining		

Key Terms

- ❑ **abutment** (ah-**BUT**-ment)
- ❑ **articulator** (ar-**TICK**-you-lay-tore)
- ❑ **bilateral** (bi-**LAT**-er-al)
- ❑ **cantilever** (**KAN**-tih-lee-ver)
- ❑ **ceramist** (sir-**AM**-ist)
- ❑ **circumferential** (ser-**kum**-fer-**EN**-shal)

- ❑ **dowel** (**DOWL**)
- ❑ **festoon** (fes-**TUNE**)
- ❑ **flange** (**FLANJ**)
- ❑ **flux** (**FLUKS**)
- ❑ **hydrocolloid** (high-droh-**KAHI**-oyd)
- ❑ **protrusion** (pro-**TRUE**-zhun)

- ❑ **retrusion** (ree-**TRUE**-zhun)
- ❑ **solder** (**SOD**-er)
- ❑ **sprue** (**SPROO**)
- ❑ **unilateral** (you-nih-**LAT**-er-al)

type of work through formal schooling or on-the-job experience. After graduation or training, the technician can become a **certified dental technician (CDT)** by passing all three examinations given by the National Board for Certification. A **denturist** fabricates dentures and is legalized by the state dental boards in some states. A **ceramist** (sir-**AM**-ist = *an expert in ceramics*) specializes in porcelain crowns and restorations.

All dental laboratory work, when not completed specifically by the dentist, must follow prescription orders from the practicing dentist. This **work order** is attached to each case sent to the lab. The amount of time required by the laboratory to complete the prescription is termed the **working days** and is included in the appointment setup.

DENTAL LABORATORY EQUIPMENT

Various items and equipment are necessary in the dental laboratory to complete the construction and fabrication procedures.

- **articulator** (ar-**TICK**-you-lay-tor = *device to imitate joint action*): machine that imitates the movement of the mandible and TMJ on mounted models. Constructed models of the patient's mouth are arranged in the patient's "bite pattern" or articulation. Figure 19-1 shows gypsum models with a denture setup placed on an articulator that imitates the opening and closing of the patient's jaw. Smaller one-time use hinge articulators can be used to hold together maxillary and mandibular casts in an articulated manner, but they are not adjustable.

- **model trimmer:** grinding, motorized, abrasive disc device used to trim or remove excess gypsum on diagnostic casts in preparation for placement on articulators or for models that may be used as visual records of mouth conditions for patient education and treatment planning.

- **gypsum mixing machine:** device used for mechanical mixing of gypsum products; the machine also has a vacuum process to eliminate air bubbles in the mixture.

- **vibrator:** small table-model appliance with a platform to hold bowls of freshly mixed gypsum; used to gently shake or vibrate air bubbles to the top of the mixture.

Figure 19-1 Gypsum models with denture setup mounted on an articulator

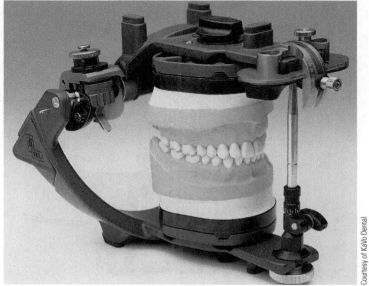

Courtesy of KaVo Dental

- **furnace:** heating device with high temperature range (up to 2000°C or 3632°F); used to melt out the wax patterns from the investment material; similar to a pottery kiln but smaller.
- **waxing unit:** heater unit to melt and hold lab wax (50–120°C, 122–248°F) in a liquid state for use in laboratory construction procedures.
- **waxing pens/pencils:** handheld electrical heating device with various insert tips used to carve and mold wax patterns.
- **oven:** hot-air heat devices to prepare materials 100–480°C (200–900°F).
- **bath:** hot oil, or water-heat device to prepare materials to 200°C (350°F) temperature.
- **hydrocolloid conditioning machine:** heating device that uses water to condition and prepare reversible hydrocolloid material for impressions. The machine has three compartments for graduated heated water baths.
- **burner:** heating device to externally heat an object not contained within it, for example, Bunsen burner or micro torch; used to heat wax for carving or sheets of baseplate wax for models.
- **vacuum formers:** device used to heat acrylic sheets and vacuum pressure them to a prepared form for construction of a custom impression tray, mouth guard, surgical template, or tooth-bleaching trays. The vacuum press in Figure 19-2 contours the acrylic sheet to the model form.
- **electroplating unit:** electrical device used to apply alloy materials to surface objects, such as dies; the alloy covering on the stone die protects the surface of the die during fabrication.
- **blowtorch:** heating device using compressed gas or chemical fuel to melt alloys for casting.
- **casting machine:** centrifugal spin device used to force melted alloy into an investment ring.

Figure 19-2 Vacuum press

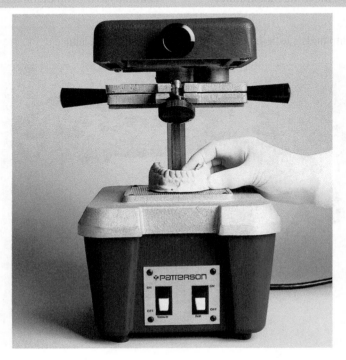

- **curing unit:** device used to heat-cure or complete the polymerization process of acrylics; may use pressurized heat or a light-curing unit for bonding materials and substances.
- **sandblasting machine:** air-abrasion machine with forced abrasive material (sand) flow to polish and clean items.
- **lathe:** electrical motor with extended rods for attachment of appliances (abrasive discs, rag wheels, bur chuck, etc.) for sanding, smoothing, and shaping of materials.
- **splash pan:** receptacle with high back that is inserted under the lathe wheel ends; the pan captures and contains the splash from the attachments and helps to maintain a clean area.
- **dust collector:** suction-powered unit to remove gypsum and acrylic dust from the lab area.
- **plating unit:** machine to electroplate gold veneers, precious metals, and semiprecious metals.
- **electric motors and handpieces:** benchtop units providing selective handpiece power for lab operations. Figure 19-3 shows a tabletop lab handpiece used for laboratory refining and adjusting procedures.

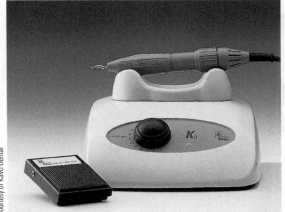

Figure 19-3 Example of a tabletop lab handpiece

Courtesy of KaVo Dental

- **welder/solder machine:** electric unit used to weld orthodontic bands or for general soldering.

DENTURE CONSTRUCTION LABORATORY PROCEDURES

Each dental laboratory procedure, whether performed in the dental office or in a commercial lab, has terminology related to the fabrication of specific items. Some terms are more general, and others are specific to a procedure. Common terms related to denture construction procedures are *denture* and *prosthesis*. A **denture** set is a replacement for a body part, also known as a prosthesis.

Types of Dentures

An assortment of denture types accommodates all of the reconstructive reasons for tooth replacement:

- **full-mouth denture set:** a complete replacement for the maxillary and mandibular arches; composed of two trays—the maxillary denture plate and the mandibular plate.
- **single denture:** a denture replacement for one arch, either maxillary or mandibular.
- **immediate denture:** a denture that is placed in the mouth at the time the natural teeth are surgically removed. After removal of the teeth and an alveolectomy to prepare the bone, the tissues are sutured, and the denture is inserted into place—not permanently attached like an implant denture.
- **overdenture:** acrylic denture prepared to fit on the bony ridge and gingiva while attached to the remaining teeth or implant devices (see Figure 19-4).

Denture Construction

Specialized terms are used to describe the materials and process of fabricating a set of dentures:

- **denture base:** pink acrylic part of the denture that fits over and covers the alveolar ridge (gum); can be shaded light or dark pink, ethnic, or clear palate.

Figure 19-4 An example of an overdenture prosthesis

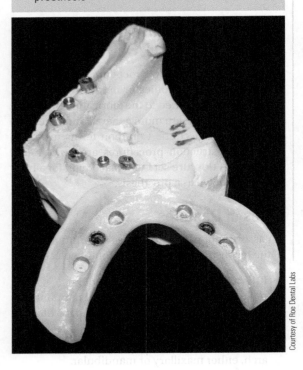

Courtesy of Roe Dental Labs

- **denture teeth:** artificial teeth used in denture construction; may be porcelain or acrylic material and supplied on anterior or posterior "cards," differing in shape, color, and material (see Figure 19-5).
- **denture flange:** extension of denture over the posterior anatomy present; used to stabilize.
- **denture post dam:** suction seal of denture that extends side to side from the rear of the denture.
- **impression tray:** may be custom made or purchased commercially as plain or perforated full arch (upper and lower), quadrant (right and left), or anterior (universal) in metal or plastic material. The trays are used to hold material for the impression procedure. Trays with holes are used for alginate material; other materials use a smooth plain tray, sometimes painted with an adhesive coating. Water-cooled trays—used to cool the material for faster setup—have hollow raised edges to help retain the hydrocolloid material and are attached by tubing to a suction unit to recover the circulating water. Examples of some impression trays may be viewed in Figure 12-4 in Chapter 12, Prosthodontics.

Figure 19-5 Denture teeth on anterior and posterior "cards"

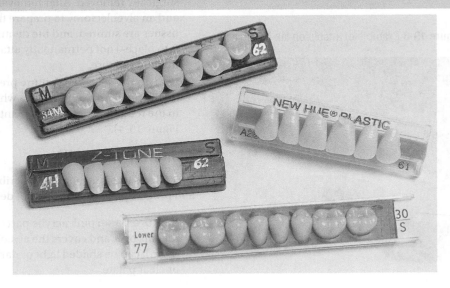

- **spacer:** material, usually baseplate wax, that is placed on the model or cast surface to allow a space for the impression material.
- **stop:** indents or holes cut out of the spacer in the tray to prevent the tray from being placed too deeply.
- **adhesive:** sticky liquid that is painted or sprayed on the surface of the smooth impression tray to help retain the impression material in the tray.
- **molding:** finger shaping of the impression material over the edge of the tray for better adaptation; also called **muscle trimming**.
- **wax setup:** sample prosthesis used to fit, adjust, and test jaw relationship of the wax denture. Made of baseplate wax, shellac, or thermoplastic material formed and constructed on a model of the patient's mouth, the baseplate will become the pattern for the denture base.
- **occlusal rims:** wax block placed on the baseplate over the residual ridge of the plate; the rims are used for placement of denture teeth while mounted on the articulator.
- **festooning:** melting, shaping, and forming of the wax rims to simulate functional and esthetic gingival tissue.

Wax Try-In Procedures

After the construction of the wax denture with the positioned denture teeth, the patient returns to the dentist for a try-in appointment. This visit is to determine the proper seating and articulation of the dentures and the correct alignment of the denture teeth. The dentist will observe and examine a number of things during this visit:

- **centric relationship:** the most retruded, unstrained position in the mandibular condyle in the glenoid fossa, or commonly stated as "biting on the posterior teeth."
- **retrusion** (ree-**TRUE**-shun): position of the mandible as far posterior as possible while in occlusion.
- **protrusion** (proh-**TRUE**-shun): position of the mandible as far anterior as possible while in occlusion.

- **lateral excursion:** sliding position of the mandible from side to side, while in occlusion.
- **vertical dimension:** space height of the denture teeth while in occlusion.
- **smile line:** amount of denture tooth space that is viewed while the patient is smiling.
- **cuspid eminence:** vertical length or height of the denture cuspid placement.

Laboratory Construction

Following the wax try-in, the technician invests the setup in a flask and removes the wax by boiling. A separating medium such as tin-foil solution is applied to the mold, the original denture teeth are replaced, and an acrylic is mixed, placed into the flask, and cured. When cured, the acrylic denture with the teeth is removed, cleaned, polished, and returned to the dentist.

REMOVABLE PARTIAL DENTURE CONSTRUCTION LABORATORY PROCEDURES

A dental prosthesis that replaces one or more teeth is a **partial appliance**. When it is fixed or cemented in the mouth, it is usually called **crown and bridgework**. When the prosthesis is able to be removed at will by the patient, it is known as a **removable partial denture**. A **bilateral** partial denture replaces the teeth and structures on both sides of the arch, whereas a **unilateral** partial denture replaces teeth and structure on only one side. Although construction of the partial denture resembles that of the complete denture, the partial has more components. Some of these components are illustrated in Figure 12-3, Chapter 12, Prosthodontics. Related terms are:

- **framework:** the skeleton of the partial prosthesis to which acrylic material and artificial teeth will be applied (see Figure 19-6).
- **abutment:** the remaining natural tooth or implanted device that supports and stabilizes the prosthesis.

Figure 19-6 An example of dental framework for a prosthesis

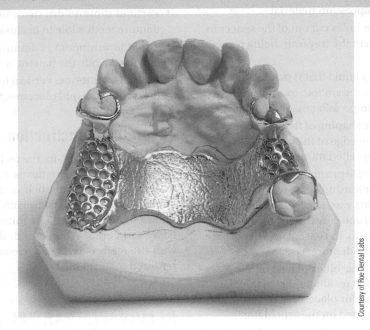

Courtesy of Roe Dental Labs

- **connector:** metal framework that unites the left and right sides of the partial appliance. Major connectors may be in the form of a bar, plate, or strap. A connector is termed **palatal** in the maxillary and **lingual** in the mandibular prosthesis. Minor connectors may unite the framework with the saddles.
- **saddle:** mesh extension of the framework that rests on the alveolar ridge. The mesh will be covered with pink acrylic material to resemble oral tissue.
- **stress breaker:** a device placed in stress-bearing areas to assist with occlusal forces.
- **retainer:** a clasp or removable partial denture attachment that is applied to an abutment tooth to provide retention; may be clasp type or an intracoronal retainer and fabricated as a cast, wrought-wire, or a combination of the two. The two styles of clasps are:
  - ○ **bar:** originates at the prosthesis base or connector border and extends upward toward the tooth undercut.

  - ○ **Circumferential** (ser-**kum**-fer-**EN**-shal = *around*): a clasp that encircles a tooth more than 180 degrees with one terminal end in the undercut of the tooth crown.
- **rest:** metal projector or clasp extension that fits into the prepared area or restoration of the abutting tooth. Rests supply support and stabilization and are described according to their surface position, such as occlusal rests or lingual rests.

FIXED PROSTHODONTIC DENTAL LABORATORY PROCEDURES

A dental prosthesis that is prepared and cemented into or onto the teeth is termed a fixed prosthesis. Examples of fixed prostheses are inlays, onlays, veneers, various crowns, and fixed bridges. These prostheses are cast and prepared in the dental laboratory from impressions or patterns supplied by the dentist. Some common terms and illustrations used to describe fixed prosthodontic items were introduced in Chapter 12, Prosthodontics. Related terms are:

- **inlay:** cast restoration that sits inside of the tooth cusps and is constructed to fit in the tooth preparation of the proximal walls and a portion of the occlusal surface.
- **onlay:** cast restoration that covers one or more of the tooth cusps and is constructed to fit the tooth preparation of proximal walls and most or all of the occlusal surface.
- **three-quarter crown:** cast restoration that is applied to a tooth prepared on all surfaces except the facial surface.
- **full crown:** cast restoration that covers the entire visible, anatomical tooth.
- **porcelain fused to metal crown (PFM):** full cast crown restoration that has a porcelain (ceramic) veneer applied to prepared surfaces. The PFM gives an esthetic, natural appearance to the metal casting.
- **veneer:** a thin, tooth-colored shell that is applied to the prepared facial surface of a tooth.
- **porcelain jacket crown (PJC):** thin metal and ceramic veneered crown for an anterior tooth.
- **post and core crown (PCC):** crown for use in an endodontically treated tooth with significant loss of tooth structure. The crown has an internal post to fit into the pulp chamber and the prepared core to give full coverage and strength.
- **temporary crown:** acrylic, aluminum, or composite crown constructed and provisionally cemented on for protection while construction of the permanent crown is completed.
- **fixed bridge:** prosthesis that replaces one or more missing teeth; usually involves adjoining teeth (abutment) to space and is therefore termed *crown and bridge prosthesis.*
- **cantilever** (**KAN**-tah-**lee**-ver) **bridge:** prosthesis in which only one side of the device is attached to the retainer or abutment tooth.
- **Maryland bridge:** conservative, prepared resin-retained prosthesis using a bonding procedure to hold to adjacent teeth; may be used in either anterior or posterior area.

Prosthesis Fabrication

Fabrication of the dental prosthesis is completed in the dental laboratory. The construction process of these dental devices also has specialized terminology:

- **occlusal records:** measurements of jaw relationships and articulation of teeth; measurements are obtained with impressions and/or articulation devices.
- **facebow:** measurement device used to record the occlusal position (see Figure 19-7). A wax-lined bite fork is placed in the mouth for a bite registration, and calipers from the facebow are inserted into the patient's ears for axis relation. The nosepiece is placed on the nasal bridge and noted. After the device is removed, all measurements are repeated on the articulator to simulate the patient's occlusal record. Computerized digital impressions of both arches combined with design software can now be used to record and plan the positioning of prostheses. Models may be fabricated and articulated using captured digital information, thereby eliminating the use of some facebow-positioning measurements.
- **die:** exact stone replica of the tooth preparation that is receiving the prosthesis; usually made of dental stone and may be electroplated for extra strength.

Figure 19-7 Facebow for recording measurement

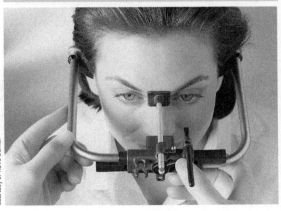

Courtesy of KaVo Dental

- **dowel (DOWL) pin:** tapered brass post that is placed into the die when the stone is poured; used as the handle of the die during the waxing and carving of the pattern.
- **wax pattern:** exact wax replica of the prosthesis to be completed; prepared by melting wax on the die and carving it to proportion. The pattern is invested (encased) in a gypsum product, then melted out to leave a form or shape for the casting of the alloy reproduction (see Figure 19-8A).
- **separating medium:** material placed upon the die before the wax is melted onto it to enable separation when completed. A thicker medium may be applied to provide **die relief**, a space in the prosthesis to accommodate the cement process.
- **sprue (SPROO) pin:** a small, plastic pin or wax channel area attached to a wax pattern to provide space in the investment for the entry of melted metal in the casting procedure (see Figure 19-8B).
- **sprue base:** a brass disc with a rounded, pyramid top used to hold the sprue pin that is attached to a wax pattern. The base receives the bottom of the casting ring, and, when all assembled, it is filled with investment material (see Figure 19-8B).
- **casting ring:** small ring, 1⅜" by 1¼", that is used to hold the invested pattern during the investing of the gypsum material and the casting of the melted metal (see Figure 19-8B, C, and D).
- **liner:** ring-lining material placed inside the casting ring to allow for the investment expansion.
- **investment:** gypsum, silica, and reducing-agent material prepared to maintain the shape of the wax pattern during casting; may be mixed and placed into the ring with a vacuum machine or by hand.
- **wax elimination:** burn or heating out of wax pattern from hardened investment material, leaving a void in the shape of the wax pattern. Wax elimination is completed in the lab furnace.
- **casting:** procedure in which melted alloy is centrifugally forced from the crucible into the casting ring to fill the void in the shape of the melted out wax pattern. It is completed with a casting machine—either electrically heated and forced or manually melting the alloy and force casting—or by throwing the melted material into the void through a spring action release.

Figure 19-8 Preparations of a gold inlay: (A) wax pattern with sprue pin attached; (B) sprue pin inserted into sprue base while investment material is being poured; (C) pattern in inverted inlay casting ring after wax pattern has been melted away; (D) casted gold inlay in investing ring before removing and polishing; (E) completed gold inlay in the prepared tooth

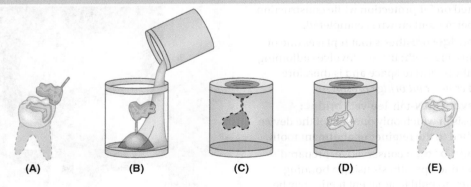

(A)   (B)   (C)   (D)   (E)

- **blowtorch:** compressed-air heating device to melt the alloy for casting; produces a flame with four heating zones exiting from the nozzle:
  - **Zone 1:** junction area when gases meet; unproductive.
  - **Zone 2:** combustion area, oxidizing, slightly green; not to be used.
  - **Zone 3:** reducing area, bluish, hottest part of flame; the desirable use zone.
  - **Zone 4:** oxidizing area, where flame meets air; coolest part of the flame.
- **pickling solution:** solution used to remove surface film from the cast restoration.

Finishing and Polishing Procedures

The finishing and polishing procedure refines the cast restoration. It may be completed with a sandblasting device or by using handpiece drills and bits along with polishing material and rag wheels on a dental lathe. The completed casting may be returned to the dentist for permanent cementation or used in a fixed appliance with other pieces.

Uniting Prosthesis Units

After the construction of each independent part or unit of the appliance, the prosthesis is completed. The separate units are united to form one piece of bridgework. The process of uniting parts or units together to form a single prosthesis has special terms associated with it:

- **soldering:** joining of two metals by the fusion of an intermediate alloy that may be silver or gold.
- **flux** (**FLUKS** = *flow*): an agent used to protect the alloy from oxidation during the heating process; may be a powder with a low-fusing melting point that forms a molten state over the area to be soldered.

- **anti-flux:** material, usually graphite, that is applied to retard the forward advance of the melted solder.
- **welding:** the direct joining of two metals by a fusion process.
- **porcelain fused to metal:** a process of bonding porcelain material to a metal sub-base, then firing it to hardness.

MISCELLANEOUS DENTAL LABORATORY PROCEDURES

Besides the construction of dentures, castings, and prostheses, the dental technician may perform other procedures, such as relining, repairing, and duplicating dentures; replacing broken teeth in dentures; fabricating mouth guards, bleaching trays, biteplanes, orthodontic retainers, and appliances; or constructing sleep and snoring abating devices, study models, and performing basic laboratory services required by the dental profession. In the cosmetic vein, some laboratories are now called on to present a before-and-after picture or model view for the prospective makeover patient; other laboratories encourage patients to visit for custom shading and finishing colors. Some dental laboratories perform all possible services, and others limit their services to specified procedures or materials.

CAD/CAM IN THE DENTAL LABORATORY

With the addition of CAD/CAM (computer-aided design and computer-aided manufacturing) technology, the dental laboratory procedures and protocol are changing. Instead of the labored impression taking, model making, waxing, and prosthesis construction, machine systems are providing a digital data image capture of the prepared site and supplying a workable fabrication model or milled restoration with minimum effort.

There are four available computer-aided systems:

1. CEREC AC with Bluecam (Sirona), a CAD/CAM unit
2. E4D Dentist (D4D Technologies), a CAD/CAM unit
3. LAVA chairside oral scanner (COS) (3M ESPE), digital impression unit (DIU)
4. iTero (Cadent), digital impression unit (DIU)

CAD/CAM Systems

The two CAD/CAM systems are:

- **CEREC AC with Bluecam:** "one-day dentistry" for inlays, crowns, onlays, and restorations. The dentist makes a tooth preparation, dusts the prep with opaque powder, and then uses a blue light scan wand to capture data image of the prepared arch and opposing quadrant (bite registration). The dentist reviews the 3D model from the system for modifications or changes until approval. In the office laboratory, the milling unit—an enclosed device with diamond surfaced burs for lathe grinding of blocks—is loaded with the correct shaded, sized material (ceramic) block, and the wireless order is relayed to the mill unit. Upon completion of milling (approximately 15–20 minutes), the restoration is tried for fit, polished, and placed in the etched and cemented prep. With CEREC Connect, the captured data may also be sent to an outside laboratory for a lab-fabricated restoration in any material.
- **E4D Dentist:** uses a laser-type wand that obtains three views (buccal, lingual, and occlusal) per tooth. Does not need contrasting powder and can exhibit multiple (up to 16) restorations on a single window. The system can produce a 3D working model for dentist approval and in-office milling or can forward the digital model to the dentist's choice

laboratory facility for final fabrication of the restoration.

DIU (Digital Impression Unit)

There are two DIU systems:

- **LAVA COS (chairside oral scanner):** uses a handheld wand with LED lights to scan over the prepared and powdered prep area, opposing arch, and buccal surfaces. The monitor indicates correct wand positioning by color view: white for acceptable, pink for data need, and black for not scanned. The dentist uses 3D glasses to review the processed 3D model and, when approved, forwards the information with a prescription inscribed on the touch screen to the system's technician, who designs the prosthesis. The manufacturer uses a resin technique (stereolithography) to construct a working model to be sent to the dentist's chosen laboratory facility to fabricate the restoration in any chosen material and return it to the dentist (see Figure 19-9).
- **iTero system:** uses a handheld laser/optical wand with wireless foot pedal to take a series of images. The machine speaks to the user (dentist/assistant) indicating which tooth surface and tooth to do. These images of the powderless prep are used to produce a 3D model that the dentist reviews and alters, if needed. After the dentist reviews and modifications are made with a wireless mouse, the data is uploaded to the iTero milling center for model fabrication from polyurethane blocks that are shipped to the dentist's laboratory of choice within 3–5 days.

There are many advantages to using computer-assisted systems in the dental laboratory, but there is a large startup expense; with the in-office milling units, there is also an inventory cost for mill blocks in various shades, sizes, and materials. The individual dentist will make the choice of which method to use in the dental laboratory arena.

Figure 19-9 Example of a processed model from a CAD/CAM impression

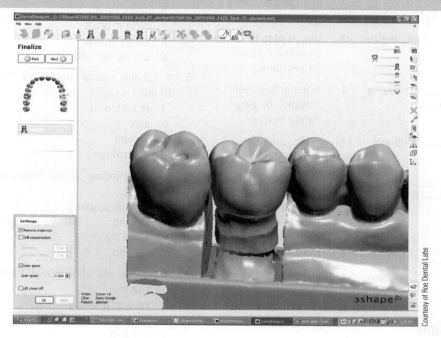

Review Exercises

Matching

Match the following word elements with their meanings.

1. _____ smile line   **A.** machine that imitates jaw and TMJ movements

2. _____ adhesive   **B.** artificial body part

3. _____ PJC   **C.** sticky material applied to trays to hold impression

4. _____ framework   **D.** amount of tooth space viewed while patient is smiling

5. _____ flux   **E.** restoration for proximal and most of occlusal surfaces

6. _____ liner   **F.** thin metal and ceramic veneered crown for anterior

7. _____ casting ring   **G.** prosthesis skeleton

8. _____ onlay   **H.** natural retaining tooth in a bridge

9. _____ wax pattern   **I.** exact reproduction of prosthesis to be constructed

10. _____ PFM	**J.**	ring-lining material to allow for casting expansion
11. _____ prosthesis	**K.**	ring used to hold investment pattern for prosthesis
12. _____ separating medium	**L.**	material to prevent oxidation of alloy during heating
13. _____ abutment	**M.**	ceramic material fused to metal process
14. _____ welding	**N.**	material placed upon die surface prior to wax placement
15. _____ articulator	**O.**	fusing union of two metals

Definitions

Using the selection given for each sentence, choose the best term to complete the definition.

1. The stabilizing extension of the denture that extends over the present posterior anatomy is the:
   a. spacer
   b. flange
   c. base
   d. saddle

2. The process of melting, shaping, and forming of the wax rims is called:
   a. pickling
   b. soldering
   c. welding
   d. festooning

3. The space height of the teeth while in occlusion is the:
   a. vertical dimension
   b. centric relationship
   c. smile line
   d. protrusive aim

4. A grinding device used to shape diagnostic casts or study models is a:
   a. dental lathe
   b. vacuum press
   c. model trimmer
   d. casting machine

5. A full-arch dental prosthesis that replaces the dentition is a/an:
   a. jacket crown
   b. denture
   c. implant
   d. full crown

6. The direct joining of two metals by a fusion heat process is:
   a. vacuum pressing
   b. pickling
   c. soldering
   d. welding

7. The milling unit of a CAD/CAM system is used for which service:
   a. vacuum pressing
   b. pickling
   c. grinding
   d. festooning

8. A material, usually graphite, used to retard the advance of melted solder is:
   a. gold
   b. silver
   c. anti-flux
   d. flux

9. A process to fuse ceramic material to a metal sub-base is called:
   a. PMF
   b. PJC
   c. PCM
   d. PFM

10. A solution used to remove surface film from a cast restoration is:
    a. pickling
    b. varnish
    c. liner
    d. acid etchant

11. A brass disc with elevated center to hold a sprued wax pattern for casting is a:
    a. casting ring
    b. sprue base
    c. sprue pin
    d. dowel

12. A cemented prosthesis that replaces one or more missing teeth, usually involving other abutting teeth, is a:
    a. retractable bridge
    b. cantilever bridge
    c. full crown
    d. fixed bridge

13. The most constructive zone of a blowtorch flame for use in dental casting is:
    a. zone 1 (injection)
    b. zone 2 combustion (green)
    c. zone 3 (reducing) bluish
    d. zone 4 oxidizing (air-flame)

14. A cast restoration applied to a tooth prepared on all surfaces except the facial view is a:
    a. porcelain jacket crown
    b. full crown
    c. three quarters crown
    d. post and core crown

15. A crown used for an endodontically treated tooth with significant surface loss is a:
    a. porcelain jacket crown
    b. full crown
    c. three quarter crown
    d. post and core crown

16. The position of the mandible as far anterior as possible while in occlusion is called:
    a. lateral excursion
    b. cuspid eminence
    c. retrusion
    d. protrusion

17. The position of the mandible as far posterior as possible while in occlusion is termed:
    a. lateral excursion
    b. cuspid eminence
    c. retrusion
    d. protrusion

18. The side-to-side sliding position of the mandible while in occlusion is called:
    a. lateral excursion
    b. cuspid eminence
    c. extrusion
    d. protrusion

19. An indent or hole cut into the spacer to prevent the tray from being place too deeply is a/an:
    a. stop
    b. separator
    c. liner
    d. setup

20. A partial denture that replaces teeth and structures on both sides of the mouth is considered which type of denture?
    a. fixed
    b. bilateral
    c. unilateral
    d. retractable

Building Skills

Locate and define the prefix, root/combining form, and suffix (if present) in the following words.

1. **interproximal**
   prefix _____
   root/combining form _____
   suffix _____

2. **reinforced**
   prefix _____
   root/combining form _____
   suffix _____

3. **technology**
   prefix _____
   root/combining form _____
   suffix _____

4. **prosthodontia**
   prefix _____
   root/combining form _____
   suffix _____

5. **unilateral**
   prefix _____
   root/combining form _____
   suffix _____

Fill-Ins

Write the correct word in the blank space to complete each statement.

1. A chairside oral scanner (COS) is used to obtain a digital _____ of the tooth preparation.

2. The dentist's orders to the laboratory to complete lab procedures in a specific manner is called a/an _____.

3. "One-day dentistry" is made possible with the use of a _____ system with an in-house mill unit.

4. A metal projection or clasp extension that fits into prepared areas or restoration that is used for support or stabilization is a/an _____.

5. A/an _____ is a mesh extension of a prosthesis that rests on the alveolar ridge.

6. The skeleton of a prosthesis is called the _____.

7. A/an _____ is a thin, tooth-colored shell that is applied to the prepared facial surface of a tooth.

8. The remaining natural tooth or implanted device used to support a prosthesis is a/an _____.

9. A/an _____ is an exact replica of a prepared tooth receiving a prosthesis.

10. A liquid used to remove the surface film from the recently casted restoration is a _____ solution.

11. A/an _____ pin is a tapered brass post inserted into the die during the setup procedure; used to hold the die during working procedures.

12. The metal framework that unites the right and left sides of the prosthesis is called a/an _____.

13. _____ wax is supplied in thin sheets and used for construction of the denture base.

14. A blue stick wax used to make wax patterns is called _____ wax.

15. Wax blocks placed upon the baseplate wax and used to hold the teeth for the denture are called _____.

16. A/an _____ is the posterior part of the denture extending from side to side and provides the denture suction.

17. Uniting two metals by fusing with another alloy is called _____.

18. _____ is the procedure where melted alloy is forced from the crucible into the casting ring.

19. The agent used to protect the alloy from oxidation during the heating process is _____.

20. A _____ median is painted on the surface of die before the wax pattern is constructed on it.

Word Use

Read the following sentences, and define the meaning of the word written in boldface letters.

1. The hygienist instructed the patient about toothbrushing and oral care with the **partial appliance**.

   _____

2. The patient requested an **immediate denture** because she did not wish to miss time where she worked.

   _____

3. When getting a crown-prep impression, most patients prefer the **CAD/CAM** digital capture system to the impression material and tray inserts.

   _____

4. The dentist advised Mr. Thomas that his new bridge would require an **abutment** on both sides of the artificial tooth replacement.

   _____

5. The prosthodontist placed the prepared model on the **articulator** to test the occlusion of the denture teeth.

   _____

20 | BUSINESS MANAGEMENT PROCEDURES

✓ Learning Objectives

On completion of this chapter, you should be able to:

1. Discuss the HIPAA concerns for patient privacy and the various avenues of communication, including oral and written methods.

2. Explain the different types of appointments and related scheduling terms and practices.

3. Identify the assorted terms used in patient recording and the methods or systems of filing and organization.

4. List and identify the different types of correspondence used in the dental facility, including the major divisions of the business letter.

5. Discuss the various types of dental insurance plans and related dental insurance terms.

6. Define the types of financial disbursements used in the dental facility, list common banking terms, and identify methods of account management.

7. Discuss the methods used in inventory control and the terms that relate to purchasing and inventory of supplies.

8. List and identify the major legal and ethical terms encountered in the dental practice.

OFFICE COMMUNICATION PROCEDURES

As a dental assistant, it will be important for you to be cross trained in all aspects of the dental office. Whether a dental facility is a large clinic or small office operation, the terms used to transact the business aspect of the practice are the same. Appointments must be made, letters written, and records maintained. Communication by oral (telephone), written (mail), and electronic (e-mail or text) means is an essential part of the business aspect of dentistry.

When working in the area of communication, the dental-care provider must follow the **Health Insurance Portability and Accountability Act (HIPAA)** privacy regulations. One of the aspects of the HIPAA bill is the protection of a patient's health and medical records. This law gives the patient the right to obtain, review, and make corrections (if appropriate) of the information collected. Doctors, dentists, hospitals, clinics, and those who provide services to the patient must give written notice of how the patient records will be safeguarded and cared for. At the initial visit, the patient signs and specifies who may have access to information. The dental facility and those who are employed there are responsible for keeping all records confidential and following the HIPAA privacy regulations when dealing with any patient matters.

Oral Communication

Oral communication involves a conversation between two or more persons either face-to-face, by phone, or through electronic automated contact. In the dental facility, much communication with others is by telephone. Often this is the first contact a patient will have with the dental facility. Related terms are:

- **incoming calls:** phone calls received by the dental facility:
  - **appointment:** call to request an appointment or information about an appointment matter.
  - **personal:** call from a personal friend, colleague, family member, and the like.
  - **inquiry:** call requesting information, such as a question about a statement or test results.
  - **emergency:** call requesting immediate attention for treatment or care.

- **professional:** call regarding particular care or concern in patient matters.
- **outgoing calls:** calls made from the dental facility personnel or an automated calling/appointment service:
  - **confirmation:** call to confirm an upcoming appointment.
  - **ordering:** call to a supplier or store to place an order.
  - **inquiry:** call to request information regarding a matter, such as the availability of product.
  - **collection:** call to arrange payment for an outstanding statement.
- **answering machine:** device used to record incoming messages when no one is available to answer the phone, including automatic routing for particular calls, mailbox recording for specific personnel, and voicemail for the office.
- **answering service:** professional service that will answer phone calls and take messages, forward messages, and advise patients of working hours and availability.
- **conference call:** telephone service in which more than two persons at different locations may converse on the phone in the same conversation.
- **video communication:** commonly referred to as teledentistry or virtual dental care; it allows patients to receive long-distance dental support. This service incorporates wireless and terrestrial communications with video conferencing and streaming media to provide the public with a dental assessment.

Written Communications

Many office communications are written, both by traditional mail, e-mail, texting, and faxing. All communications represent the dental practice and must be neat and accurate. Related terms are:

- **first-class mail:** letters, postcards, statements, business reply, and larger marked envelopes.

- **second-class mail:** periodicals, magazines, and newspapers.
- **third-class mail:** catalogs, circulars, books, and printed material weighing less than one pound.
- **fourth-class mail:** printed matter or parcels weighing more than a pound; also called parcel post.
- **certified mail:** postal fee service that records mail delivery by dating, numbering, and recording mailed pieces. The sender may track the progress of the mail using the receipt number.
- **C.O.D. mail (cash on delivery):** fee service in which a postal employee collects money at the time of delivery.
- **express mail:** fast, 24-hour delivery of mail.
- **priority mail:** mail delivery within two to three days.
- **insured mail:** postal fee service insures item sent for a set price declared by the sender.
- **registered mail:** postal fee service to record and protect mail to delivery sites; postal office supplies proof (card) that material has been received; generally used for important papers.
- **restricted delivery:** mail delivered only to the specified person.
- **signature confirmation:** requires signature of recipient upon delivery.
- **special delivery:** swift delivery of mail by the post office when received at the local station; fee for service.
- **special handling:** special USPS service that is required for specific types of shipments that need extra care when being mailed, such as live specimens.
- **e-mail:** communication by means of computer.
- **fax:** communication by telephone line connection.
- **text message:** immediate delivery of written text by means of telephone communication.
- **ground package service:** parcels or packages containing dental cases, returns, items to be repaired, and so forth may be sent by FedEx,

UPS, or USPS. Pickup service can be arranged. USPS provides package delivery using priority, parcel, media, or library rates and flat-rate boxes and containers of varying size and expense.

- **online postal services:** includes stamp purchase, calculation of postage, printing of labels, proof of delivery, and tracking of postal matters.
- **incoming mail:** mail that has been delivered to the dental facility:
  - **invoice:** printed from supplier regarding orders received by a facility; may or may not be a demand for payment.
  - **statement:** request for payment for services, products, or material received by a facility.
  - **miscellaneous:** may include lab reports, general information or correspondence, meeting information, samples, or advertisements.
  - **packages:** may be from dental laboratories, suppliers, or sample products.
  - **personal:** mail meant for a specific individual, not general business communications.
  - **payment:** envelopes containing checks as payment for statement or treatment received.
- **outgoing mail:** mail that is sent from the facility; may be sent as first class, special delivery, priority, registered, or certified.
- **ZIP code:** specific numbers assigned by the postal office to designated areas of the country.

APPOINTMENT CONTROL

The appointment book is the center or hub of the dental practice. Proper scheduling helps the practice run smoothly. Improper scheduling or deviation from the usual routine can be a source of frustration and increase the workload, as well as stress among the staff. See Figure 20-1 for an example of the appointment sheet for a day. Terms related to appointment control are:

- **appointment:** period of time set aside for a scheduled patient.
- **appointment card:** printed reminder of patient's next appointment day and time.
- **appointment entry:** recording patient's name, procedure, phone number, and other required data into a computer program or schedule book for a specific time and day.
- **buffer period:** open unit or block of time that is maintained on the schedule page; used for emergencies or to make up time when running behind schedule.
- **call list:** list of patients willing to be summoned at first available opening or when cancellations occur.
- **daily schedule:** copy of schedule of patients and procedures for the day. Copies are placed in strategic places for easy reference.
- **dovetail scheduling:** process in which appointment times may be scheduled into the day's procedures at a "down" period of another appointment. For example, suture removal for one patient may be scheduled during the waiting period of anesthesia onset of another patient.
- **matrix:** pattern of work periods available for appointment scheduling. Nonworking hours, meetings, holidays, vacations, or any time the practice will not be in service are marked off the schedule.
- **recall list:** system of monitoring patients' return to the dental facility. Patient is listed in the month of the desired service and called or notified at that time to make an appointment.
- **unit:** section of an hour; may be 10, 15, or 20 minutes. Each procedure is allotted a specific amount of units for scheduling purposes.

PATIENT RECORDS AND FILING PROCEDURES

Patient records are legal recordings of treatment and care received. These records comprise a variety

Figure 20-1 A typical appointment day schedule for the dental office

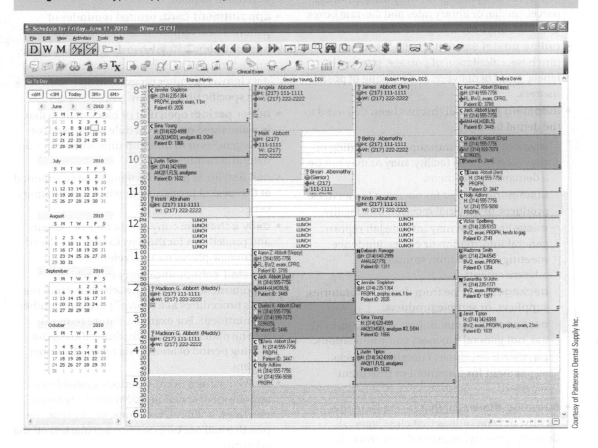

of different forms and items. When preparing and working with these patients' forms and records, neatness and accuracy should be maintained.

At the initial visit, the patient will be requested to complete forms that will supply the information to be put in the patient's file folder or placed on the computer. Some facilities give the patient a tablet PC to check themselves in and sign electronically at the conclusion. Information recorded consists of:

- **patient information chart:** questionnaire filled out by the patient, giving necessary data for office records; usually divided into general or personal, medical, insurance, and financial information queries. This information inquiry

is also called a *patient registration form* (Figure 20-2A).

- **clinical chart:** printed chart showing anatomical drawings and diagnostic results of clinical observations; also may record procedures, fees charged, and payments received.
- **consent form:** printed form signed by patient or guardian of a minor giving permission for treatment.
- **health history form:** printed questionnaire regarding patient's present and past health history, medications taken, allergies, and other health matters (Figure 20-2B).

Figure 20-2 (A) Patient registration form

PATIENT REGISTRATION

ID: _____   Chart ID: _____

First Name: _____ Last Name: _____ Middle Initial: _____

Patient Is: ☐ Policy Holder   Preferred Name: _____
☐ Responsible Party

Responsible Party (if someone other than the patient)

First Name: _____ Last Name: _____ Middle Initial: _____

Address: _____ Address 2: _____

City, State, Zip: _____ Pager: _____

Home Phone: _____ Work Phone: _____ Ext: _____ Cellular: _____

Birth Date: _____ Soc. Sec: _____ Drivers Lic: _____

○ Responsible Party is also a Policy Holder for Patient   ○ Primary Insurance Policy Holder   ○ Secondary Insurance Policy Holder

Patient Information

Address: _____ Address 2: _____

City: _____ State / Zip: _____ Pager: _____

Home Phone: _____ Work Phone: _____ Ext: _____ Cellular: _____

Sex: ○ Male   ○ Female   Marital Status: ○ Married   ○ Single   ○ Divorced   ○ Separated   ○ Widowed

Birth Date: _____ Age: _____ Soc. Sec: _____ Drivers Lic: _____

E-mail: _____ ☐ I would like to receive correspondences via e-mail.

──── Section 2 ────   ──── Section 3 ────

Employment Status: ○ Full Time   ○ Part Time   ○ Retired   Spouse Name: _____

Student Status: ○ Full Time   ○ Part Time   Spouse Employer: _____

Medicaid ID: _____ Pref. Dentist: _____   Spouse Phone: _____

Employer ID: _____ Pref. Pharmacy: _____

Carrier ID: _____ Pref. Hyg.: _____

Primary Insurance Information

Name of Insured: _____ Relationship to Insured: ○ Self   ○ Spouse   ○ Child   ○ Other

Insured Soc. Sec: _____ Insured Birth Date: _____

Employer: _____ Ins. Company: _____

Address: _____ Address: _____

Address 2: _____ Address 2: _____

City, State, Zip: _____ City, State, Zip: _____

Rem. Benefits: _____ .00   Rem. Deduct: _____ .00

Secondary Insurance Information

Name of Insured: _____ Relationship to Insured: ○ Self   ○ Spouse   ○ Child   ○ Other

Insured Soc. Sec: _____ Insured Birth Date: _____

Employer: _____ Ins. Company: _____

Address: _____ Address: _____

Address 2: _____ Address 2: _____

City, State, Zip: _____ City, State, Zip: _____

Rem. Benefits: _____ .00   Rem Deduct: _____ .00

Figure 20-2 (B) Patient medical history form

MEDICAL HISTORY

PATIENT NAME _____ Birth Date _____

Although dental personnel primarily treat the area in and around your mouth, your mouth is a part of your entire body. Health problems that you may have, or medication that you may be taking, could have an important interrelationship with the dentistry you will receive. Thank you for answering the following questions.

Are you under a physician's care now? ◯ Yes ◯ No   If yes, please explain: _____

Have you ever been hospitalized or had a major operation? ◯ Yes ◯ No   If yes, please explain: _____

Have you ever had a serious head or neck injury? ◯ Yes ◯ No   If yes, please explain: _____

Are you taking any medications, pills, or drugs? ◯ Yes ◯ No   If yes, please explain: _____

Do you take, or have you taken, Phen-Fen or Redux? ◯ Yes ◯ No   _____

Are you on a special diet? ◯ Yes ◯ No   _____

Do you use tobacco? ◯ Yes ◯ No

Do you use controlled substances? ◯ Yes ◯ No

Women: Are you
Pregnant/Trying to get pregnant? ◯ Yes ◯ No   Taking oral contraceptives? ◯ Yes ◯ No   Nursing? ◯ Yes ◯ No

Are you allergic to any of the following?
☐ Aspirin   ☐ Penicillin   ☐ Codeine   ☐ Acrylic   ☐ Metal   ☐ Latex   ☐ Local Anesthetics
☐ Other   If yes, please explain: _____

Do you have, or have you had, any of the following?

AIDS/HIV Positive	◯ Yes ◯ No	Cortisone Medicine	◯ Yes ◯ No	Hemophilia	◯ Yes ◯ No	Renal Dialysis	◯ Yes ◯ No
Alzheimer's Disease	◯ Yes ◯ No	Diabetes	◯ Yes ◯ No	Hepatitis A	◯ Yes ◯ No	Rheumatic Fever	◯ Yes ◯ No
Anaphylaxis	◯ Yes ◯ No	Drug Addiction	◯ Yes ◯ No	Hepatitis B or C	◯ Yes ◯ No	Rheumatism	◯ Yes ◯ No
Anemia	◯ Yes ◯ No	Easily Winded	◯ Yes ◯ No	Herpes	◯ Yes ◯ No	Scarlet Fever	◯ Yes ◯ No
Angina	◯ Yes ◯ No	Emphysema	◯ Yes ◯ No	High Blood Pressure	◯ Yes ◯ No	Shingles	◯ Yes ◯ No
Arthritis/Gout	◯ Yes ◯ No	Epilepsy or Seizures	◯ Yes ◯ No	Hives or Rash	◯ Yes ◯ No	Sickle Cell Disease	◯ Yes ◯ No
Artificial Heart Valve	◯ Yes ◯ No	Excessive Bleeding	◯ Yes ◯ No	Hypoglycemia	◯ Yes ◯ No	Sinus Trouble	◯ Yes ◯ No
Artificial Joint	◯ Yes ◯ No	Excessive Thirst	◯ Yes ◯ No	Irregular Heart Beat	◯ Yes ◯ No	Spina Bifida	◯ Yes ◯ No
Asthma	◯ Yes ◯ No	Fainting Spells/Dizziness	◯ Yes ◯ No	Kidney Problems	◯ Yes ◯ No	Stomach/Intestinal Disease	◯ Yes ◯ No
Blood Disease	◯ Yes ◯ No	Frequent Cough	◯ Yes ◯ No	Leukemia	◯ Yes ◯ No	Stroke	◯ Yes ◯ No
Blood Transfusion	◯ Yes ◯ No	Frequent Diarrhea	◯ Yes ◯ No	Liver Disease	◯ Yes ◯ No	Swelling of Limbs	◯ Yes ◯ No
Breathing Problem	◯ Yes ◯ No	Frequent Headaches	◯ Yes ◯ No	Low Blood Pressure	◯ Yes ◯ No	Thyroid Disease	◯ Yes ◯ No
Bruise Easily	◯ Yes ◯ No	Genital Herpes	◯ Yes ◯ No	Lung Disease	◯ Yes ◯ No	Tonsillitis	◯ Yes ◯ No
Cancer	◯ Yes ◯ No	Glaucoma	◯ Yes ◯ No	Mitral Valve Prolapse	◯ Yes ◯ No	Tuberculosis	◯ Yes ◯ No
Chemotherapy	◯ Yes ◯ No	Hay Fever	◯ Yes ◯ No	Pain in Jaw Joints	◯ Yes ◯ No	Tumors or Growths	◯ Yes ◯ No
Chest Pains	◯ Yes ◯ No	Heart Attack/Failure	◯ Yes ◯ No	Parathyroid Disease	◯ Yes ◯ No	Ulcers	◯ Yes ◯ No
Cold Sores/Fever Blisters	◯ Yes ◯ No	Heart Murmur	◯ Yes ◯ No	Psychiatric Care	◯ Yes ◯ No	Venereal Disease	◯ Yes ◯ No
Congenital Heart Disorder	◯ Yes ◯ No	Heart Pace Maker	◯ Yes ◯ No	Radiation Treatments	◯ Yes ◯ No	Yellow Jaundice	◯ Yes ◯ No
Convulsions	◯ Yes ◯ No	Heart Trouble/Disease	◯ Yes ◯ No	Recent Weight Loss	◯ Yes ◯ No		

Have you ever had any serious illness not listed above? ◯ Yes ◯ No   If yes, please explain: _____

Comments: _____
_____
_____
_____
_____

To the best of my knowledge, the questions on this form have been accurately answered. I understand that providing incorrect information can be dangerous to my (or patient's) health. It is my responsibility to inform the dental office of any changes in medical status.

SIGNATURE OF PATIENT, PARENT, or GUARDIAN _____ DATE _____

- **insurance information form:** printed questionnaire regarding insurance policy, numbers, type, and any other data supplied on the insurance card.
- **credit card/credit insurance registration:** patients who plan on using credit card services or CareCredit insurance plans may want to record data and provide signatures. Others may want to make financial arrangements at this time or in the future.
- **patient file envelope:** large file envelope used to gather and hold together all of the patient records in one central location. Folders may be color-coded to aid in file placement and retrieval. With the use of the "paperless" computer system, many offices now keep all records and patient matters stored in the office computer and backup storage discs. When a specific matter needs adjusting, the

particular file image is called up, inscribed, and then saved. All matters regarding that patient are combined in one file and at hand when needed. If some matter needs to be transferred or given to the patient, a "hard" copy (paper sheet) may be printed out immediately.

Care of Patient Records

Patient records are legal documents that belong to the dental practice; however, the patient can obtain copies and information from these records upon request. Electronic patient management and record keeping can be done by computer, but some offices still maintain paper copies of patients' charts and information as a backup protection as well as the electronic storage (see Figure 20-3). When caring for bulk amounts of patient or business records, some basic rules apply. Generally, records and

Figure 20-3 Example of a patient chart

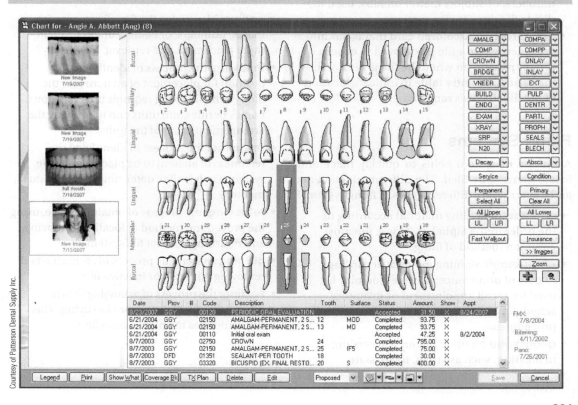

Courtesy of Patterson Dental Supply Inc.

relative materials are placed in a central location. To avoid confusion and to maintain a system of easy retrieval, the records are filed or arranged in an order.

Filing Materials

An assortment of filing materials is needed to maintain dental records:

- **file cabinet:** horizontal or vertical drawer cabinets that hold files; also, open-faced cabinets with clear access to records and more visible color-coding, and space-saving rotary files that rotate records for retrieval access.
- **file folder:** thick envelope or tabbed folder used to contain patient records and notes or other grouping of items. Tab positions may be arranged with three divisions (left, middle, right) or four divisions, called *cuts*.
- **file guide:** heavy cardboard sheet with letter, numbers, or subject matter on tabs; used to divide file drawer into sections.
- **out card:** bright-colored card that is put into the place where a file is removed to ensure proper placement when the file is returned; may also have entry table to indicate location of the file that was removed.

Filing Systems

A routine or system helps to quickly place and locate items to be filed. The different documents and items require different types of filing systems:

- **alphabetical:** filing material according to the order in the alphabet. This is the most common method of filing.
- **chronological:** filing material according to date of occurrence; this method may be used for recall appointment or inventory scheduling and other time-related procedures.
- **geographical:** filing material according to location, such as street, town, state.

This method may be used in large cities or practices with branch offices.

- **numerical:** assigning material to a number and filing according to number sequence. This method may be used for procedures or study models. The system requires a numerical access book, listing numbers with names.
- **subject:** filing material according to subject matter, such as utility bills or products.
- **color-coding:** using color folders or tabs to indicate status, department, or any other separation desired.

Filing Method

When not using a computer storage system practice, a standard method of filing is followed when placing or retrieving an item during filing. Complying with this standard makes it easier to use and work with files in any setting. Related filing terms are:

- **coding:** identifying the file alignment with marks, numbers, or color changes to aid in rapid placement and retrieval.
- **indexing:** the process of identifying the position for placement of an item into the file system. Indexing requires breaking down names or titles into units and identifying the arrangement order of the units.
- **releasing:** the process of identifying the readiness of an item to be placed into a file system. Each facility determines its individual method.
- **retrieving:** the process of obtaining a file, using the procedural method of locating, removing, and returning, for that file system.
- **purging:** systematic process of reviewing and removing outdated or inactive files.
- **sorting:** the process of arranging files in preparation for indexing or classifying. This step simplifies the placement effort.

- **transferring:** the task of moving a file folder from one file system to another, for example, from the active file to the inactive file station.

BUSINESS CORRESPONDENCE

Correspondence from a dental facility represents the practice and establishes the image of the office. Attention should be given to all materials that are sent out, including the following:

- **letters:** written correspondence between two or more parties. The content of the letter may be of assorted subjects such as insurance reviews, referrals, thank-yous, inquiries regarding supplies or statements, case studies, news announcements, birthday regards, recalls, and other items.
- **postcards:** small, heavy paper card that carries a message on one side and the name and address of the person receiving the card on the other; used for recalls, birthday greetings, and announcements.
- **memos:** written correspondence that is less formal than letters and is a frequent means of communication within a practice or in a group setting. Date, message sender, and referenced subject matter appear at the top, followed by comments.

Parts of the Business Letter

The business letter is composed in a structured manner that is common throughout the commercial world and requires adherence to the letter standards. The parts or divisions of a letter are shown in Figure 20-4 and described here:

- **dateline:** on letterhead, stating date of correspondence. If letterhead paper is not used, the address of the sender is inserted above the dateline.
- **inside address:** name, title, street, and city with state and ZIP code of person who will receive the correspondence.

- **salutation:** greeting (Dear Sir or Madam).
- **body of letter:** paragraphs that state the nature of the correspondence.
- **complimentary close:** ending line such as "Sincerely yours."
- **signature line:** printed name of the person who is sending and signing the letter.
- **title line:** title of person sending letter; placed immediately below the printed signature line.
- **reference initials:** initials of person sending the letter (in large case letters) and initials of person preparing the letter (in small case letter). Initials are separated by a slash or colon. Some offices include only the initials of the preparer and the sender's signature.
- **enclosure line:** line that indicates material enclosed with letter; multiple enclosures are so marked (e.g., Enclosures: 3).

Styles of Business Letters

Letters may be composed in different styles. The style chosen is a matter of choice. Two standard letter styles are the block style and the modified block style, both shown in Figure 20-4 and described here:

- **block letter style:** all parts of the letter (with possible exception of preprinted letterhead) are placed on the left margin; paragraphs are not indented.
- **modified letter style:** all divisions of the letter, with the exception of the dateline, complimentary close, and signature line, are placed on the left margin; paragraphs may or may not be indented.

DENTAL INSURANCE TERMS

Dental insurance is a cooperative arrangement of three parties involved in the dental care of a patient:

- The patient—subscriber or insured person
- The provider, or dentist
- The insurance company, carrier

Figure 20-4 The parts and styles of a business letter

(A) Block Style

```
Sender's Street Address
Sender's City, State, ZIP        (Return Address)
Date of Letter

Receiver's Name and Title
Receiver's Street Address        (Inside Address)
Receiver's City, State, ZIP

Dear Name:                       (Salutation)

xxxxxxxxxx  BODY OF LETTER  –  FIRST PARAGRAPH  xxxxxxxxxx
xxxxxxxxxxxxxxxxxxxxxxxxxxxxxxxxxxxxxxxxxxxxxxxxxxxxxxxxxxx
xxxxxxxxxxxxxxxxxxxxxxxxxxxxxxxxxxxxxxxxxxxxxxxxxxxxxxxxxxx
xxxxxxxxxx.

xxxxxxxxx  BODY OF LETTER – SECOND PARAGRAPH  xxxxxxxxxx
xxxxxxxxxxxxxxxxxxxxxxxxxxxxxxxxxxxxxxxxxxxxxxxxxxxxxxxxxxx
xxxxxxxxxxxxxxxxxxxxxxxxxxxxxxxxxxxxxxxxxxxxxxxxxxxxxxxxxxx
xxxxxxxxxx.

xxxxxxxxxx  BODY OF LETTER – THIRD PARAGRAPH  xxxxxxxxxx
xxxxxxxxxxxxxxxxxxxxxxxxxxxxxxxxxxxxxxxxxxxxxxxxxxxxxxxxxxx
xxxxxxxxxxxxxxxxxxxxxxxxxxxxxxxxxxxxxxxxxxxxxxxxxxxxxxxxxxx
xxxxxxxxxx.

Sincerely,              (Closing)

Signature Line

Enclosure Line

Reference Line
```

(B) Modified Block Style

```
                              (Return Address)    Sender's Street Address
                                                  Sender's City, State, ZIP
                                                  Date of Letter

Receiver's Name and Title
Receiver's Street Address      (Inside Address)
Receiver's City, State, ZIP

Dear Name:                     (Salutation)

    xxxxxxxx  BODY OF LETTER – FIRST PARAGRAPH  xxxxxxxxxx
xxxxxxxxxxxxxxxxxxxxxxxxxxxxxxxxxxxxxxxxxxxxxxxxxxxxxxxxxxx
xxxxxxxxxxxxxxxxxxxxxxxxxxxxxxxxxxxxxxxxxxxxxxxxxxxxxxxxxxx
xxxxxxxxxx.

    xxxxxx  BODY OF LETTER – SECOND PARAGRAPH  xxxxxxxxx
xxxxxxxxxxxxxxxxxxxxxxxxxxxxxxxxxxxxxxxxxxxxxxxxxxxxxxxxxxx
xxxxxxxxxxxxxxxxxxxxxxxxxxxxxxxxxxxxxxxxxxxxxxxxxxxxxxxxxxx
xxxxxxxxxx.

    xxxxxxx  BODY OF LETTER – THIRD PARAGRAPH  xxxxxxxxxx
xxxxxxxxxxxxxxxxxxxxxxxxxxxxxxxxxxxxxxxxxxxxxxxxxxxxxxxxxxx
xxxxxxxxxxxxxxxxxxxxxxxxxxxxxxxxxxxxxxxxxxxxxxxxxxxxxxxxxxx
xxxxxxxxxx.

           (Closing)            Sincerely,

                                Signature Line

Enclosure Line

Reference Line
```

The financial arrangements and benefits in insurance coverage differ from one plan to another, from company to company, and from program to program. Various types of benefit plans are offered. The most common ones are described in the following subsections.

Prepaid Insurance Plans

Prepaid dental insurance plans are those in which the subscriber pays a specific amount (premium) of money for covered services. The subscriber has a choice of dental providers and services and pays for any service that the plan does not fully cover. The payment plans from the insurance companies are determined in a specific manner, based on several factors:

- **usual, customary, reasonable fee (UCR):** benefits are percentages of the UCR determined through survey and research of local dentists' fees. For example, 80% of three surface amalgam restorations would be 80% of the regional UCR fee for that procedure.
- **table of allowance:** insurance company policy establishes a specific amount for a specific service. The patient is responsible for any difference in fees between the cost of the service and the table of allowance fee.
- **fixed fee:** fixed schedule of fees for specific services determines the amount of benefits received. The provider agrees to accept this amount as full cost. Fixed fees are usually federally mandated, for example, Medicaid.

Capitation

A capitation dental insurance plan involves subscribers who are members of groups or organizations that enter into a contract for dental services. There are three principal types of capitation plans:

- **Health maintenance organization (HMO):** The provider and patient must belong to the plan that offers specific services to members and a stipulated payment allotment to the provider regardless of the amount of procedures completed; also called *closed panel dentistry*.
- **Preferred provider organizations (PPO):** The employer, group, or organization contracts with the provider for lower-than-usual rates on dental services. The group or organization in return publicizes and encourages members to avail themselves of this program. The provider receives more patients and increased clientele in exchange for discounted fees.
- **Exclusive provider organization (EPO):** The EPO is similar to the PPO program with the exception that the subscriber is offered service from *only* dentists who are members of the provider network.

Government Insurance Programs

The federal and state governments provide some health care, including dental services, to qualified persons. Occasionally, some procedures, such as oral surgery, may be covered. The government offers the following health plans:

- **Workers' compensation:** covers employees injured at the working site or in fulfillment of their occupation; individual state regulated and administered.
- **Medicaid:** low-income and qualified persons receive medical treatment or care, with prior authorization, except in emergencies, in which case treatment is provided without waiting for approval; state-administered program, and each state sets its own guidelines.
- **Medicare:** health care for patients over age 65 who have registered for care. Medicare is available in four parts:
  - **Part A:** hospital care—inpatient services in hospital, skilled-care facilities, hospice, and home health care.
  - **Part B:** physician care—doctor service, outpatient care, some preventive care; patients may be responsible for a deductible amount; some doctors accept assigned fees.

- ○ **Part C:** Medicare-Advantage—provides extra health-care coverage with additional patient premium costs; provides benefits under plan A and B, emergency care, and urgent care; some offer vision, dental, and wellness, and may also offer HMO, PPO, and Private Fee for Services (PFFS) plans.
- ○ **Part D:** covers pharmacy costs in two manners: Medicare Prescription Drug Plan (PDP) or Medicare Advantage Plan (HMO or PPO); must have parts A and B. Restorative dentistry and most other dental care is not covered by Medicare, with the exception of some hospital surgical care and some prescription needs.
- **Civilian Health and Medical Program of the Uniformed Services (CHAMPUS):** provides care for dependents of military personnel; usually received in military or public-health facilities. This program is now called TRICARE, but both names are appropriate.

Terms Used in Dental Insurance

When working with dental claims and insurance matters, knowledge of related terms is necessary, and a good understanding of the insurance-coding practice can be valuable. Some dental offices employ individuals who do nothing but complete the insurance claims for the practice. They use the proper number application given to each treatment procedure, and there are many numbers. An improper or incomplete application of these code numbers can make the difference in the benefit amount paid to the claim.

Each division of dentistry is given a class number, and all treatment plans in that division are given a specific number in that class. There are reference books and classes to teach the proper method to file an insurance claim. One might say that payment terminology is listed in numbers while benefit matters are listed in insurance terminology. Listed next are the more commonly used insurance terms. (Additional insurance terminology is listed in an insurance glossary located in the appendix.)

- **approved services:** all services covered by a dental plan.
- **assignment of insurance benefits:** policyholder's authorization to pay allowable claim benefits to the care provider (dentist). If not signed, the benefits will be sent to the policyholder.
- **authorization to release information:** permission from the patient or patient's guardian to release patient record data and treatment record to a specified party.
- **beneficiary:** person entitled to receive the policy's payment of claim.
- **benefit:** amount paid by insurance company to the policyholder or specified provider of care.
- **birthday rule:** standards to determine the primary insurance policy when two or more policies are involved, as with children of parents who each have a different policy or company. Primary policy is determined by the earliest birthday of the two policyholders in the calendar year. If the birth dates are the same, the oldest policy is considered the primary policy.
- **calendar year:** one year beginning with January 1 and extending to December 31st.
- **carrier:** insurance company or institution that does the insuring.
- **certificate of eligibility:** official card identifying the individual covered by a company or group.
- **claim:** a listing of rendered services, fees charged, and dates of service that is sent to the insurer.
- **claim form:** preprinted or computer programmed form that contains information about the insurer, provider, services, codes, and fees to be submitted for benefit payment.
- **coordination of benefits:** plan by different insurance companies where both pay on the claim. The primary company makes the first payment, and any remaining claim balance is sent to the secondary company. Both payments together may not exceed 100% payment of fees.

- **contract year:** period of time for which a contract is written that may not begin on January 1st. The contract year lasts from the date of issuance to the following anniversary date; also called *policy year.*
- **copayment:** a specific amount or percentage of each claim for which the policyholder pays, per plan agreement.
- **customary fee:** average fee range for procedures completed by the care providers in a given area or geographical section.
- **deductible:** specified amount to be paid by the policyholder in an allotted time (calendar year or policy year), which must be paid before benefits from insurance company begin.
  - **individual deductible:** requires each member to meet a specific amount per year before payments begin.
  - **family deductible:** requires a group total amount from the entire family to meet requirements.
- **dependent:** person who is carried as a member of the policy other than the holder; may be spouse, child, or elder parent relying on the policyholder's financial assistance.
- **dual coverage:** a patient's having two dental policies at the same time; may be individual or family policy.
- **effective date:** date on which the contract becomes in force and benefits begin.
- **exclusion:** dental service or procedure not listed under the benefit plan.
- **fee schedule:** listing of payable amounts for specific procedures performed; also called *Schedule of Benefits.*
- **fiscal year:** any 12-month period set by an agency or company for accounting and scheduling; many banks and government agencies start the year on July 1 and end on June 30th.
- **group policy:** insurance policy covering a specific group or business group, in which only members of that group or business may belong to that plan. An individual company may have a multitude of policies for various levels of employees.
- **insured:** policyholder; the one who pays the premiums or enters into the contract.
- **maximum benefits:** largest possible amount of payment permitted during a specified time, such as within a calendar or policy year or for the life of the policy.
- **participating provider:** health-care giver who belongs to a specific organization's care plan and agrees to accept benefits for allowed care procedures. The insured will not be charged except policy-stated copayment fees, uncovered services, or deductibles.
- **preauthorization:** request sent to insurance company to determine if the policy covers specified procedures or treatments and the amount of payment that will be received, also called *predetermination,* usually sent on a claim form and marked "Pre-Treatment Estimate." After approval and completion of services, the form is resubmitted as a statement of actual services by the dentist.
- **premium:** amount of money payment required of policyholder to keep the policy in force; may be required monthly, quarterly, or yearly.
- **procedural code:** code system constructed to provide a specific number to each treatment or procedure performed; used to file claims and determine benefits.
- **provider:** the party who renders professional services; each provider has an identification number.
- **reasonable fee:** amount determined by the insurance company from a survey of providers in the area or region.
- **release of information statement:** statement or form signed by the patient or patient's guardian to authorize confidential information to be sent to a third party.
- **schedule of benefits:** allotted benefits for specific procedures; same as fee schedule.

- **signature on file:** area or space on initial registration form indicating continued permission for payment and release of information; saves signature for each claim submission.
- **subscriber:** insured person; the policyholder.
- **superbill:** preprinted form listing procedure numbers and services rendered to the patient.
- **third party:** organization or person who makes payment but is not part of the provider–patient contract.
- **usual fee:** average fee charged by a provider for a specific service.

FINANCIAL MANAGEMENT

A dental practice or facility will incur income and expenses necessary for its operation. The recording of these transactions is an important aspect of the duties of the office manager or front-desk receptionist. Each office determines which method is used to maintain financial records. The more popular ways are:

- **manual:** use of ledger books, receipt slips, entry charges, and payments from the patient's records. Statement information is reviewed, and monthly statements are sent to those with balances. This method is seldom used, as it is not as effective and time saving as the other techniques.
- **one-write system:** using a collection of papers arranged in sequential order, one written entry can be recorded for various office records. After the entry is made, all records reflect the same amount with less room for transposing errors (see Figure 20-5).
- **computer entry:** automatic and "paperless" method of recording financial records. Entries are placed on patient records, and machines transfer information to the proper selected accounts and terminals for easy and quick reference of patient accounts, statements, office records, credit reports, and so forth.

Disbursement records can follow the same chosen procedure as the income system. There

Figure 20-5 Example of a one-write system

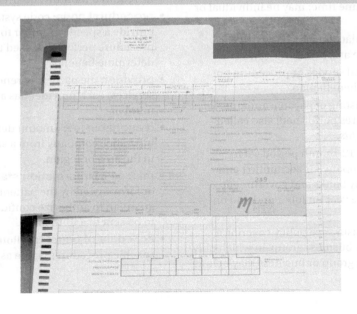

is a vocabulary of important terms relative to the disbursement and record keeping of monies handled by any business, including a dental practice:

- **account:** record of transactions, charges, fees paid, and any adjustments; may be an individual or a family account. An *aged* account is one that has been outstanding for a specified period of time, such as 30, 60, 90, or 120 days.
- **bookkeeping:** structured method of maintaining records of financial transactions.
- **charge slip:** paper form used to show the procedure performed, fees charged, and need for follow-up appointment. The slip travels with a patient throughout treatment and to the front office for posting.
- **collection:** request for payment of an aged account; may be attempted with a phone call, letter, or with assistance of a collection agency.
- **day sheet:** daily record of appointments, services, and business activities of the day; also called a *daily journal sheet*. It may also be the basis for a daily pegboard bookkeeping system.
- **ledger card:** a record-keeping sheet of services, charges, and payments for a person or a family.
- **pegboard bookkeeping:** a system for recording financial activities of the dental practice day. All forms are strategically layered over each other, allowing a written entry to be recorded on several documents; also called a *one-write system*.
- **statement:** form sent to an individual or a responsible party requesting payment for services.

Disbursements

Disbursements are monies leaving the facility. These payments are made using the practice's checking account, which provides a legal record of the transaction for bookkeeping and tax purposes. Some disbursements are fixed, and some are variable. Fixed expenses are those that occur regularly, such as utilities and rent. Variable expenses occur with use, such as supplies.

Checks

A check is a written order to the bank for a draft or transfer of funds. It is payable to the person or business named on the check. The different types of checks are:

- **canceled:** a check that represents a completed transaction and is returned to the account holder.
- **cashier's:** a check written on the bank's account and signed by a bank treasurer or official. The purchaser determines the name of the payee, supplies the money for the check, and pays a fee for the procedure.
- **certified:** a check that has been endorsed by the bank to be valid. The bank removes and holds the amount of the check from the account to ensure that the transaction is covered. The bank charges a fee for this service.
- **traveler's:** a check in which the bank sells agency checks in specified amounts ($10, $20, $50, etc.). The purchaser signs the face of the check once at the time of purchase and again at the time of use. A fee is charged for this service, but traveler's checks are usually accepted more readily than a personal check when a person is traveling.
- **voucher:** a check with an attached stub indicating payment information, such as a payroll check with hours worked, gross and net pay, deductions, and yearly totals. The stub is removed when the check is cashed.
- **money order:** similar to a check, as it is a written order, but may be issued by stores or business establishments and post offices. The purchaser denotes the amount and the name of the person to be placed on the check. The purchaser pays the issuer the money for the amount of the money order, plus an additional fee for the service.

Miscellaneous Payment Terms

Other forms of payment and terms that may be used when working with checks and disbursements include the following:

- **electronic transfer of funds:** paperless method to transfer monies. The payee may call or contact the banking institution, provide identification, and place an order to transfer funds to another account or business.
- **automatic payment:** arrangement by payee authorizing specified parties to automatically deduct specific funds to cover fixed or other monthly charges such as utilities. The funds are withdrawn and the transaction is noted on the monthly statement.
- **credit card transaction:** using a credit card to cover an expense. Verification of credit line and determining that the charge amount is not overextended may be established at the time of the service. The patient submits a payment to the credit company, who forwards the amount less a fee to the dentist. The patient is credited the entire cost of the treatment charge paid.
- **loan transaction:** a patient may make arrangements for a loan to cover a specific procedure.

Some loan institutions, such as CareCredit, in cooperation with participating dentists, have a health loan available with a credit card style payment system of monthly installments. No interest is charged if the payment plan is paid in full in the 6-, 12-, or 24-month time frame. If a payment is late, an interest fee calculated from the purchase date is charged.

Miscellaneous Banking Terms

The following are miscellaneous terms related to banking transactions:

- **deposit slip:** a form for recording submitted cash and checks, included with monies deposited into the business account. A deposit may be made in person at the bank, through the mail, or placed in a night deposit vault after banking hours.
- **endorsement:** payee's signature placed on the back of the check to show that the payee has cashed the check. The three types of endorsements are:

  - **blank endorsement:** signature of the payee only; may be cashed by anyone.
  - **restricted endorsement:** signature of the payee following a restriction line such as "For deposit only"; it can be deposited only in the payee's account.
  - **third-party endorsement:** signature of the payee following instructions to pay the check amount to a third person, such as "Pay to order of Delta Dental Supply Co." This type of endorsement is also called *endorsement in full* and is difficult to cash.

- **petty cash:** a fund setup in an office to pay for incidental office purchases. A record of expenditures is kept, and the fund is replenished when needed.
- **reconciliation:** determining if the checkbook balance agrees with the bank balance; done monthly when the statement and canceled check records are returned to the office. Any deposits or checks that were written and not yet received or recorded by the bank at the statement date are called "outstanding."
- **nonsufficient funds (NSF):** designation for a check written for more money than is present in the account; commonly called "a bounced check." The bank charges the check writer a fee for returning the check, and the person receiving the check may also charge an extra fee.
- **stop payment:** payee order to the bank not to honor or cash a specific check. If processed before the check has cleared the bank, a fee is charged to the payee.

INVENTORY CONTROL

To run an efficient dental practice, the office must maintain the proper supply of materials and functioning equipment. One of the duties of the receptionist or office manager is to see that all supplies and materials are on hand, up to date, and in good working order. The best way to accomplish this task is to maintain an accurate inventory list that is updated when making purchases and repairs. Inventory control terms are:

- **back order:** an item that was not included in an order and will be shipped at a later date.
- **capital supply:** items of major cost that are used on an ongoing basis, such as dental chair, autoclave, or radiograph developer.
- **expendable supply:** items that are used up or consumed during procedures, such as cements, tissues, and gloves.
- **invoice:** listing of materials or items included in an order; may also include demand for payment.
- **nonexpendable supply:** items that are used more than once but not of major cost, such as dental instruments.
- **purchase order:** printed order for materials or equipment that is used mainly in large institutions; may need authorization before being processed.
- **packing slip:** list of items and quantity of items enclosed in the order; may also include item price (one item), unit price (price per group of items, such as 12), and bulk price (discounted price for a specific amount of items or units).

- **reorder point:** minimum quantity or amount of an item that is necessary to have on hand before another order is necessary.
- **lead time:** amount of time between the reorder of a supply and its arrival.
- **inventory or order control card:** printed card listing major supply, reorder point, and information regarding source, price, and quantity needed.
- **shelf life:** expected amount of time a material can be retained before it loses its effectiveness or before a product's expiration date.
- **barcode:** electronic order system of bar markings per item. Necessary item's barcode is swiped by barcode wand, which feeds information to the computer. Quantity and date are added to the order, which are electronically sent to the supply house (Figure 20-6).

Each office facility completes business management procedures in its own particular style. Some may make book-entry recordings, others may use a setup with some computer involvement, and still others may have a complete software system that can perform practically any necessary

Figure 20-6 An example of an assistant using a barcode scanner for inventory

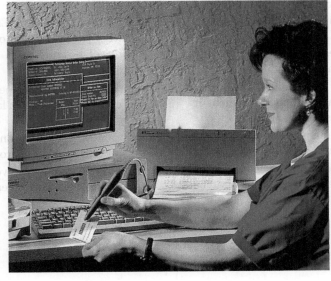

Courtesy of Patterson Dental Supply Inc.

transactions, such as recording payments and disbursement, statement preparation, filing insurance claims, making patient records, calling recalls and confirmations, routing, business trends, end-of-day reports, and so on. A knowledge of the preceding terms will help you understand and be ready to put to use any system required in your workstation.

LEGAL AND ETHICAL TERMS

All dental professionals should be aware of the ethical and legal aspects associated with providing treatment and care. Each State Board of Dental Examiners regulates the dental practice and those performing the services. Federal laws control records privacy, work conditions, and the distribution of drugs; local zoning or municipal statues also affect practices. Dental professionals should understand the terminology regarding ethical and legal relationships involved with patient care, such as the following:

- **abandonment:** lack of follow-through by the provider in the care of an established patient.
- **abuse:** any care or relationship that harms, pains, or causes mental anguish to another.
- **breach of confidentiality:** unauthorized release of confidential data, either spoken or written.
- **confidentiality:** respect for the privacy of another's status, data, or condition.
- **consent:** patient's agreement to treatment; may be written, oral, or implied. A patient or guardian gives consent for a minor.
- **contract:** an agreement between two or more parties for the performance of services or care.
- **defamation:** a false statement causing damage to a person's reputation or resulting in ridicule.

- **defendant:** accused or person named in a lawsuit.
- **deposition:** testimony given under oath regarding specific event or occurrence.
- **ethics:** rules and standards of conduct set forth by the profession.
- **felony:** serious crime, with stricter penalties than a misdemeanor or petty crime.
- **fraud:** deliberate misrepresentation of facts or information.
- **incompetent:** not mentally able; one who lacks skills or abilities.
- **judgment:** final decision by the court.
- **liability:** responsibility for the course of action.
- **licensure:** certification of a candidate's ability and knowledge in a chosen profession.
- **litigation:** lawsuit.
- **malpractice:** failure to provide proper care and treatment; indication of a lack of proper skill or ability, such as failing to remove a broken off root tip in oral surgery.
- **negligence:** failure to provide reasonable skill, care, and judgment, for example, improper sterilization of instruments.
- **plaintiff:** injured person or guardian in a lawsuit; the party who initiates or files a lawsuit.
- ***res ipsa loquitur:*** (Latin for "the deed speaks for itself"): the cause.
- ***respondeat superior:*** (Latin for "the master answers"): responsibility of the employer for the actions of the employees.
- **statute:** law.
- **statute of limitations:** period of time following the event during which a lawsuit or legal action may be instituted.
- **subpoena:** legal summons requiring a person to report to a trial or to provide testimony.
- **testimony:** statement, given under oath, regarding details of an event or occurrence.

Review Exercises

Matching

Match the following word elements with their meanings.

1. _____ unit
2. _____ indexing
3. _____ capital supply
4. _____ letter
5. _____ consent form
6. _____ back order
7. _____ subscriber
8. _____ ethics
9. _____ call list
10. _____ felony
11. _____ check
12. _____ fixed expense
13. _____ exclusion
14. _____ account
15. _____ appointment

A. scheduled treatment time
B. list of patients willing to accept last-minute appointment
C. services or procedures not listed in a benefit plan
D. written correspondence
E. written draft or demand of payment from a bank account
F. record of services, transactions, charges, fees paid
G. usual monthly charge, rent
H. section of hour, used for scheduling appointment purposes
I. item of major cost
J. part of supply order to be shipped at a later date
K. aligning position for file placement using names, dates, and so on
L. serious crime
M. insured person, policyholder
N. code of conduct set by a profession
O. form signed by patient/guardian giving permission for care

Definitions

Using the selection given for each sentence, choose the best term to complete the definition.

1. A payee order to a bank not to honor a specific check is a:
   a. cashier check
   b. endorsement
   c. stop order
   d. cancelled check

2. Mail that is mostly composed of magazines and printed matter is:
   a. first-class mail
   b. second-class mail
   c. third-class mail
   d. parcel post

3. A paperless method of transferring money is considered which financial system?
   a. pegboard
   b. electronic
   c. third party
   d. accounting

4. A utility bill receipt may be filed under "Utility," which is an example of which filing system?
   a. alphabetical
   b. chronological
   c. numerical
   d. subject

5. A mailed letter is considered which type of office communication?
   a. oral
   b. conference
   c. written
   d. electronic

6. A fund of money used to pay for small items purchased for office needs is:
   a. petty cash
   b. recount money
   c. voucher check
   d. draft

7. Process of arranging items for filing, using names, dates, numbers, or subjects:
   a. sorting
   b. coding
   c. transferring
   d. retrieving

8. One of the HIPAA law's purposes is to protect:
   a. patient procedure
   b. patient time
   c. patient fees
   d. patient privacy

9. A serious or major crime, such as arson or murder, is considered a:
   a. misdemeanor
   b. petty crime
   c. tort
   d. felony

10. Which of the following selections is not considered an outgoing call?
   a. collection
   b. ordering
   c. new patient appointment
   d. confirmation

11. A listing of services provided, fees charged, and service dates sent to the carrier is a/an:
   a. claim
   b. authorization form
   c. inquiry
   d. contract

12. Purposeful misrepresentation of facts or knowledge is a case of:
   a. fraud
   b. libel
   c. slander
   d. felony

13. A requirement for the family or individual to pay the first $100 is called a:
   a. primary carrier
   b. coordination of benefits
   c. split-fee
   d. deductible

14. Which government health plan offers benefits to military personnel?
   a. Medicare
   b. CHAMPUS
   c. Medicaid
   d. Workers' Comp

15. Marking off holidays and setting up a new appointment book is the making of a/an:
   a. cross-file
   b. index
   c. matrix
   d. appointment schedule

16. An autoclave is considered which type of expense?
   a. disposable
   b. capital
   c. nonexpendable
   d. expendable

17. Keeping records secret and private is an act of:
   a. negligence
   b. screening
   c. legality
   d. confidentiality

18. January 1st to December 31st is considered which type of year in insurance terminology?
   a. annual
   b. calendar
   c. policy
   d. account

19. A payment of money required of the policyholder to keep a policy in force is a:
    a. benefit
    b. copayment
    c. premium
    d. deductible

20. What kind of check is written on a person's account and guaranteed by the bank?
    a. voucher
    b. traveler's
    c. certified
    d. cashier's

Building Skills

Locate and define the prefix, root/combining form, and suffix (if present) in the following words.

1. **preauthorization**
   prefix _____
   root/combining form _____
   suffix _____

2. **disbursement**
   prefix _____
   root/combining form _____
   suffix _____

3. **nonexpendable**
   prefix _____
   root/combining form _____
   suffix _____

4. **malpractice**
   prefix _____
   root/combining form _____
   suffix _____

5. **misrepresentation**
   prefix _____
   root/combining form _____
   suffix _____

Fill-Ins

Write the correct word in the blank space to complete each statement.

1. A telephone call placed by the assistant from the facility is a/an _____ call.

2. The amount of money the patient pays to keep the policy in force is called the _____.

3. A rendering of a patient's account that is sent monthly to the patient is a/an _____.

4. A six-month checkup appointment is termed a/an _____ appointment.

5. When a child's parents both have dental insurance, the child is considered to have _____ coverage.

6. A service or procedure covered by the insurer is a/an _____ service.

7. A private letter to the doctor would be considered _____ mail.

8. _____ is the dividing of a name or item in preparation for filing.

9. A _____ is a request sent to insurance companies to determine if the policy will cover an upcoming treatment.

10. A letter with all parts placed against the left margin is considered a _____ style letter.

11. Radiographs that need to be filed are numbered and placed in a _____ file.

12. The greeting "Dear Sir" is the _____ part of the letter.

13. The time span from the start of the policy to a year later is called the _____ year.

14. Many institutions use a _____ to place orders for supplies.

15. A _____ form gives permission for treatment for the patient or the patient's minor.

16. An open unit in the appointment book used for catching up or for emergencies is called a _____ period.

17. The act of harming a person bodily or mentally is called _____.

18. A/an _____ is a legal finding of a court.

19. A/an _____ is placed in the file cabinet in place of the removed file folder.

20. A/an _____ is a short interdepartmental or facility correspondence.

Word Use

Read the following sentences, and define the meaning of the word written in boldface letters.

1. Some people prefer to be placed on a **call list** when they are not sure of their work schedule.

   _____

2. The **disbursement** sheet for the petty cash fund showed a small balance, so additional funds were added.

   _____

3. When preparing an order for gypsum material, the assistant inquired about the **bulk** price.

   _____

4. In the insurance contract system, the dentist is considered the **provider**.

   _____

5. One of the usual monthly duties at the front desk is the **reconciliation** of the office checking account.

   _____

APPENDIX A | WORD ELEMENTS

PREFIXES

A

a-, an-	without, away from
ab-	away from, absent, negative
acro-	end extremity
ad-	toward, in the direction of
albus-	white
ambi-	both, both sides
ankylo-	fused/growing together
ante-	before, in front of
anter/o-	before, in front of
anti-	against, counteracting
aqua-	water
aud-	hear
auto-	self

B

bene-	good, well
bi-	two, both
bio-	life
brachy-	short
brady-	slow

C

cent-	hundred
circum-	around, surrounding
co-, com-	with
con-	with
contra-	against, opposite
cut/o-	skin
cyan/o-	blue
cry/o-	cold

D

de-	down, loss, without
demi-	half
dexi/o-	right
dextr/o-	right
di-	twice, double

dia-	complete through
diplo-	double
dis-	separate, absent
dors-	back
dys-	pain, difficulty

E

e-	without
ec-	out, out from
ecto-	external, outside
endo-	within, inside
epi-	over, upper
eu-	normal, good, true
ex-	outside, away from
exo-	out
extra-	beyond, outside

F

fore-	in front of, before

G

gene-	origin, start
gyne-	woman

H

hemi-	half
homo-	same
hyper-	above, excessive, more than
hypo-	low, deficient, less than

I

im-	not
in-	not, into
infra-	beneath, under, below
inter-	between, among
integra-	forming into one
intra-	within, inside
iso-	equal

J

juxta-	besides

L

later/o-	side
leuk/o-, leuc/o-	white

M

macro-	large
mal-	bad
med-	middle
mega-	large
melan/o-	black
mes/o-	middle
micro-	small
mid-	middle
mono-	one, single
multi-	many
myna-	muscle, slime

N

neo-	new
non-	no, not
normo-	usual, normal

O

ob-	against
ortho-	straight

P

pachy-	thick
pan-	all
para-	beside, beyond
per-	through
peri-	around
poly-	many
post-	behind, after

pre-	before, in front of
prima-	first
pro-	forward
pseudo-	false

Q

quad/quat-	four

R

re-	back
retro-	after, behind

S

semi-	half, partial
sinistro-	left
sta-	standstill, stop
sub-	under
super-	over, above
supra-	over, above
sym-	with, together
syn-	together, union

T

tachy-	fast, rapid
trans-	across, through
tri-	three

U

ultra-	excess, beyond
un-	not
uni-	one

V

ventro-	body front

X

xanth-	yellow

ROOT WORDS/COMBINING FORMS

A

abdomin/o	abdomen
acanth/o	thorny, spiny

acr/o	extremities
aden/o	gland
adren/o	adrenal gland
alveo	tooth socket bone

ambl/o	dull, dim
angi/o	vessel
ankyl/o	looped, crooked, stationary
anter/o	before, in front of
aorto	aorta
apic/o	apex
arteri/o	artery
arthr/o	joint
audi/o	sound
aut/o	self
axill/o	armpit

B

bifid/o	split, cleft, in two parts
bil/o	bile
blast/o	developing cell
blepharo	eyelid
bride	debris
brachi/o	arm
bronch/o	bronchial tubes
brux/o	gland, chew
bucc/o	cheek
burs/o	bursa (cavity)

C

carcin/o	cancer
cardi/o	heart
cari/o	decay, rot
carpo	wrist
caud/o	tail
cement/o	cementun
cephal/o	head
cerebr/o	cerebrum
cervic/o	neck
cheil/o	lip
chir/o	hand
chol/o	gall, bile
cholecyst	gallbladder
chondr/o	cartilage
chrom/o	color
cocc/i, cocc/o	round, spherical bacteria
col/o	colon, large intestine
coll/i	neck
coron/o	crown
cost/o	rib

crani/o	skull
cry/o	cold
cutane/o	skin
cyst/o	fluid-filled sac, bag, bladder
cyt/o	cell

D

dacry/o	tear duct
dactyl/o	fingers, toes
decidu	falling off, shed
degrade	break down
dent/i, dent/o	tooth
derm/o	skin
dextr/o	right
diaphor/o	sweat
digit	finger
dipl/o	double
dips/o	thirst
dors	back
duc/o	hard, dura mater
duct/o	lead, carry
duoden/o	duodenum

E

edemat/o	swelling
edentul/o	toothless
electr/o	electric current
embry/o	embryo, to be full
emet/o	vomit
enam/o	enamel
encephal/o	brain
enter/o	intestine
epsi/o	vulva
eryther/o	red
esophag/o	esophagus
erthesi/o	feeling
ete/o	cause of disease
excis/o	cutting out

F

faci/o	facial
fasci/o	fibrous, band
femur	femus
fet/o	fetus, unborn
fibr/o	fibrous, tissue

fibrilla	irregular rhythm
fiss/o	crack
flu/o	flow
foramin/o	opening
foss/o	shallow depression
furca-	branch
freno	connecting band
fronto	forehead

G

gangli/o	nerve plexus
gastr/o	stomach
gen	birth, coming
gene	to become
genit/o	birth, reproductive organs
germ	microorganism
geront/o	old age
gingiv/o	gum
glen/o	socket, pit
gloss/o	tongue
glott/i/o	back of tongue
glac/o	sugar
gnatho	jaw
gnos/o	knowledge
graphy	picture
gynec/o	woman, female

H

halo/o, halit/o	breath
hemo, hemat/o	blood
hepart/o	liver
hered/o, heredit/o	inherited
herni/o	hernia
hist/o	tissue
hydr/o	water
hypno/o	sleep
hyster/o	uterus

I

illumina	light
immune/o	immune, protected
implant	man-made
incis/o	cutting into
infect	invade
iri/o	iris
isch/o	deficiency, blockage

J

jejun/o	jejunum (intestine)
jugul/o	throat

K

kal/o	potassium
kerat/o	cornea, hard, horny
kin/o	movement
kyph/o	hump

L

labi/o	lips
lacrim/o	tears, lacrimal duct
lact/o	milk
lamina	layers
lapar/o	abdomen
laryng/o	larynx
leuk/o	white
ligament	tough fibrous band of tissue
lingu/o	tongue
lip/o	fat
lith/o	strong, calculus
lob/o	lobe
lord/o	bent forward
lucent	through
lymph/o	lymph

M

mamm/o	breast
mastic/o	chew
masticat/o	chew
maxill/o	maxilla, upper jaw
meat/o	meatus, opening
mechan	machine
melan/o	black
men/o	menstruation
mening/o	meninges
mesi/o	middle
metric	measuring
muc/o, mucus/o	mucus
my/o	muscle
myc/o	fungus
myel/o	spinal cord, bone marrow

N

nar/i	nose, nostrils
narc/o	stupor
nat/o	birth
necr/o	death
nephr/o	kidney
neur/o	nerve
noct/o	night
numer	number

O

occlud/o	shut, close up
ocul/o	eye
odont/o	tooth
oleg/o	scanty, few
oma	tumor
oophor/o	ovary
ophthalm/o	eye
or/o	mouth
orchis/o	testes
ortho	straighten
oste/o	bone
ot/o	ear
ovario	ovary
ovi/o	egg
ox/o	oxygen

P

pachy/o	thick
palat/o	palate, roof of mouth
papill/o	nipple
pariet	parietal bone
part/o	birth, labor
path/o	disease
pector/o	chest
ped/o	child, foot
phag/o	swallow
pharyng/o	pharynx, throat
phas/o	speech
phleb/o	vein
phob/o	fear
plastic	resin
plated	thin layer
pleur/o	relating to the side, usually lung membrane
pneum/o	lung, air

pod/o	foot
proct/o	rectum
proxi	joining
psych/o	mind, soul
pulm/o	lung
pyel/o	kidney
py/o	pus

R

radi/o	radius
rect/o	rectum
ren/o	kidney
retin/o	retina
rhin/o	nose
rhythm	pattern
rhytid/o	wrinkles

S

salping/o	oviduct, tube
sclera/o	hardening
scoli/o	twisted
seb/o	oil, sebum
semin/i	seed
sensi	capable of feeling
sept/o	poison, infection
somat/o	body
somm/o	sleep
son	sound
spir/o	breath, breathe
splen/o	spleen
spondyl/o	spine
squam/o	scaly
stabiliza	firm, solid, steady
stat/i	standstill, stop
sten/o	contracted, narrow
stern/o	sternum
stomat/o	mouth
stric/o	narrowing
symmetr/y	same, similar
syring/o	fistula, tube

T

tars/o	ankle
tax/o	order, arrangement
tempor/o	temporal bone

tend/o	tendon, stretch out
tens/o	stretch, strain
therm/o	heat
thromb/o	clot
thorac/o	chest
thym/o	thymus
thyr/o	thyroid
ton/o	tension, pressure
tox/o	poison
trache/o	windpipe, trachea
trick/o	hair
tympan/o	eardrum, middle ear

U–Z

ungu/o	nail

ur/o	urine, urinary
urethra/o	urethra
urin/o	urine
uter/o	uterine
valvul/o	valve
vas/o	vessel
ven/o	vein
ventila	air vent
vesic/o	bladder, sac
viscer/o	viscera, internal organ
volt	unit of measure
xanth/o	yellow
xer/o	dryness
zygoma/o	cheekbone

SUFFIXES

A

-a, -an, -ary	pertaining to
-able	capable of
-ac	pertaining to, relating to
-al	pertaining to, relating to
-algesia	pertaining to pain
-algia	pertaining to pain
-ant	promoting action or process
-ar	pertaining to
-ary	pertaining to
-ase	enzyme

C

-cele	swelling, hernia
-cente	puncture
-centesis	surgical puncture to remove fluid
-cide	kill
-cise	cut
-clast	break up
-cle	small
-crine	secrete
-crit	separate
-cule	small
-cyte	cell

D

-derma	skin
-dema	swelling

-desis	surgical fixation
-dyne or -dynia	pain

E

-ectasis	dilation
-ectomy	surgical removal of
-ectopy	displacement
-edema	swelling
-ema	condition of
-emesis	vomiting
-emia	blood condition
-ent	agent or specialist
-er	agent or person concerned
-esis	condition or state of
-esthesia	sensation

F

-ferous	producing
-fida	split
-form	shape, resembling
-fuge	driving away, pushing
-fusion	come together

G

-genic	originated
-grade	to go
-gram	picture, record
-graph	picture, record

-graphy	recording a picture, recording a record

H

-hood	condition, state of being, or group

I

-ia	pertaining to, condition of
-iasis	in the presence of, abnormal condition
-ic	pertaining to
-ical	pertaining to
-icle	small
-id	condition
-ile	pertaining to
-ine	pertaining to
-ion	small
-ism	condition of
-ist	agent or specialist
-itis	inflammation
-ium	small, little, tissue
-ity	condition or state of
-ization	process/procedure
-ize	take away, remove

K

-kinesis	movement

L

-lapse	slide, fall
-lepsy	seizure
-lith	stone
-logist	specialist
-logy	study of
-lucent	shine, clear
-lysis	destruction

M

-malacia	abnormal softening
-mania	obsessive preoccupation
-megaly	large, enlargement
-meter	measuring instrument
-ment	action or state of
-mission	sending

-mortem	death
-motor	movement

O

-oid	resembling
-ola	small
-ole	small, little
-ology	study of
-oma	tumor
-one	hormone
-opia	vision
-or	agent
-orrhagia	hemorrhage
-orrhaphy	suture
-orrhea	flow
-ose	sugar
-osis	condition of
-ostomy	create a surgical opening
-otia	ear
-otomy	cutting into
-ous	pertaining to
-oxa	oxygen

P

-para	bring forth
-paresis	weakness
-parous	giving birth, bearing
-pathy	disease
-penia	few, decrease, deficiency
-pepsia	digestion
-pexy	fixation
-phage	ingest, swallow
-phasia	speech
-phil	attraction
-phobia	fear
-plasia	development, formation
-plasty	surgical repair
-plegia	paralysis
-pnea	breathing
-ptosis	organ drooping, drooping
-ptysis	spitting

R

-rrhage	abnormal flow, excessive flow
-rrhaphy	to stitch, to suture

-rrhea	flow, discharge
-rrhexis	rupture

S

-sarcoma	tumor, cancer
-scopy	to scan, to visualize
-sclerosis	hardening
-sis	state of
-sol	solution
-somnia	sleep
-spadia	cut, tear
-spasm	involuntary muscle move, twitch
-sphysia	pulse
-stalsis	constriction, contraction
-stasis	constant level
-stenosis	stricture, abnormal narrowing
-stomy	surgical opening

T

-thorax	chest
-thymia	condition of the mind

-tic	pertaining to
-tion	condition or state of
-tivity	condition
-tome	cutting instrument
-tomy	incision, surgical cutting
-tresia	opening
-tripsy	crush
-trophy	nourishment
-tropia	to turn

U

-ular	relating to
-ule	small
-ulus	small
-um	pertaining to
-uria	pertaining to urine

Y

-y	the act, result of an act

ANSWERS TO CHAPTER 1 EXERCISES

EXERCISE 1-1

1. an = without
2. hemi = half
3. quat = four
4. pri = first
5. an = without
6. mono = one
7. an = without
8. bi = two
9. tri = three
10. poly = many
11. uni = one
12. tri = three
13. semi = half
14. deci = ten
15. mono = one

EXERCISE 1-2

1. E
2. D
3. G
4. F
5. A
6. A
7. B

EXERCISE 1-3

1. macro = large
2. iso = equal
3. hyper = elevated, over, excess
4. hypo = under, below
5. micro = small, minute
6. pan = all around
7. ultra = extreme, beyond

EXERCISE 1-4

1. around = peri-
2. outside = ecto-
3. behind = retro-
4. under = sub-
5. toward = ad-
6. mid/among = mes-
7. apart = ana-
8. through = trans-
9. together = syn-
10. down from = de-
11. right = dexi-
12. after = post-
13. before = pre- or ante-
14. both sides = ambi-
15. into = in-
16. away from = ab-
17. out from = ex/o-
18. within = endo-
19. above = supra-
20. complete = dia-

EXERCISE 1-5

1. I
2. M
3. K
4. E
5. J
6. C
7. B
8. G
9. H
10. F
11. D
12. A
13. L

EXERCISE 1-6

1. gingiva
2. labia, cheilo
3. apical
4. glossa
5. maxilla
6. stoma
7. mesial
8. mucosa
9. distal
10. coronal

EXERCISE 1-7

1. -form
2. -ic
3. -gram
4. -oid
5. -eal
6. -ior
7. -lar
8. -ous
9. -al
10. -ac
11. -graph
12. -ary

EXERCISE 1-8

1. -ity = acidity
2. -sion = incision
3. -ium = bacterium
4. -oma = lipoma
5. -tion = mastication
6. -tic = necrotic
7. -pathy = myopathy
8. -ule = molecule
9. -ism = bruxism
10. -olus = alveolus

EXERCISE 1-9

Answers may be of student's choice.

EXERCISE 1-10

1. gingivoplasty = -plasty, surgical contouring of the gingiva
2. fibromyalgia = -algia, painful disease of the fiber muscles
3. germicide = -cide, chemical agent used to kill microbes

4. stethoscope = -scope, instrument used to hear chest and body sounds
5. hemorrhea = -rrhea, discharge of blood
6. cauterize = -ize, to burn
7. frenectomy = -tomy, surgical procedure of the frenum
8. apicoectomy = -ectomy, surgical removal of the apex of a tooth
9. rotate = -ate, circular movement of an object
10. claustrophobia = -phobia, fear of enclosing areas
11. carcinoma = -oma, cancer, or malignant growth
12. prognosis = -gnosis, medical estimate of future outcome
13. biopsy = -opsy, laboratory view of tissue subject
14. leukocyte = -cyte, white blood cell
15. histology = -ology, microscopic study of tissue

EXERCISE 1-11

1. matrices
2. mamelons
3. frena
4. radii
5. sulci
6. irises
7. axillaries
8. diagnoses
9. gingivae
10. stomatas

GLOSSARY

Note: Some terms are provided in Spanish. The Spanish term is shown in **_purple type_**.

abandonment (ah-**BAN**-dah-ment)—lack of follow-through by the provider for the care of an established patient (**_abandono_**)

abducens (**AB**-due-senz)—away from; sixth cranial nerve that controls lateral eye movement

abfraction (ab-**FRACK**-shun)—loss of tooth surface in cervical area; caused by tooth grinding and compression

abrasion (ah-**BRAY**-shun)—scrape from; wearing away of a tooth surface from abnormal causes (**_abrasión, rasgurío_**)

abscess (**AB**-cess)—collection of pus in the periodontal tissues (**_absceso_**)

absent (**AB**-sent)—not present, missing (**_ausente_**)

absorption (ab-**SORP**-shun)—drug substance transfer from the administration site by body fluids (**_absorción_**)

abuse (ah-**BUSE**)—any care relationship that harms, pains, or causes mental anguish to another (**_abusar (v), abuso (n)_**)

abutment (ah-**BUT**-ment)—natural tooth or teeth prepared to hold a bridge retainer in position (**_pilar, contrafuerte_**)

accessory, accessory nerve (ack-**SESS**-ore-ee)—auxillary; XI (eleventh) cranial nerve assisting with spinal movements (**_accesarios_**)

account (ah-**COUNT**)—a record of business, procedural, and financial transactions (**_cuenta_**)

acellular (ay-**SELL**-you-lar)—not made up of or containing cells

acetaminophen (ah-seat-ah-**MIN**-oh-fen)—used as an aspirin replacement for children (**_acetaminofeno_**)

acid etchant (acid **ETCH**-ent)—material to prepare cavity margins for retention of bonding materials

acidity (ah-**SID**-a-tee)—condition of being sour; makes litmus paper red (**_acidez_**)

acquired pellicle (**PEL**-ih-kal)—little skin, thin covering on teeth, plaque (**_pelicula adquirida_**)

acronym (**ACK**-roh-nim)—word formed from initials, such as **DDS** or **HIV** (**_acrónemo_**)

acrylic (ah-**KRIL**-ick)—synthetic resin material used in fabrication of appliances (**_acrilico_**)

activator (**ACK**-tih-vay-tor)—substance that reacts with the initiator to start polymerization (**_activador_**)

acute (ah-**CUTE**)—sharp or severe (**_grave, agudo (a)_**)

acute radiation exposure—radiation resulting from a massive short-term, ionizing dose, such as in an accidental exposure or explosion of radiation material

addiction (ah-**DICK**-shun)—compulsive, uncontrollable dependence on some habit (**_la adicción_**)

adenoid (**ADD**-eh-noyd)—lymphatic tissue found in the nasopharynx area (**_adeniodeo_**)

adhesive (ad-**HEE**-sive)—sticky or adhering material or substance (**_adhesivo, pegajoso_**)

adjacent (ah-**JAY**-cent)—nearby or adjoining (**_advacentes_**)

adjunctive orthodontics (ad-**JUNC**-tive)—necessary procedures taken to correct or restore function (**_coavudante othhodóico_**)

adrenocorticosteroids (ah-dren-oh-**kor**-tih-koh-**STARE**-oyds)—byproducts from the adrenal cortex

adverse effect (ad-**VERSE** ee-**FECT**)—response to a drug that is not desired; an effect could be too intense, weak, toxic (**_efectos adverso_**)

aerobes (**AIR**-ohbs)—microorganisms that cannot survive without oxygen; may be facultative (adaptable) or obligate (strict)

aerobic (air-**OH**-bick)—requiring oxygen to live; needing oxygen (*aeróbico*)

aerosol spray (**AIR**-oh-sol spray)—drug solution suspended in and delivered by a propellant (*aerosol*)

airway (**AIR**-way)—device inserted into the mouth and down the throat to provide air passage to the windpipe (*respiratorias*)

ala-tragus line (ah-la-**TRAY**-gus line)—imaginary line from the ala (wing) of the nose to the ear meatus (center of ear) (*la línea de ala-trago*)

-algia (**AL**-jee-ah)—suffix meaning *pain* or *ache*

alginate (**AL**-jih-nate)—seaweed; agar-based elastic impression material (*algas/alginato*)

allergic reactions (ah-ler-**JIC** re-**ACT**-shun)—sensitivity to an antigen present within the body, resulting in various symptoms (*reaccioones alérgicas*)

allograft (**AL**-oh-graft)—human bone graft from a person other than the patient (*aloinjerto*)

alloy (**AL**-oy)—a mixture of metals (*aleación*)

alternating pulse sound (all-ter-**NATE**-ing sound)—alternations of weak and strong pulsations (*alterno del sonida de pulso*)

alveolar (al-**VEE**-oh-lar)—pertaining to the alveolus (*alveolar*)

alveolectomy (al-vee-oh-**LECK**-toe-mee)—surgical removal of alveolar bone crests (*alveolectomia*)

alveolitis (al-**vee**-oh-**LIE**-tiss)—infection or inflammation of the alveolar bone; a dry socket

alveolus (al-**VEE**-oh-lus)—bone growth on the border of the maxilla and mandible (*alvéolo*)

alveoplastomy (al-vee-oh-**PLASS**-toe-me)—surgical reshaping or contouring of the alveolar bone

amalgam (ah-**MAL**-gum)—soft alloy mass containing mercury, which hardens into restoration (*amalgama*)

amalgam carrier (ah-**MAL**-gam **CARE**-ier)—hand instrument used to carry plastic (movable) amalgam to restorative site (*portador de amalgama*)

amalgamation (ah-**mal**-gah-**MAY**-shun)—blending or pulverizing an alloy with mercury (*amalgamación*)

AMBU bag (am-bu bag)—bag device placed over the nose and mouth of the patient to apply pressure-forced air into the lungs

ameloblast (ah-**MEAL**-oh-blast)—enamel-forming cell; encourages cell growth for enamel tissues (*ameloblastos*)

amelogenesis imperfecta (ah-**meal**-oh-**JEN**-ih-sis im-purr-**FECK**-tah)—incomplete or improper development of enamel tissue (*amelogénesis imperfecta*)

amoxicillin (ah-mocks-ih-**SILL**-in)—antibiotic drug (e.g., Amosil, Larotid) (*amoxicilina*)

ampicillin (am-pih-**SILL**-in)—antibiotic type drug (e.g., Polycillin, Omnipen) (*ampicilina*)

anaerobic (an-ah-**ROH**-bick)—bacteria that do not need oxygen for survival; facultative anaerobes grow best without oxygen but do not require its absence

analgesia (an-al-**JEE**-zee-ah)—without pain; feeling of a lack of pain (*analgésia*)

analgesic (an-al-**JEE**-zick)—drug that relieves pain (*analgésico*)

anaphylactic (an-ah-fih-**LACK**-tick)—shock arising from reaction to body allergen (*shock anafiláctico*)

anaphylaxis (an-ah-fill-**ACK**-sis)—allergic reaction to a drug or food (*anafiliaxia*)

aneroid (**AN**-er-oyd)—dial-type blood-pressure device using air-pressure readings (*aneroide*)

anesthesia (**an**-ess-**THEE**-zee-ah)—without sensation (topical anesthesia is in a specific place, the surface; local anesthesia is limited to one place; block anesthesia produces a regional loss of sensation; general anesthesia involves loss of consciousness)

aneurysm (**AN**-you-rizm)—dilation of a blood vessel due to wall weakness, possible rupture (*aneurisma*)

angina pectoris (an-**JYE**-nah **PECK**-tore-iss)—pain or pressure around the heart (*angina de pecho*)

angle of the mandible (**ANG**-ule **MAN**-di-ble)—area from where the ramus ascends on the lower border of the mandible (*angulo de la mandicule*)

ankyloglossia (**ang**-key-loh-**GLOSS**-ee-ah)—shortness of the lingual frenum; "tongue-tied" (*anquiloglosia*)

ankylosed (**ANG**-kih-lowzd)—stiff joint; tooth fixation; retention of a deciduous tooth (*anquilosis*)

ankylosis (ang-kill-**OH**-sis)—a stiff joint or tooth fixation, or retention of a deciduous tooth

anneal (ah-**NEAL**)—purification by placement into flame; heated in flame until red

anode (**ANN**-ode)—positive pole in X-ray tube that serves as the target for the electron force

anodontia (an-oh-**DON**-she-ah)—absence of teeth; partial or total loss of teeth (*ausencia de dientes*)

anomalies (ah-**NOM**-ah-lees)—out of the normal range, development, or general rule (*anomalias*)

anopia (an-**OH**-pee-ah)—blindness (*le cegura (n), ciego (adj)*)

anosmia (an-**OZ**-me-ah)—loss of sense of smell (*perdida del olfato*)

answering machine—device that records calls received when the phone is not answered (*contestador automático*)

answering service—professional service to answer calls, forward calls, and take messages (*responder servicio*)

antagonism (an-**TAG**-oh-nizm)—opposite or contrary action of a drug (*antagonisno*)

antagonist (an-**TAG**-oh-nist)—opposing tooth; tooth that occludes or counteracts (*antagonista*)

ante- (**AN**-tea)—prefix meaning *before* or *forward*

antecubital fossa (an-tee-**CUE**-bee-tal **FAH**-sah)—anterior depression or bend in the elbow; blood pressure site (*fosa antecubital*)

anterior (an-**TEE**-ree-or)—before or in front of; front of mouth from canine to canine (*anterior*)

anterior band slitter—orthodontic instrument used to slit the anterior band

anti- (**AN**-tie)—prefix meaning *opposed to, against,* or *counteracting*

antianxiety drug (an-tie-ang-sigh-ah-**TEE**)—drug used to produce sedation (*sedación de drogas, droga de anti-angustia*)

antibody (**ANN**-tih-bod-ee)—protein material that destroys antigens; part of the immune system (*anticuerpos*)

anticoagulants (an-tie-koh-**AGG**-you-lants)—drugs that delay or prevent the clotting of blood (*anticuerpos*)

anti-flux (ann-**TIE**-flux)—material, usually graphite, applied to retard the forward advance of the melted solder (*antifundente*)

antifungal drug (ann-tie-**FUN**-gal)—agent that will destroy or hamper the growth or multiplication of fungus (*droga de antifüngicos*)

antigens (**AN**-tih-jens)—foreign substances introduced into or produced by the body (*antigeno*)

antihistamines (**an**-tie-**HISS**-tah-means)—drugs that counteract the effects of histamines in the body (*antihistaminico, antialérgico*)

antihyperlipids (an-tie-high-per-**LIP**-ids)—drugs that decrease or prevent high blood lipid plasma

antihypertensives (an-tie-**high**-per-**TEN**-sives)—drugs to lower or decrease high tension (*antihypertensivos*)

anti-infective drug (an-tee-in-**FECT**-ive)—agent that will act against or destroy infections (*medicamento anti-infecciosos*)

anti-inflammatory drug (ann-tee-in-**FLAM**-ah-tory)—drug that relieves inflammation (*anti-inflamatories*)

antimicrobial (an-tie-my-**KROH**-bee-al)—a substance used to kill or destroy microbes (*anti-microbiano*)

antipyretic (an-tee-pye-**RET**-ick)—drug used to reduce a fever (*antipirético*)

antiseptic (an-tih-**SEP**-tick)—usually a diluted disinfectant; inhibits growth of microbes (*antiséptico*)

antiviral drug (ann-tee-**VIE**-ral)—drug used to destroy or suppress the growth of viruses (*droga anti-viral*)

aorta (ay-**ORE**-tah)—main artery that exits from the heart (*aorta*)

aperture (**AP**-er-chur)—opening or port in a collimator disk to regulate the size of an X-ray beam (*aberatur*)

apex (**AY**-pecks)—root end of tooth (*ápice*)

apexification (ay-pecks-ih-fih-**KAY**-shun)—treatment of a nonvital tooth to stimulate closure (*apexificacíon*)

apexogenesis (ay-pecks-oh-**JEN**-ih-sis)—treatment of vital pulp to continue natural development (*apexogénesis*)

aphthous ulcer (**AF**-thuss **UHL**-cer)—small ulcer; also called canker sore (*(afta) úlcera aftosa*)

apical (**AY**-pih-kahl)—pertaining to the apex of the tooth

apicoectomy (ay-pih-koh-**ECK**-toh-mee)—surgical amputation of the apex of the root (*apicectomia*)

aplasia (ah-**PLAY**-zee-ah)—failure of an organ or body part to develop properly (*aplasia*)

apnea (**AP**-nee-ah)—cessation of breathing, usually temporary (*dejar de respirar, apnea*)

appointment (ah-**POINT**-ment)—time period set aside for a scheduled patient and procedure to be performed (*cita*)

appointment card (ah-**POINT**-ment kard)—printed reminder of a patient's appointment scheduled time (*tarjetas de cita*)

appointment entry (ah-**POINT**-ment kard)—recording the patient's name and other data needed for the appointment (*la entrada de cita*)

appointment matrix (may-**TRICKS**)—pattern of work schedule with days off and times not covered (*matriz de cita*)

apposition (ap-oh-**ZIH**-shun)—addition of parts in the fourth stage of tooth development (*aposicíon*)

approved services—all services covered by the dental plan (*servicios aprobados*)

arch (**ARE**-ch)—curved or bow-like, one half of the mouth; may be maxillary or mandibular (*arco*)

arch-forming plier—orthodontic plier used to form and contour the arch wire (*alica de formar arco*)

arch wire (**ARE**-ch wire)—orthodontic wire, horseshoe in shape; helps shape the arch during movement (*arco de alambre*)

armamentarium (ar-mah-men-**TARE**-ee-um)—layout of dental material and equipment (*armamentario*)

arrested caries (ah-**RES**-ted **KARE**-eez)—decay showing no progressive tendencies (*caries detenida*)

arrhythmia (ah-**RITH**-mee-ah)—absence of rhythm of the heart; irregular heartbeat (*latido irregular del corazón, arritmia*)

arteriosclerosis (ar-teer-ee-oh-skleh-**ROH**-siss)—small artery closing possibly due to plaque

artery (**ARE**-ter-ee)—vessel that carries blood from the heart to the tissues of the body (*la arteria*)

arthrotomy (ar-**THRAH**-toh-me)—cutting into a joint, or surgical joint repair (*artrotomia*)

articular eminence (ar-**TICK**-you-lar **EM**-ih-nense)—forms anterior boundary of the glenoid fossa and helps keep the mandible in position (*eminencia articular*)

articulate (are-**TICK**-you-late)—coming together in a pattern or design (*articular*)

articulating paper (are-**TICK**-you-lay-ting)—color paper strip to test the level of occlusion (*papel de articular*)

articulation (are-tick-you-**LAY**-shun)—movement of teeth of lower jaw in an up and down tooth configuration (*articulatión*)

articulator (ar-**TICK**-you-lay-tor)—mechanical device that stimulates jaw joint actions (*articulador*)

artificial acquired immunity—immunity obtained from inoculation or vaccination to a disease (*la immunidad adquirida artificial*)

artificial teeth—teeth made of porcelain or acrylic material for use in dentures and appliances (*dientes artificials*)

art portion of study model—flat base that is added to impression to make models esthetic (*porción artistica de modelo de estudio*)

asepsis (ay-**SEP**-sis)—condition of being germ-free (*asepia*)

aseptic (ay-**SEP**-tick)—without disease; a condition without pathogens (*aséptic*)

asphyxiation (ass-**fick**-see-**AY**-shun)—cessation of breathing because of loss of oxygen supply (*asfixia*)

assignment of insurance benefits—policyholder's authorization to pay benefits to a provider (*asignación de los beneficios del seguro*)

asthma (**AZ**-mah)—shortness of breath accompanied by wheezing sounds caused by swollen or spastic bronchial tubes or mucous membranes

astringent (ah-strin-**JENT**)—agent that has a binding effect or constricts (*astringente*)

asymmetric (ay-sim-**ET**-rick)—lack of balance of size and shape on opposite sides (*asimétrica*)

asymmetrical (ay-sim-**EH**-trih-kal)—imbalance in size and shape on opposite sides

ataxia (ah-**TACKS**-ee-ah)—eye muscle incoordination (*ataxia*)

atherosclerosis (**ath**-er-oh-skleh-**ROH**-sis)—narrowed arteries caused by a buildup of plaque

atrioventricular (**ay**-tree-oh-ven-**TRICK**-you-lar)—a valve situated between the atrium and the ventricle

atrium (**AY**-tree-um)—upper chamber of the heart, one on each side (pl., atria) (*atrico*)

attenuated (ah-**TEN**-you-**ate**-ed)—diluted or reduced virulence of a pathogenic microbe (*atenuado (a)*)

attrition (ah-**TRISH**-un)—chafing or abrasion of tooth; final stage of tooth development (*desgaste, atrición*)

auditory meatus (aud-ah-**TORY** mee-**AY**-tus)—large opening in temporal bone for auditory nerve passage (*meato auditivo, conducto auditivo*)

auditory ossicles (**AHS**-ih-kuls)—small bones in the ear; not considered part of the face or skull (*huesecillos del oido*)

augmentation (awg-men-**TAY**-shun)—buildup of gingival and bone tissue in collapsed areas, resulting from tooth extraction or disease (*aumento*)

aura (**AW**-rah)—awareness of oncoming physical or mental disorder (*aureola*)

aural (**ORE**-ahl)—pertaining to the ear (*oido*)

aural temperature (**ORE**-ahl)—pertaining to the ear; site for ear temperature (*temperature auditiva*)

ausculate (awe-**SKUL**-ate)—to listen to movement

authorization to release information—permission from the patient or the patient's guardian to release patient record data and treatment record to a specified party

autoclave (**AWE**-toh-klave)—apparatus for sterilization by means of pressurized steam (*auticlave*)

autogenous (**awe**-toh-**JEE**-nus)—in transplantation, to move one's tooth from one area to another area (*autógeno*)

autograft (**AW**-toh-graft)—bone graft from another site in the same patient (*autoinjerto*)

auxiliary springs (aux-il-lor-**EE** springs)—stainless steel attachments used to apply force for directional pull (*resortes auxillares*)

avulsion (ah-**VULL**-shun)—pulling away from, tearing, or knocking out (*avulsión*)

axial surface (**AX**-ee-al)—long length surface of a tooth

axillary (**ACK**-sih-lair-ree)—under-the-armpit site for taking temperature (*axilar*)

back order—item that was not shipped in the present order and will be shipped later

bacteria (back-**TEER**-ee-ah)—one-celled microorganisms lacking chlorophyll

bactericide (back-**TEER**-ee-ah-side)—agent that kills or destroys bacteria (*bactericida*)

bacteriostatic (back-tee-ree-oh-**STAT**-ick)—inhibiter or retarder of bacterial growth (*bacteriostático*)

balm (**BALM**)—oil-based and water-based suspended emulsion (*bálsam*)

band—orthodontic circle made of stainless steel to be cemented onto the tooth surface (*banda*)

band and loop—type of space maintainer used to hold an area open (*banda y lazo*)

band pusher—orthodontic instrument used to push bands upon the teeth; also termed band driver

band removing plier—orthodontic instrument used to remove orthodontic bands

bar—solid-line construction, usually made of metal, uniting one side of an appliance to the other side, such as a palatial bar (maxillary) and a lingual (mandibular) bar

barbiturate (bar-**BIT**-you-rate)—antianxiety drug (e.g., Surital, Nembutal, Seconal) (*barbitúrico*)

barrier control (**BARE**-ee-er control)—an obstacle or impediment; rubber dam to prevent saliva, germ infection (*control de barrera*)

barrier technique—method to avoid contamination by applying material between germs and object (*técnia de barrera*)

basal cell carcinoma (**BAY**-sal cell **CAR**-sin-nova)—malignant epithelial cell growth (*carcinoma de célular basales*)

base—barrier against chemical and thermal irritation to pulp (*basa. fundamento*)

baseplate wax—supplied in sheets; may be used to make denture baseplates (*placa base de cera*)

beaver-tail burnisher (**BURR**-nish-er)—double-ended hand instrument with a round edge and a flat blade, which is used to smooth out (round head) or to carry material (flat blade)

Bell's palsy (Bell's **PAUL**-zee)—sudden but temporary unilateral facial paralysis from unknown cause

benign (bee-**NINE**)—not malignant (*benignos*)

benzocaine (**BEN**-zoe-kane)—anesthetic drug (e.g., Hurricane and Solarcaine topicals) (*benzocaína*)

benzodiazepine (ben-zoe-dye-**AZ**-eh-peen)—antianxiety drug (e.g., Librium, Valium) (*benzodiazepina*)

bevel (**BEV**-el)—slanted edge; a technique to prepare the tooth surface for a prosthetic device (*bisel*)

bicuspidization (bye-cuss-pih-dih-**ZAY**-shun)—surgical division of a tooth with both sides retained

bifurcation (**bye**-fer-**KAY**-shun)—branching into two parts, such as lower molar roots (*bifurcación*)

bilateral (bi-**LAT**-er-al)—two sides

binary (**BYE**-nar-ee)—alloy made up of two different metals (*binario*)

biodegradable (**bye**-oh-dee-**GRADE**-ah-bull)—metabolic material for breakdown of protein material

biofeedback (bye-oh-**FEED**-back)—method of learning to control one's body functions in relation to stress

biofilm (**BYE**-oh-film)—bacterial cells adhering to moist surfaces in a protective slime or covering (*biópelicula*)

biohazard container—receptacle to hold discarded biohazardous trash and items (*receptáculo de riesgo biológico*)

biomechanical (bye-oh-meh-**KAN**-ih-kuhl)—RCT procedure using biological (chemical) and mechanical (twisting) means (*biomecanica*)

biopsy (**BYE**-op-see)—a tissue sample for microscopic study (*biopsia*)

bird beak pliers—orthodontic pliers used to bend and shape the appliance wires

birthday rule—method to determine which of two or more effective contracts pays benefits (*regal de cumpleaños*)

bisecting angle technique—a method in which the central X-ray beam is directed perpendicularly at an imaginary line that is bisecting the angle between the film placement and tooth surface

biteblock—a device used to hold radiation film in the mouth for exposure to the film (*bloque de mordida*)

bite loop tab—loop that encircles periapical film; used by patient to hold film in mouth

biteplane—acrylic appliance constructed to correct simple crossbites (*plano de mordida*)

bite registration—impression of teeth in a biting; occlusal position aides for study model position (*registro de mordida*)

bitestick—wooden stick used to push appliances on the teeth; may "seat" appliances (*palo de mordida*)

bitewing film exposure—X-ray of crowns of the maxillary and mandibular teeth while in occlusion; also called interproximal X-ray or commercial size 3 film

bitewing survey—X-ray scan of teeth and their interproximal areas (**BWX**)

bitewing window—area or designated space in X-ray mount for placement of processed film (*ventana de aleta de mordida*)

blepharoplasty (**BLEF**-er-oh-plas-tee)—plastic surgery of the eyelid

block style of letter—all divisions of the letter are placed next to the left margin (*estilo bloque de la carte*)

blood pressure—indication of the pulsating force of blood circulating through the blood vessels; a vital sign (*presión arterial*)

blowtorch—a compressed air-heating device used to melt alloy for castings (*soplete*)

body of letter—paragraphs that state the nature of the correspondence (*parte principal de carte*)

bonding agent—used to unite some restorative agents to tooth surface and underlying materials (*agente adhesivo*)

bone file—larger hand instrument with serrated edges; used to smooth larger areas of bone (*raspa de hueso*)

bone graft—transplanting bone to restore bone loss resulting from periodontal disease (*injerto óseo*)

bookkeeping—structured method of maintaining records of financial transactions

boxing pour method for study models—use of a wax strip around an impression seated in an impression tray to make a box to receive mixed gypsum for a study model

boxing wax—supplied in strips and used to box or wrap around an impression prior to pouring gypsum material

bracket (**BRACK**-et)—holding device used to support and stabilize arch wires in place

bradycardia (bray-dee-**KAR**-dee-ah)—slow pulse rate, under 60 beats per minute (*pulso lento*)

brand name—drug name registered with the U.S. Patent Office (*nombre de marca*)

breach of confidentiality (con-fa-dent-she-**AL**-ah-tee)—relating personal and confidential matters to others (*violación de la confidencialidad*)

bridge—prosthesis used to replace one or more missing teeth (*prótesis dental*)

broach (**BRO**-ch)—a thin, barbed, sharp-ended **RCT** instrument inserted in the pulp canal to remove pulpal tissue (*aguja*)

bruxism (**BRUCK**-sizm)—grinding of teeth, especially in sleep or habitually (*rechinar los déntes*)

buccal (**BUCK**-al)—pertaining to the check; surface of posterior tooth touching the cheek (*mejella, bucal*)

buccal tube—orthodontic device cemented onto the tooth; fitted to hold the arch wire in place

buccinator (**BUCK**-sin-ay-tore)—principal cheek muscle; gives name to buccal surface (*buccinador*)

buffer period (**BUFF**-er period)—open time unit set aside to be used for emergencies or to make up lost time (*periódo regulador*)

bupivacaine (boo-**PIV**-ah-kane)—anesthetic type of drug (e.g., Marcaine) (*bupivocaina, droga anestética*)

burnish (**BURR**-nish)—to smooth or rub out (*puler*)

burnisher (**BURR**-nish-er)—hand instrument with a rounded head of various shapes, which is used to smooth out surfaces

button (**BUTT**-on)—orthodontic device added to bands to help support or supply addition directional force (*butón*)

CAB (**CAB**)—(c = compressions, a = airway, b = breaths)

cabinet (cab-ah-**NET**)—operatory storage unit composed of various sized drawers and divisions (*armario*)

calcification (kal-sih-fih-**KAY**-shun)—hardening, deposit of lime salts; fifth stage of tooth development (*calcificación*)

calcination (cal-**SIN**-nay-shun)—preparation of gypsum products

calculus (**KAL**-kyou-luss)—deposit of hard mineral salts on the tooth surfaces (*cálculo*)

calendar year—one year, from January 1 to December 31 (*año calendario*)

call list—list of patients willing to be summoned at the first available opening or cancellation (*lista de llamados*)

canaliculi (**kan**-ah-**LICK**-you-lie)—small channels or canals, which may be present in the cementum (*canaliculos*)

canceled check—check that has completed the transaction and is returned to the account holder (*cheque cancelodo*)

candidiasis (kan-dih-**DYE**-ah-sis)—infection of the mouth; thrush (*tordo, micosis*)

cantilever bridge (**KAN**-tih-lee-ver)—prosthesis in which only one side of the device is attached (*voladizo*)

capillary (**KAP**-ih-lair-ee)—minute blood vessel that transport blood from veins to arteries (*capilar*)

capital supply—item of major cost that is used more than once, such as a dental chair (*capital de la oferta*)

capsule (**CAP**-sul)—drug encased in a gelatin shell to dissolve in the stomach (*cápsula*)

carcinoma (kar-sih-**NO**-mah)—tumor of connective-tissue origin (*carcinoma*)

cardiac (**CAR**-dee-ack)—pertaining to the heart (*cardiaco*)

cardiogenic shock (kar-dee-oh-**JEN**-ick)—shock arising from improper heart action (*shock cardiogénico*)

cardiopulmonary resuscitation—act of providing air and heartbeat to a patient (*reanimación cardiopulmonar*)

cardiovascular drug (**CAR**-dee-oh-vas-que-lar)—agent employed for treatment of heart and blood vessels (*drogas cardiovascula*)

caries (**CARE**-eez)—tooth decay (*caries*)

cariogenic (care-ee-oh-**JEN**-ick)—start of decay; causes of decay (*cariogénico*)

carious lesion (**CARE**-ee-us **LEE**-shun)—decay area (*lesion cariosa*)

carotid (care-**OT**-id)—large artery arising from the aorta of the heart to branch into the internal and external carotid arteries (*carótid*)

carpule (**CAR**-pule)—glass vial container for anesthetic solution; also called cartridge (*cartucho*)

carrier—third-party company that does the insuring

carrier infection—disease passed on by either animal or human contamination (*portador de la infección*)

carver (**CAR**-ver)—thin-bladed hand instrument to remove decay or carve newly placed restorative material

cashier's check (cash-**EARS** check)—a purchased check written on a bank's account and signed by the bank treasurer (*cheque de cajero*)

casting (**CAST**-ing)—metal reproduction of a wax pattern (*fundición*)

casting ring—small ring, 1-3/8″ by 1-1/4″, which is used to hold the invested pattern during (*anillo de fundición*)

casting wax—square sheet of various thicknesses; used for construction of patterns for cast (*cera de fundición*)

catalyst (**CAT**-ah-list)—substance that speeds up a chemical reaction (*catalizator*)

cathode (**KATH**-ode)—negative pole in X-ray tube that serves as an electron source (*catodo*)

cellulitis (sell-you-**LYE**-tiss)—inflammation of cellular or connective tissue (*celulitis*)

cementation (see-men-**TAY**-shun)—bonding or uniting two or more items (*cementación*)

cementoblasts (see-**MEN**-toh-blasts)—cementum-forming cells; encourages growth of cementum cells

cementoclasts (see-**MEN**-toh-klasts)—germ cells that destroy tooth cementum

cementoenamel junction (see-**MEN**-toh-ee-**NAM**-el)—tooth area where cement and enamel tissues meet (*union del esmalte y cemento*)

cementum (see-**MEN**-tum)—tissue covering the root of a tooth

centric relationship (**SEN**-trick)—occlusal relationship of the teeth occurring when biting on rear teeth; a seated mouth closure (*relación céntrica*)

cephalometric (seff-ah-low-**MEH**-trick)—pertaining to the head; in X-ray, a cephalometric film is a view of the entire head (*medida de la cabeza*)

cephalometric film (seff-ah-loh-**MEH**-trick)—large radiographic film for exposure of the head (*radiografía cefalométricia*)

cephalostat (**SEFF**-ah-loh-stat)—pin used to center and stabilize the head during X-ray exposure

ceramist (sir-**AM**-ist)—an expert in construction of dental ceramic appliances (*ceramista*)

cerebrovascular accident (sare-ee-broh-**VASS**-kyou-lar)—stroke; result of insufficient blood supply to the brain (*accidente cerebrovascular*)

certificate of eligibility—official identification of an individual covered by a carrier (*ceertificado de eligibilidad*)

certified check—a personal check that has been endorsed to be valid by the bank (*cheque certificado*)

cervical (**SIR**-vih-kul)—pertaining to the neck (*cervical*)

cervical line—cementoenamel junction (*linea cervical*)

cervical traction—orthodontic appliance worn on the head; attaches to the facebow and applies external force to the bands

cervix (**SIR**-vicks)—neck of a tooth (*cuello*)

chain of infection—method for or cause of infection; a break in the barrier against disease (*cadena de infección*)

chamfer (**SHAM**-fur)—tapered margin at the tooth cervix; a preparation for a crown replacement (*chaflán*)

charge slip—paper form used to show procedures performed and fees charged (*cuenta*)

cheilosis (kee-**LOH**-sis)—inflammation of the lips, particularly at the corners (*inflamación de los labios*)

chelator (**KEY**-lay-tor)—chemical ion softener used to soften dentin walls during an **RCT** (*quelante*)

chemical vapor sterilization—total sterilization by means of chemical vapor under pressure (*sterilizacion por vapor de quimica*)

cherubism (**CHER**-you-bizm)—enlargement of cheek tissue; a familiar trait (*querubismo*)

chest thrust—quick pressure upon the chest to force air upward and clear the windpipe (*compresiones del pecho*)

Cheyne-Stokes respiratory sound—respirations gradually increase with volume until climax, then subside and cease for a short time period, and start again; noted in the dying

chisel (**CHIS**-el)—instrument with narrow, straight blade with cutting edge; used to break away enamel (*cinsel, escoplo, formón*)

chronic (**KRON**-ick)—not acute; drawn out, lasting (*crónica*)

chronic radiation exposure—accumulated radiation effects from continual or frequent exposures (*exposicón crónica a la radiación*)

cingulum (**SIN**-gyou-lum)—smooth, convex, or rounded bump on lingual of maxillary anteriors (*cingulo*)

circumferential (ser-**KUM**-fer-en-shal)—clasp that encircles a tooth more than 180 degrees with one terminal end in the undercut of the tooth crown

circumvallate (sir-kum-**VAL**-ate)—largest, V-shaped papillae, situated on the dorsal aspect of the tongue; sense bitter tastes

claim—a listing of rendered services, fees charged, and dates of services; request for payment (*demanda*)

claim form—form used to submit information to insurance company for payment

clasp—extension of a partial appliance that grasps the adjoining teeth to provide support (*cierre*)

cleft lip—tissue fissure or incomplete junction of maxillary lip tissues (*labio leporino*)

cleft palate—congenital fissure in the roof of the mouth with an opening into the nasal cavity; can be unilateral (one sided) or bilateral (two sided), complete or incomplete

cleft tongue—bifid tongue, usually split at the tip (*lingua hendida*)

cleoid/discoid carver (**KLEE**-oyd/**DISK**-oyd)—double-ended instrument used for excavating or carving

clinical chart—printed chart with tooth drawings and diagnostic results of clinical observations (*historia clinica*)

clonic (**KLAHN**-ick)—alternate contraction and relaxation of muscles (*clónicas*)

closed bite registration (reg-ah-**STRAY**-shun)—registration taken while teeth are in occlusion (*registro de mordida cerrada*)

coagulant (koh-**AG**-you-lant)—agent that causes blood to congeal (*coagulante*)

codeine (**KOH**-deen)—drug used to depress the central nervous system (e.g., Tylenol 3, Empirin 3) (*codena*)

coding—identifying the file alignment with marks, numbers, or color changes to aid in filing (*codificación*)

cognitive (cog-nah-**TIVE**)—use of memory, reasoning, perception, and judgment when applied to uncomfortable situations

collection (co-**LEC**-shun)—request for payment; may be sent by letter, statement, or call (*colección*)

collimator (**KAHL**-ih-may-tore)—device used to regulate the exit of an X-ray beam from the tube (*colimador*)

commensal (koh-**MEN**-sahl)—an organism living in or on another without harming its host (*flora comensal*)

commissure (**KOM**-ih-shur)—corner of the mouth where the lips meet (*comisura dela boca*)

complex cavity—decay involving more than two surfaces of a tooth (*cavidad compleja*)

complimentary close—ending line of a letter, such as Sincerely or Sincerely yours (*cerca complementarias*)

composite (cahm-**PAH**-zit)—resin material used for dental restorative purposes (*composite*)

compound (**CAM**-pound)—nonelastic impression material used in edentulous impressions (*compuesto*)

compound cavity—decay involving two surfaces of a tooth (*cavidad compuesta*)

compression (com-**PRESS**-shon)—force upon the chest to provide pressure upon the heart to initiate the heartbeat (*compresión*)

conchae (**KONG**-kee)—small bones in the interior of the nose (plural form of concha) (*concha*)

concussion (kun-**CUSH**-un)—injury caused by being shaken violently or a head blow, such as a sports injury or an accident-injured tooth

condensation (kon-den-**SAY**-shun)—the act of compressing or plugging soft matter into a mass (*condensación, compresión*)

condenser (kon-**DENSE**-or)—instrument with a thick, rounded or oval-shaped flat head, which is used to pack (*condensador*)

conduction anesthesia (kon-**DUCT**-shun an-ah-**STEE**-jah)—nerve block anesthesia given at the base of the mandible in the condyle neck (*conducción dela anestesia*)

condylar inclination (**KAHN**-dih-lahr in-klih-**NAY**-shun)—angular movement of the mandible depending upon placement and function of condyle of the mandible (*inclinacióm condilar*)

condyle (**KON**-dial)—posterior bone growth of the mandible; part of the temporomandibular joint (*cóndilo*)

condyloid (**KON**-dih-loyd)—posterior growth on the ramus of the mandible (*condilea*)

cone cutting—placement error in X-ray exposure, resulting in an incomplete film exposure

conference call—telephone conversation of two or more persons at different locations (*llamada de conferencia*)

congenital (kahn-**JEN**-ih-tahl)—occurring or present at birth; one factor in malocclusion (*cogenital*)

connector (kahn-**ECK**-tore)—device used to unite or attach two or more parts together (*conector*)

conscious sedation (**KON**-cious see-**DAY**-shun)—calming of nervous anxiety without the loss of consciousness (*sedación consciente*)

consent (con-**SCENT**)—the patient or guardian agrees to treatment via written, oral, or implied consent (*consentimiento*)

consent form (con-**SCENT** form)—printed form signed by the patient or the guardian giving permission (*formulario de consentimiento*)

contact area (con-**TACT** area)—surface point where two teeth meet, side by side (*área de contacto*)

contact infection (con-**TACT** in-**FECT**-shun)—direct passage of disease through intimate relationship via saliva, blood, or mucus (*infección de contacto*)

contouring pliers (con-**TOUR**-ing **PLY**-ers)—orthodontic pliers used to contour bands for convex or concave fit (*alicates de contorno*)

contract (con-**TRACT**)—an agreement between two or more parties for a performance of services or care (*contrato*)

contrangle (con-tra-**ANG**-el)—motorized handpiece with angled head

contrast (con-**TRAST**)—variations in shade from black to white (*contraste*)

Controlled Substances Act (1970)—government act to set the schedule for drug types

copayment—plan where the policyholder pays a specific amount or percentage of each claim (*copago*)

coping (**KOH**-ping)—a thin covering that is placed over remaining tooth surfaces in bridgework (*afrontamiento*)

core buildup—use of synthetic material to enlarge the tooth core area to provide support (*nucleo acumulación*)

coronal suture (**KOR**-oh-nal)—suture at the junction of the frontal and parietal bones (*sutura coronal*)

coronoid (**KOR**-oh-noyd)—anterior growth on the ramus of the mandible

corrective orthodontics—procedures taken to reduce or eliminate malocclusion (*ortodoncia correctiva*)

cortical plate (cor-**TEA**-cal plate)—outer bone layer growth of the alveolar bone (*placa cortical*)

cotton forceps—tweezer-like pinchers used to transport materials to or from the mouth

coulomb (**COO**-lum)—international electromagnetic measurement

cranium (**KRAY**-nee-um)—portion of the skull that encloses the brain (*cráneo*)

cream—oil-based and water-based emulsions capable of carry a medicament (***crema***)

crepitus (**KREP**-ih-tus)—grinding, joint abrasion

cribriform plate (**KRIB**-rih-form)—thin lining of the alveolar socket; also called lamina dura

criothyrotomy (kry-oh-thigh-**ROT**-oh-mee)—incision or cut into the thyroid and crioid cartilage

crossbite—when midsagittal alignment between central incisors is not in agreement (***mordida cruzada***)

crown—top part of the tooth; portion of tooth covered by enamel (***corona***)

Crozat appliance—removable orthodontic appliance with a molar clasp

cumulative effect (**CUEM**-la-tive e-**FECT**)—long-term effect of radiation resulting from multiple exposures (***effecto acumulativo***)

cure process—hardening of material through an auto- (chemical) or a light-activated method

curettage (**CURE**-eh-tahj)—scraping of a cavity; or in a prophylaxis, scraping of the cementum deep in a periodontal pocket (***raspado***)

curette (kyou-**RETT**)—round-tipped blade instrument with a longer extended neck and two cutting edges (***cureta***)

cusp (**KUSP**)—elevation or mound on the biting surface of a tooth (***cúsp***)

cuspid (**KUSS**-pid)—third tooth posterior of the midline; also called canine or eye tooth (***cúspide***)

cuspid eminence (**KUSS**-pid **EM**-ih-nence)—vertical length or height of cuspid placement in denture construction (***eminencia canino***)

cuspidor (**KUSS**-pih-dore)—cutting edges

cusp of Carabelli (**KUSP** of care-ah-**BELL**-ee)—extra cusp present on the lingual surface of the maxillary first molar

customary fee (**KUSS**-toe-marry)—average fee range for procedures completed by care providers in a given area (***tarifa habitual***)

cuticle (**KYOU**-tih-kul)—tissue layer covering the tooth surface; also called the Nasmyth membrane (***cuticula***)

cyanosis (sigh-ah-**NO**-sis)—bluish color of facial skin resulting from lack of oxygen (***cianosis***)

cyst (**SIST**)—abnormal, closely walled sac present in or around tissues (***quiste***)

daily schedule—copy of the schedule of patients and procedures for the day (***horario diario***)

dateline—independent line in a letter, stating the date of correspondence (***fecha***)

day sheet—daily record of appointments, services, and business activities of the day (***hoja de dia***)

debridement (deh-**BREED**-ment)—removal of damaged tissue or foreign matter (***eliminación del tejido dañado***)

deciduous (deh-**SID**-you-us)—primary teeth; first set of teeth (***caduco***)

defamation (def-**AH**-may-shun)—false statement causing damage to a person's reputation or causing ridicule (***difamación***)

defendant (dee-**FEN**-dent)—the accused or person named in the lawsuit (***demandado***)

defibrillation (dee-fib-rih-**LAY**-shun)—reversal of cardiac standstill; reinstatement of cardiac rhythm

deficit (**DEF**-ih-sit)—lower pulse rate at wrist site than at heart site; "heart flutter" (***deficit de pulso***)

definition (def-ah-**NISH**-on)—sharpness and clarity of the outline of the image on the radiograph (***definición***)

degenerative (dee-**JEN**-er-ah-tiv)—disease resulting from natural aging, such as arthritis (***degenerarivo***)

deglutition (dee-glue-**TISH**-un)—the act of swallowing (***deglución***)

dehydration (dee-high-**DRAY**-shun)—water loss or deprivation (***dehidratación***)

demand-valve resuscitator—device on the oxygen mask to apply pressure to oxygen flow

dens in dente (**DENZ** in **DEN**-tay)—tooth in tooth; usually found on linguals of maxillary laterals

density (**DENZ**-sah-dee)—film blackening resulting from the percentage of radiation transmitted through the film (*densidad*)

dental chair—chair appliance; power driven with the capability to assume assorted positions (*sillón dental*)

dental dam (**rubber dam**)—a thin sheet of rubber used as a mask to isolate the work area (*presa dental*)

dental dam clamp (**rubber dam clamp**)—small retaining device to hold dam material on the tooth (*abrazadera presa dental*)

dental dam forceps (**rubber dam forceps**)—device used to spread open and transport the dam clamp

dental dam frame (**rubber dam frame**)—a device used to maintain the dam material in place

dental dam ligature (**rubber dam ligature**)—floss, thread, or small pieces of dam material or a device used to tie or hold down the clamp and dam material

dental dam punch (**rubber dam punch**)—used to place measured holes in the dam material

dental lamina (**LAM**-ih-nah)—membrane band containing organs of future teeth (*lamina dental*)

dental sac—pocket covering, derived from the mesoderm and making up the tooth covering (*saco dental*)

dental unit—power and suction appliance with handpiece; water control and suction (*unidad dental*)

dentated (**DEN**-tay-ted)—bur with extra cutting teeth in a crosscut pattern

denticles (**DEN**-tih-kuls)—small tooth growths, also known as pulp stones

dentifrice (**DEN**-tih-friss)—a tooth powder or paste used to clean teeth (*dentifrico*)

dentigerous (den-**TIJ**-er-us)—having or containing teeth

dentin (**DEN**-tin)—main tissue of the tooth, present in the root and the crown; surrounds the pulp (*dentine*)

dentinogenesis imperfecta (den-tin-oh-**JEN**-eh-sis im-per-**FECK**-tuh)—inadequate formation of tooth resulting in weak teeth

dentition (den-**TISH**-un)—tooth arrangement; set of teeth (*dentición*)

denture (**DEN**-chur)—a removable appliance to replace an entire arch of missing teeth; partial denture is an appliance that replaces a few missing teeth in an arch

denture base—acrylic part of denture prosthesis that substitutes for the gingival tissue (*dentadura baso*)

denturist (**DEN**-ture-ist)—person who independently specializes in denture construction

dependence (dee-pen-**DENSE**)—physical (chemical) and psychological (desire) need or dependence (*dependientes*)

dependent (dee-pen-**DENT**)—person, other than the policyholder, who is carried as a member of the claim

deposition (dep-oh-**SIH**-shun)—testimony given under oath regarding a specific event or occurrence (*deposición*)

deposit slip—form for recording submitted cash and checks into an account (*ficha de depósito*)

desiccant (**DES**-ih-kant)—chemical to dry the prep area, remove matter (*desecante*)

desquamative (des-**KWAM**-ah-tiv)—shedding or scaling off; tissue loss (*pérdida de lejido*)

detail—point-to-point delineation or the view of minute structures in a radiographic image (*detalle*)

developing process—action used to produce the latent image on a radiographic film (*proceso de desarrollo*)

diabetic coma (di-ah-**BET**-ick)—loss of consciousness due to severe untreated or unregulated diabetes (*como diabético*)

diagnosis (die-agg-**NO**-sis)—term denoting the name of a disease (*diagnosis*)

dialysis (die-**AL**-ih-sis)—solute material passage through a membrane (*diálisis*)

diamond rotary instrument—diamond-surfaced bur used for rapid, gross tooth removal

diaphragm (stethoscope) (**DYE**-ah-fram)—layer over the disc end of a stethoscope; enlarges or amplifies pulse sounds

diaphragm (X-ray tubehead) (**DYE**-ah-fram)—device used to regulate the size of the X-ray beam

diastema (dye-ah-**STEE**-mah)—an opening or gap between two teeth (*apertura de diente*)

diastolic (dye-ah-**STAHL**-ick)—the force of the pulse blood while at rest (*diastólica*)

die—reproduction of a prepared tooth (*molde*)

differentiation (diff-er-en-she-**AY**-shun)—growth stage of tooth development causing changes in shape (*diferenciación*)

digital sensor exposure—radiographic exposure of a sensor rod placed in the oral cavity and then transmitted to a computer monitor for viewing and recording

diplopia (die-**PLOH**-pee-ah)—double vision (*vision doble*)

direct bond—the technique of cementing brackets directly onto the tooth surface

direct dentin stimulation—scratching of dentin to obtain pain reaction; a method of locating and diagnosing pulpal conditions

discloid/cleoid (**DISK**-oyd/**KLEE**-oyd)—double-ended hand instrument with discloid (disc-shaped) end and a cleoid (pointed blade) on the other end; used to remove decay and carve materials

disclosing dyes (dis-**CLOSE**-ing)—food coloring material that is placed in the mouth to dye matter and plaque (*colorantes*)

disease—pathological change in body or body functions (*infermedad*)

disinfectant (dis-inn-**FECK**-tant)—chemical that kills many microbes but not spore-forming bacteria (*disinfectante*)

disinfection (dis-inn-**FECK**-shun)—application of chemicals to kill, reduce, or eliminate germs (*disinfectante*)

dissipate (**DISS**-ih-pate)—to scatter, spread out; to let heat escape (*disipar*)

distal (**DISS**-tahl)—pertaining to the far or away side; side farthest from the midline of the face (*hacia la parte posterior*)

distal end cutter—an orthodontic cutting instrument used to cut arch wire in a buccal tube

distal shoe maintainer—orthodontic space maintainer

distoclusion (dist-toh-**KLOO**-zhun)—class II malocclusion, or the lower jaw in a retruded position

distribution (dis-tra-**BU**-shun)—process of dividing and circulation of the absorbed drug to the desired site (*didtribución*)

diuretics (dye-you-**RET**-icks)—drugs that increase secretion of urine (*diurético*)

dorsal (**DOOR**-sal)—back, pertaining to the rear (*dorsal*)

dosimeter (doh-**SIH**-meh-ter)—measures the amount of stray or secondary X-ray exposure (*dosimetro*)

double pour method in study models—after filling in the impression area with gypsum, mix another gypsum batch, and place the first poured onto the mixed pile of gypsum

dovetail scheduling—appointment times scheduled into the day's procedures at a down time

dowel pin (**DOWL**)—tapered brass post placed into a die to use as a handle during construction

droplet infection—infection from pathogens released from the mouth or nose of infected person (*infección por gotitas*)

drug interaction—effect resulting from combination of two or more drugs at one time (*intracción farmocológica*)

dry heat sterilization—sterilization by means of a dry heat oven; hot-air bake (*esterilización por calor seco*)

duct (**DUCT**)—narrow vessel or opening that allows secretions from glands to enter the body (*conducto*)

ductility (duck-**TILL**-ih-tee)—ability to be drawn or hammered into a fine wire without breaking (*ductilidad*)

duplication of films—process to duplicate or make a copy of a radiographic film (*duplicación de la pelicula*)

duration—lasting effect of a drug (*duración*)

dys- (**DIS**)—prefix meaning *bad, difficult,* or *painful*

dysphagia (dis-**FAY**-jee-ah)—difficulty swallowing (*dificultad de tragar*)

dyspnea (**DISP**-nee-ah)—air hunger, out of breath; difficult or labored breathing (*dificultad de respirar*)

ectoderm (**ECK**-toh-derm)—outer layer of development

-ectomy (**ECK**-toh-me)—suffix meaning *surgical removal of*

ectopic (eck-**TAH**-pick)—out of place; one factor in malocclusion (*fuera de lugar*)

edema (eh-**DEE**-mah)—swelling (*edema*)

edentulous (ee-**DENT**-you-luss)—without teeth (*sin dientes*)

edentulous survey—radiographic survey of entire oral cavity that lacks teeth

edgewise pliers—orthodontic pliers used to hold or adjust arch wires

effective date (ee-**FECT**-tive date)—date on which the contact becomes in force and benefits begin (*fecha de efectiva*)

efficacy (**EFF**-ih-kah-see)—intensity of a drug (*eficacia*)

elastic (ee-**LAS**-tic)—band with an elastic ability to apply pressure by attachment to opposing brackets (*elástico*)

elasticity (ee-las-tiss-ih-tee)—ability of a material to be stretched and resume its original shape (*elasticidad*)

elastomeric (ee-las-toh-**MARE**-ick)—having properties similar to rubber

electromagnetic (**EE**-lec-tro-**MAG**-net-ick)—physical force generating electricity produced by a magnetic current

electronic mail (**e-mail**) (ee-lect-**TRON**-ic mail)—communication by means of the Internet (*correo electrónio*)

electroplate (ee-**LECK**-troh-plate)—thin metal covering applied to a surface through electrolysis (*galvaniza*)

elixir (ee-**LICK**-sir)—sweetened, aromatic, water-alcohol solution (*droga*)

elongation (ee-lon-**GAY**-shun)—radiographic placement error resulting in an extended length of the tooth image; ability of a metal to stretch before permanent deformation begins

embolism (**EM**-boh-lizm)—floating clot lodging in an artery (*embolia*)

embrasure (em-**BRAY**-zhur)—V-shaped tooth gap area beneath contact area and gingival crest (*alféizar*)

emergency call list (ee-**MER**-gen-see call list)—important phone numbers that may be necessary in an emergency (*lista de llamadas de emergencia*)

emergency tray—tray assembled with materials and items necessary for emergencies (*bandeja de emergencia*)

eminence (**EM**-in-ence)—high place, projection, or prominence (*eminenciáe*)

emulsion (ee-**MULL**-shun)—mixture of two liquids that are not mutually soluble (*emulsión*)

enamel (eh-**NAM**-el)—outer covering of the crown of a tooth (*esmalte*)

enamel hypoplasia (high-poh-**PLAY**-zee-ah)—underdevelopment of the enamel tissue (*esmalte subdesarrollados*)

enamoplasty (ee-**NAM**-oh-plas-tee)—selective reduction of enamel tissue to reduce fissures and pits (*reducción del esmalte*)

enclosure line (en-**CLOS**-shur)—line that is printed at the bottom of a letter to indicate that material is enclosed (*recinto de la linea*)

endemic (en-**DEM**-ick)—disease occurring in the same population or locality (*endémicas*)

endo- (**EN**-doe)—prefix meaning within or inside

endocardium (en-doh-**KAR**-dee-um)—inner layer of the heart, lining the four heart chambers (*endocardio*)

endodontia (en-doh-**DAHN**-she-ah)—dental specialty dealing with diseases of pulp tissue

endodontic (en-doh-**DAHN**-tick)—pertaining to the area within a tooth, pulp tissue (*endodoncia*)

endodontist (en-doh-**DAHN**-tist)—dentist specialized in the treatment of the diseased pulp

endogenous (en-**DAH**-jeh-nuss)—arising from within the cell or organism; illness from within (*endógeno*)

endorsement (en-**DOORS**-ment)—signature placed on the back of a check to show that the payee has cashed the check (*aprobación firma*)

endosseous (en-**DOSS**-ee-us)—within the alveolar bone, such as an implant into the bone (*endóseo*)

endosteal (en-**DOSS**-tee-ahl)—type of implant placement within the bone (*endostal*)

endotoxins (en-doh-**TOCKS**-inz)—a poison within or internal (*endotoxina*)

enflurane (**EN**-floh-rane)—volatile general anesthetic liquid (*enfluoros*)

enteral (**EN**-ter-ahl)—taken into the gastrointestinal system (*adoptades en el sistima gastrointestinnal, entéerico, via enteral*)

enteric-coated drug (en-**TARE**-ick)—specially coated pill that prevents release and absorption of its contents until reaching the gastrointestinal tract

enzyme (**EN**-zime)—body-produced chemical that breaks down food (*enzima*)

epicardium (epp-ih-**KAR**-dee-um)—outer serous layer of the heart (*la capa externa del corazon*)

epidemic (ep-ah-**DEM**-ick)—among people, widespread, occurring in many places (*epidemia*)

epilepsy (**EP**-ih-lep-see)—seizure; disease with recurrent attacks of disturbed brain functioning (*epilepsia*)

epistaxis (ep-ih-**STACK**-sis)—nosebleed (*hemmorragia nasal*)

epithelium (ep-ith-**EE**-lee-um)—tissue lining or layer (*epithelium*)

epulis (ep-**YOU**-liss)—a gumboil or fibrous tumor of oral tissue (*bola de cañón, epulis*)

erosion (ee-**ROE**-zhun)—gnaw away, destruction of tooth tissue caused by disease, chemicals (*la erosión*)

eruption (ee-**RUP**-shun)—breaking out of teeth; growth stage in which tooth enters oral cavity (*erupción*)

erythema (air-ith-**EE**-mah)—skin redness that may be a result of radiation or allergy (*rojez de la piel*)

erythema dose—radiation exposure that produces a temporary redness of the skin

erythromycin (ah-rith-row-**MYE**-sin)—antibiotic drug (e.g., E-mycin, **ERYC**, Erycette)

erythroplakia (air-rith-throw-**PLAY**-key-ah)—red patch on tissue; may be precancerous

esthetic (ehs-**THET**-ick)—pertaining to beauty; act of making something appealing (*estheteesteta*)

ethics—laws of conduct set forth by the profession (*la ética*)

ethmoid (**ETH**-moyd)—spongy bone forming part of the anterior nasal area of the skull

etiology (ee-tee-**AHL**-oh-jee)—the cause of a disease or beginning of an illness (*etiologia*)

excavator (**ECKS**-kah-vay-tore)—hand instrument used to remove decayed matter from the prep site (*excavadora*)

exclusion (ecks-**CLUE**-shun)—dental service or procedure not listed under the dental plan (*la exclución*)

excretion (ecks-**KREE**-shun)—process of eliminating waste products from the body (*excreción*)

excursion (ecks-**KER**-zhun)—lateral movement of the mandible (*excursión*)

exfoliate (ecks-**FOH**-lee-ate)—to shed or fall off

exfoliation (ecks-foh-lee-**AY**-shun)—shedding or falling off (*exfoliación*)

exodontia (ecks-oh-**DAHN**-shah)—extraction of teeth (*extracción del diente*)

exogenous (ecks-**AH**-jeh-nuss)—produced outside; disease occurring from causes outside the body (*exógenos*)

exolever (**ECKS**-oh-lee-ver)—device used in oral surgery to raise and elevate a tooth or root tip

exostosis (ecks-ahs-**TOH**-sis)—bony outgrowth

exothermic (eeks-oh-**THER**-mick)—giving off heat, as in some chemical union reactions (*emiten calor, exotérmico*)

expander (ecks-**PAN**-der)—device used to expand or enlarge the maxillary jaw (*expansor*)

expectorate (ex-**PECK**-toh-rut)—to spit or empty the mouth (*expectorar, escupir*)

expendable supply (ex-pen-**DAH**-ble supply)—item used or consumed during procedures, such as cements, gloves (*suministro de fungibles*)

expiration (ecks-purr-**AY**-shun)—expulsion of air from the lungs (*exhaler*)

explorer (ecks-**PLOR**-er)—sharp pick end instrument of various shapes and angles; used to detect small caries (*explorador*)

exposure time (ex-**POSE**-ure time)—duration of the interval that the electric current will pass through the X-ray tube (*tempo de exposición*)

express mail—fast, 24-hour delivery of mail (*correo urgente*)

ex-pro—instrument with combination ends: one an explorer end and one a periodontal probe end

extirpation (ecks-ter-**PAY**-shun)—to root out; removal of nerve and pulp in **RCT** (*extirpación*)

extraction (ecks-**TRACK**-shun)—surgical removal of a tooth or teeth (*extracción*)

extraoral film—radiographic film placed and exposed outside of the oral cavity (*pelicula extraoral*)

extrinsic (ex-**TRIN**-sick)—outer, as in stains on the outside of the tooth (*extrinseco*)

extruded (ecks-**TRUE**-ded)—pushed out of normal position (*extruido*)

extruder gun/syringe (ecks-**TRUE**-dur)—device to measure and blend two materials into a homogenous mixture

extrusion (ecks-**TROO**-zhun)—movement of tooth out of the alveolus; orthodontic movement

exudate (**EX**-you-dayt)—passing out of pus (*que pasa de pus*)

facebow—metal orthodontic arch bow device that attaches to intraoral buccal tubes; headgear

facial (**FAY**-shal)—pertaining to the surface of the cheek and lips (face) (*facial*)

facultative anaerobes—bacteria that grow best without oxygen but do not require its absence

fauces (**FOH**-seez)—constricted opening leading from the mouth and oral pharynx, composed of tissue pillars; area where tonsils are located

febrile pulse sound (**FEEB**-ril)—normal pulse rate becoming weak and feeble upon illness or prostration (*el sonida del pulsa febril*)

Federation Dentaire Internationale—one method of tooth numbering, in which each quadrant has a specific starting number to designate that area

felony (fell-**OH**-nee)—serious crime, more punishable than a misdemeanor or petty crime (*delito*)

festoon (fes-**TUNE**)—to trim and finish off (*guirnalda*)

fiber (**FIGH**-ber)—thread-like film element (*fibra*)

fibroblasts (**FIE**-broh-blasts)—fiber-forming cells that develop the parieodontium

fibroma (fie-**BROH**-mah)—benign tumor of the connective tissue

filament (**FILL**-ah-ment)—tungsten coil in the cathode focusing cup to generate the electrons (*filamento*)

file—a thin, rough, serrated instrument used in RCT/*legajo ficha*; a business device for records arrangement (*de archivos*)

file cabinet—furniture used to hold business files; files differ in size and shape (*contenedor de archivos*)

file folder—thick envelope folder with tab used to contain patient records and other data (*carpeta de archivos*)

file guide—heavy cardboard sheet used to divide file drawer into (*guia de archivos*)

filiform (**FIL**-ah-form)—smallest, hair-like papillae covering the tongue's entire dorsal aspect

film holding instrument—device used to hold radiographic film in place during exposure (*soporte de pelicula*)

film safe container—lead-lined container used to hold X-ray film before or after exposure

film speed—comparison rate of exposure time needed by the film for proper exposure (*velocidad de la pelicula*)

filter—aluminum disc placed between the collimeter attachment and the exit spot to filter X-rays (*filtrante*)

finger sweep—placement of a finger into the mouth to locate and wipe out airway obstruction

first-class mail—letters, postcards, statements, business reply, and larger marked envelopes (*correo de primera clase*)

fiscal year—any twelve-month period set by an agency or company for accounting scheduling

fissure (**FISH**-er)—groove or natural depression; slit or break (*fisura*)

fistula (**FISS**-tyou-lah)—pathway for pus escape; opening in tissue for pus drainage (*fistula*)

fixed fee—fixed schedule of fees for a specific service that provider agrees to accept (*tasa fija*)

fixing—a chemical process of making a radiographic image permanent

flagella (flah-**JELL**-ah)—small, whip-like hairs providing movement for some bacteria (*flagelo*)

flange (**FLANJ**)—projecting rim or lower edge of a prosthesis (*reborde*)

floss—string or thread composed of silk, nylon, Teflon, or synthetic materials; used to remove plaque buildup (*hilo dental*)

floss holder—device used to hold floss; useful for people with limited use of hands (*sostenedor de la seda*)

fluoride—decay preventive, natural element that strengthens teeth tissues (*fluoruro*)

fluorosis (floor-**OH**-sis)—reaction to over fluoridation; also called mottled teeth

flux (**FLUCKS**)—agent employed to protect alloy from oxidation during the heating process (*flujo*)

focal spot (**FOE**-cull spot)—target or area where the X-ray beam is projected (*punto focal*)

fog—clouded, darkened, or blemished X-ray film result; caused by multiple factors (*velar*)

foliate (**FOH**-lee-ate)—tissue bits located on the posterior, lateral edges of the tongue (*foliar*)

fomes (**FOH**-mez)—inanimate objects that absorb and transmit infection, such as a doorknob

fomites (**FOH**-mights)—plural of fomes (*fomitas*)

fontanel (fon-tah-**NELL**)—literally "little fountain"; baby's soft spot on the skull (*fontanela*)

foramen (foh-**RAY**-men)—an opening or hole in the bone for passage of nerves and vessels (*foramen, orficio*)

forceps (**FOUR**-ceps)—plier-like instrument used to remove teeth (*fórcep*)

forensic dentist (for-**EN**-sick)—specialist in pathological evidence for legal procedures (*dentista forense*)

foreshortening (fore-**SHORE**-ten-ing)—error in radiographic placement resulting in shortened tooth image on film surface (*escorzo*)

fossa (**FAH**-sah)—shallow, rounded, irregular depression or concavity found on lingual surface of anterior teeth and on occlusal surface of posterior teeth

fourth-class mail—printed matter and parcels weighing over a pound; also called parcel post (***paquetes postales***)

fracture (**FRAC**-ture)—a breakage; in a tooth, a root or crown (or both) may be fractured (***fracturae***)

framework—metal skeleton or spine onto which a removable prosthesis is constructed (***estructura***)

Frankfort plane—imaginary line from the tragus of the ear to the floor of the orbit that is used to align the maxillary arch parallel to the floor

fraud—deliberate misrepresentation of facts or information (***el fraude***)

frenectomy (freh-**NECK**-toh-me)—surgical removal or resectioning of frenum

frenum (**FREE**-num)—tissue fold that connects two parts of the mouth (pl., frena) (***frenillos***)

frequency of pulse sound—pulse count (***pulsa contaje***)

friction grip bur—smooth-ended bur that slips into the friction grip handpiece and is held by friction grip

frontal (**FRON**-tal)—the anterior area bone that makes up the forehead

full mouth survey—multiple exposures of radiographs resulting in a view of entire area

fungiform (**FUN**-jih-form)—small, dark red papillae on the middle and anterior dorsal surface and along the sides of the tongue; sense sweet, sour, and salty tastes

fungus (**FUNG**-us)—division of chlorophyll-lacking plants that includes slimes and molds (pl., fungi) (***hongases***)

furcation (fur-**KAY**-shun)—branching off; area where the tooth roots branch apart (***furcación***)

furrow (**FER**-oh)—shallow, concave groove located on either the crown or the root (***surco***)

fusion (**FEW**-zhun)—joining together; union of tooth buds resulting in large crown or tooth (***la fusión***)

galvanic (gal-**VAN**-ick)—electrical charge emitted from meeting and reaction of two dissimilar metals (***choque galvánico***)

Gasserion ganglion (**GANG**-lee-un)—nerve bundle or union center of trigeminal nerve branches

gastric distension (gas-**TRICK** dis-**TEN**-shun)—condition resulting from air forced into the abdomen instead of the lungs

Gates-Glidden drill—latch-type bur with flame-shaped tip; used to open and access during **RCT**

generic (**JIN**-air-ick)—drug name conferred by the U.S. Adopted Name Council (***genéricos***)

genioplasty (**JEE**-nee-oh-plas-tee)—plastic surgery of the chin or cheek (***cirugia de mentón***)

germicide (**JER**-miss-eyed)—substance that destroys germs (***germicido***)

germination (germ-ih-**NAY**-shun)—single tooth germ separating to form two crowns on one root (***germinación***)

gingiva (**JIN**-jih-vah)—mucous tissue that surrounds the teeth; attached gingiva is firm, bound (***teijido de las encias***, ***gingiva***)

gingival crest—lip edge of free gingiva, also called the gingival margin (***cresta gingival***)

gingival margin trimmer—bladed hand instrument with cutting edge to adapt to tooth margin

gingivectomy (jin-jih-**VECK**-toh-me)—surgical excision of unattached gingival tissue

gingivitis (**jin**-jih-**VIE**-tis)—inflammation of gingival tissues (***gingivitis***)

gingivoplastomy (jin-jih-voh-**PLAS**-toh-me)—surgical recontour of the gingival tissue

glenoid fossa (**GLEE**-noyd **FAH**-sah)—depression in the temporal bone; location of the condyle (***fosa glenoidea***)

glossa (**GLAHS**-ah)—the tongue (***tongue***, ***la lengua***)

glossitis (glah-**SIGH**-tiss)—inflammation of the tongue (***inflamación de la lengua***)

glossopalatine arch (gloss-oh-**PAL**-ah-tine)—anterior tissue pillar in throat; tonsil location

glossopharyngeal (gloss-oh-fair-en-**JEE**-al)—**IX** ninth cranial nerve

glucose (**GLUE**-kohs)—a blood sugar (*glucosa*)

gnarled (**NARLD**) **enamel**—enamel rods twisting and curving within the enamel tissue

gold foil—thin sheet of gold used for restorations (*llamina de óro*)

gomphosis (gahm-**FOH**-sis)—the holding and anchoring action of a tooth in its socket

grand mal seizure—noticeable epileptic attack (*convulsion tónico-clónica generalizada, ataque*)

granule (**GRAN**-you-ll)—a minute mass; small, grain-like body

granuloma (gran-you-**LOH**-mah)—granular tumor or growth, usually in the root area

groove—a rut, furrow, or channel; may be a developmental or surface groove (*surco*)

gutta-percha point (gut-**TA** per-**CHA** point)—endodontic canal point made of a rubber-like, thermoplastic material

gypsum (**GYP**-sum)—calcium sulfate product of various grits, speed, strengths, and colors; used for models and dies (*yeso*)

halothane (**HAL**-oh-thane)—volatile general anesthetic liquid (*halotano*)

hamulus (**HAM**-you-luss)—hook-like end of bone that serves as a site for muscle attachment

handpiece—motor-driven drill; available in different speeds, shapes, and types

hardness—ability of a material to withstand penetration (*dureza*)

hatchet (**HATCH**-et)—hand instrument with hatchet-like edge; used to break away decayed tooth tissue (*hacha*)

Hawley appliance—removable orthodontic appliance worn to maintain space after correction

headgear—ortho appliance worn on the head to support and apply forces to internal appliance

health history form—printed questionnaire regarding patient's present and past health history (*formulario de la historia de saluda*)

Health Maintenance Organization (**HMO**)—plan offering specific services to its members and a stipulated payment allotment to the provider

Heimlich maneuver—abdominal thrusts to force air to expel or dislodge an obstruction in the airway

hemangioma (he-man-jee-**OH**-mah)—tumor of dilated blood vessels

hematoma (hee-mah-**TOE**-mah)—blood swelling or bruise (*moretón, hinchazón*)

hemiarthroplasty (**HEM**-ee-are-throw-plas-tee)—surgical repair of a joint with a partial joint implant

hemiplegia (hem-ih-**PLEE**-jee-ah)—paralysis on only one side of the body (*hemiplejia*)

hemisection (**HEM**-ih-seck-shun)—cutting a tissue or organ in half (*reducir a la mitad*)

hemorrhage (**HEM**-or-reege)—blood burst; excessive bleeding (*sangrado excesivo, hemmorrogia*)

hemostasis (hee-moh-**STAY**-sis)—stabilizing blood with anesthesia

hemostat (**HE**-moh-stat)—device or drug used to arrest the flow of blood (*hemostático*)

herpes—**Herpes Simplex Virus** (**HSV**) (**HER**-peez)—recurrent virus disease of vesicles or watery, crusty pimples; cold sore (*herpes*)

herringbone effect—exposure error resulting in an image of the lead backing on the X-ray

heterodont (**HET**-er-oh-dont)—teeth of various shapes

heterogeneous (het-er-oh-**JEE**-nus)—placement of a tooth from a source other than self

high-volume evacuator (**HVE**)—mouth-suction device with hand instrument tip (*aspiración de la boca*)

histodifferentiation (his-toh-dif-er-en-she-**AY**-shun)—branching into different parts

hoe (**HO**)—smaller bladed hand instrument with an angled cutting tip resembling a garden hoe (*azada*)

holding solution—a disinfectant solution with a biodegradable chemical; used to soak items

homogenous (hoh-**MAH**-jeh-nus)—same or alike; uniform material

homonym (**HAHM**-oh-nim)—a word that sounds the same as another word

hormonal (**HOR**-mow-nal)—pertaining to hormones (*hormonal*)

How or Howe pliers—orthodontic pliers used to make arch wire adjustment

Hutchinson incisors—rounded, small teeth caused by maternal syphilis during tooth

hydrocolloid (high-droh-**KAHL**-oyd)—agar impression material capable of changing forms (*material de impression de agar*)

hydromorphine (high-dro-**MORE**-fene)—depresses the central nervous system (e.g., Dilaudid)

hydrophilic (high-droh-**FIL**-ick)—capability to attract and hold water (*hidrofilico*)

hydrophobia (high-droh-**FOH**-bee-ah)—fear of water; giving off or shedding of water (*hidrofobia*)

hygroscopic (high-groh-**SKAH**-pick)—submersion into or addition of water to material prior to the initial set (*expansión higroscópia*)

hyoid (**HIGH**-oyd)—small bone in the neck area called the "Adam's apple" (*hioides*)

hyper- (**HIGH**-per)—prefix meaning above, excessive, or beyond

hypercementosis (high-per-see-men-**TOH**-siss)—overgrowth of cementum from stress or trauma (*cemento excesiva*)

hyperdontia (high-per-**DAHN**-she-ah)—excess of teeth number; supernumerary teeth (*cantidad, excesiva de las dientes*)

hyperemia (high-per-**EE**-mee-ah)—increase in blood and lymph because of irritation (*aumento en la sangre, hiperemia*)

hyperextension (high-purr-eck-**STEN**-shun)—condition in which a tooth arises out of its socket (*hiperextensión*)

hyperglycemia (high-per-glaye-**SEE**-me-ah)—condition where there is an excessive of blood sugar (*azúcar en la sangre excesive, hiperglucemia*)

hyperkinetic (high-purr-kih-**NET**-ick)—overly energetic; low ability to stand pain

hyperplasia (high-per-**PLAY**-zee-ah)—excessive tissue, swollen gingiva (*hiperplástico*)

hypersensitivity (high-per-sen-sih-**TIV**-ih-tee)—abnormal sensitivity, reaction to pain or stimuli (*hipersensible*)

hyperthermia (high-per-**THER**-mee-ah)—body temperature over 104°F (40°C) (*hipertermia*)

hypertrophy (high-per-**TROE**-fee)—increased inspiration resulting in a CO_2 decrease (*hipertrofia*)

hyperventilation (high-per-ven-tih-**LAY**-shun)—increased inspiration resulting in carbon dioxide decrease (*hiperventilación*)

hypocalcification (high-poh-kal-sih-fih-**KAY**-shun)—underbonding or incomplete calcification, resulting in weak, susceptible teeth (*hipocalcificación*)

hypodontia (high-poh-**DAHN**-she-ah)—congenital missing of teeth; lack of teeth (*la falta de dientes*)

hypoglossal (high-poh-**GLOSS**-al)—**XII**-twelfth cranial nerve

hypoglycemia (high-poh-gly-**SEE**-me-ah)—condition in which blood sugar is abnormally low (*bajo azúcar en la sangre, hipoglucemia*)

hypokinetic (high-poh-kih-**NET**-ick)—high pain tolerance ability; under sensitive or underactive response to pain (*baja respuesta al dolor, hipocinético*)

hypoplasia (high-poh-**PLAY**-zee-ah)—underdevelopment of tissue; lack of enamel covering (*falta de desarrollo de los tejidos, hipoplasia*)

hyposulfite (**HIGH**-poh-sul-fite)—chemical used in X-ray film processing to remove silver grains from exposed film (*hiposulfito*)

hypothermia (high-poh-**THER**-mee-ah)—body temperature under 95°F (35°C) (*hipotermia*)

hypoxia (high-**POCK**-see-ah)—lack of oxygen, as in tension (*la falta de oxigeno, hipox*)

ibuprofen (eye-byou-**PROH**-fenn)—anti-inflammatory medication (e.g., Advil and Motrin) (*ibuprofeno*)

ID—intradermal drug route (*intradérmica*)

identification dot—raised bump on film that indicates the side of film to place facing X-ray source (*punto de indentificación*)

idiosyncrasy (id-ee-oh-**SIN**-krah-see)—effect from unusual and abnormal drug response (*idiosincrasia*)

IH—inhalation drug route (*inhalación*)

IM—intramuscular drug route (*intramuscular*)

imbibition (im-bih-**BISH**-un)—taking on of moisture or fluid absorption (*teniendo en liquidas*)

immediate denture—denture that is placed into the mouth at the time of teeth extraction

immunity (im-**MEW**-nah-tee)—resistance to organisms due to previous exposure or conditions (*immunidad*)

immunocompromised (im-you-no-**KAHM**-proh-mizd)—having a weakened immune system resulting from drugs or other outside forces

immunoglobulin (im-you-no-**GLOB**-you-lin)—plasma-made proteins that can act as antibodies

impaction (im-**PACT**-shun)—a covering or interference with normal growth; may be bone, tissue, or both (*diente impactado*)

implant (im-**PLANT**)—device that is inserted into the alveolar bone to anchor a prosthesis device; also, a drug planted under the skin for sustained slow release

implantation (im-plan-**TAY**-shun)—placing or inserting an implant device (*implantaciación*)

implant scaler/curette—special metal-coated or plastic-coated hand instrument used to scale or clean off implant posts

368

implode (im-**PLODE**)—burst inward as in ultrasonic cavitration (*implosionar*)

impregnated (im-**PREG**-nay-ted)—saturated or filled with a solution or substance (*impregnado*)

impression tray—tray device used to hold material that records the impression

incipient caries (inn-**SIP**-ee-ent)—beginning decay of tooth tissue (*inicio de la dental, incipiente*)

incisal (in-**SIGH**-zal)—cutting edge of anterior teeth (*incisal*)

incisive papilla (in-**SIGH**-siv pap-**PILL**-la)—tissue growth situated in the anterior of the palate behind the maxillary centrals (*papilla incisiva*)

incisive suture (in-**SIGH**-siv)—suture located in the anterior area of pre-maxilla, palatine processes (*incisiva suture*)

incisor (in-**SIGH**-zore)—cutting, anterior tooth (*incisivo*)

incoming call—phone calls received by a facility or station (*llamada entrante*)

incompetent (in-**KOMP**-ah-tint)—not mentally able or one who lacks the skills or abilities (*incompetente*)

incontinence (in-**CON**-tin-ense)—loss of bladder control (*incontinenciae*)

increment (**IN**-kreh-ment)—increase or addition in small amounts (*incremento*)

incus (**INK**-uss)—ossicle of the middle ear; "anvil" (*yunque*)

index (in-**DECKS**)—measurement of conditions or standards (pl., indices) (*indice de*)

indexing (in-**DECKS**-ing)—the process of identifying the position for placement of an item into the file system

indicator (in-dah-**KAY**-tor)—as in sterilization, tape showing that sterilization conditions have been met (*indicador*)

indirect infection—infection caused by improper handling of materials or contamination of items leading to infection (*infección indirecta*)

infarction (in-**FARK**-shun)—decreased blood supply causing necrosis of the heart (*ataque del corazón*)

inferior conchae (**KONG**-kee)—lowest of three scroll-like bones on both sides of the nasal cavity (*concha inferior*)

infiltration (in-fill-**TRAY**-shun)—injection of anesthetic into the gingival and alveolar (*infiltración*)

infra- (**INN**-frah)—prefix meaning beneath, below, inferior to

infraorbital (in-frah-**OR**-bih-tahl)—growth process from the zygomatic bone articulating with the maxilla to form the lower side of the eye orbit

ingestion (in-**JEST**-shun)—taking a substance into the gastrointestinal tract (*ingestión*)

inguinal (**ING**-guee-nal)—pertaining to the abdomen or groin (*inguinal*)

inhalation (in-hah-**LAY**-shun)—breathing vapor or gas into the lungs (*inhalación*)

inhibitor (in-**HIB**-ih-tore)—substance that prevents polymerization (*inhibidor*)

initial set—period of time when the material assumes the shape but remains pliable (*conjunto inicial*)

initiator (ih-**NISH**-ee-ay-tore)—agent capable of starting the polymerization process (*iniciador*)

injection (in-**JECT**-shun)—forced placement into the body or vessel, tissue, or cavity (*inyección*)

inlay (**IN**-lay)—a solid, casted, or milled restoration made in the shape of the prep and cemented into place (*incrustación*)

inlay wax—hard, stick wax that is melted onto a die and carved to become a wax pattern (*cera de incrustación*)

inoculation (inn-ock-you-**LAY**-shun)—injection of a serum or toxin into the body to produce immunity (*inoculación*)

inscription (in-**SCRIP**-shun)—part of the prescription giving drug name, dose form, and amount of drug (*inscripción*)

inside address—part of letter giving the name, title, and address of the receiving person (*dirección interior*)

inspiration (in-spur-**AY**-shun)—breathing in (*inspiración*)

instrumentation (in-strew-men-**TAY**-shun)—use of machines or appliances (*instrumentación*)

insulation (in-sue-**LAY**-shun)—setting apart; preventing the transfer of heat (*aislamiento*)

insulin (**IN**-sue-lin)—hormone released by the pancreas (*la insulina*)

insulin shock—condition resulting from overdose of insulin resulting in lower blood sugar levels (*choque de insulina*)

insurance information form—printed questionnaire regarding insurance and other data (*formulario de informaciónde seguro*)

insured—policyholder; one who pays the premiums and makes the contract (*asegurado*)

insured mail—postal company insures delivery for a set price declared by sender and for a fee (*correo certificadoto*)

intensifying screen (in-tense-sah-**FIE**-ing)—fluorescent-treated cassette screen to reduce patient's radiation exposure (*la pantalla de intensificación*)

interceptive orthodontics—procedures taken to lessen the severity of existing malfunctions

interdental aids—appliances or devices that assist in the cleansing of the teeth (*ayudantes interdental*)

interferon (in-ter-**FEAR**-on)—proteins produced by cells exposed to viruses; aids immunity (*interferón*)

interleukins (in-ter-**LOO**-kins)—chemicals produced by the white blood cells that elicit response (*interlucinas*)

interpulpal injection (inn-ter-**PUHL**-puhl)—anesthetic injection directly into pulpal area (*inyección interpupal*)

intolerance (inn-**TAHL**-er-anse)—inability to endure a drug, or the incapacity for a drug (*intolerancia*)

intra- (**INN**-trah)—prefix meaning within

intradermal (in-trah-**DER**-mal)—implanted under the skin for sustained slow release (*implante vajo la piel*)

intraligamentary injection (in-trah-ligg-ah-**MEN**-tah-ree)—injection of anesthetic into periodontal ligament (*inyección intraligamentaria*)

intramuscular injection (in-tra-**MUSS**-kyou-lahr)—injection given within the muscle parenterally administered (*inyección intramuscular*)

intraosseous injection (in-trah-**OSS**-ee-us)—injection of anesthetic material into the bone (*inyecta en el hueso*)

intraperitoneal (in-trah-pare-ih-toh-**NEE**-ahl)—within the peritoneal cavity

intrapulpal (in-trah-**PUL**-puhl)—anesthetic injection given within the pulp (*dentro de la pulpa*)

intrathecal (in-trah-**THEE**-kal)—within the spinal cavity

intravenous injection (in-tra-**VEE**-nus)—injection within a vessel (*intravenosa inyección*)

intrinsic (in-**TRIN**-sick)—stain from within the tooth (*intrinseca*)

intrusion (in-**TROO**-zhun)—tooth movement into the alveolus during orthodontic treatment (*intrusión*)

inventory or order control card—printed card listing major supply, reorder point, and data (*arjeta de inventario*)

invert (in-**VERT**)—to turn toward or reverse material; turning in the edges of a dental dam (*invertir*)

inverted pour method for study models—filled impression material is turned over a gypsum pile

investment (in-**VEST**-ment)—gypsum used to surround and hold the denture or appliance form until pouring or casting

invoice (in-**VOICE**)—printed form from supplier regarding orders received by that facility (*factura*)

irrigation (ear-ah-**GAY**-shun)—use of liquid material or substances to wash or bathe an area (*riego*)

ischemia (iss-**KEE**-me-ah)—holding back blood (*reteniendo la sangre*)

isoflurane (eye-soh-**FLUR**-ane)—volatile general anesthetic liquid

isolation (eye-so-**LAY**-shun)—the process of separating or detaching from others or other areas (*aislamiento*)

IT—intrathecal drug route within the spinal area (*en la espina, intratecal*)

-itis (**EYE**-tis)—suffix meaning *inflammation of*

IV—intravenous drug route (*intervenoso*)

jugular (**JUG**-you-lur)—large vein that carries blood from the brain back to the heart (*vugular*)

juvenile diabetes—onset of diabetes condition in persons under 15 years of age (*la diabetes juvenil*)

Kaposi's sarcoma—skin disease or growth caused by a virus

keratinized (**KARE**-ah-tin-izd)—hard tissue; also called masticatory mucosa (*los tejidos duras*)

kilovolt power (**KILL**-oh-volt)—1000-volt unit in radiation (kVp)

labia (**LAY**-bee-ah)—lips (Latin), labium is singular (*labios*)

labial (**LAY**-bee-ahl)—pertaining to the lips; anterior surface of the anterior teeth (*labial*)

lacrimal (**LACK**-rih-mal)—two bones at the inner side of the orbital cavity

lacuna (lah-**KYOU**-nah)—a small, open space in the cementum (*laguna*)

lambdoid suture (**LAM**-doyd)—located between the parietal and upper border of the occipital bone (*lambdoidea*)

lamellae (lah-**MEL**-ah)—developmental imperfections of the enamel, extending to the dentin (*laminilla*)

lamina dura (**LAM**-ah-nah **DUR**-ah)—thin plate or layer; the applying of a thin layer to another object

laminagraphy (lam-in-**AUG**-rah-fee)—technique in which tissue images are collected and measured in slices or sections

laminate (**LAM**-ih-nate)—thin plate or layer (*laminado*)

latch-type bur—rotary bur that fits into right-angled or contra-angled handpiece (*torno*)

lateral (**LAT**-er-ahl)—side, position on the side; second tooth from midline (*lateral*)

lateral excessive/deficient—excessive bone in one direction and deficient bone in another

lateral excursion (ecks-**KERR**-zhun)—measurement of side-to-side mandible movement

lead apron/thyrocervical collar—radiation protection device placed upon the patient (*delantal de plomo*)

ledger card—record-keeping sheet for recording services, charges, and payments (*tarjetla de libros*)

Lentulo-spiral drill—thin, endodontic, latch-type, rotary instrument used to spin and spread calcium hydroxide or cement into the canal

lesion (**LEE**-zhun)—injury or wound (*lesión*)

letter—written correspondence between two or more parties (*carta*)

leukocytes (**LOO**-koh-sites)—white blood cells (*glóbulos blancos*)

leukoplakia (loo-koh-**PLAY**-key-ah)—precancerous, white patches on oral tissues (*mancha blanca*)

liability (lie-ah-**BILL**-ah-tee)—responsibility for the course of action

licensure (**LIE**-sen-sure)—certification of a candidate's ability and knowledge in a chosen profession (*licencia*)

ligature (**LIG**-ah-chur)—a material used to tie or hold down (*ligadura*)

ligature cutter—orthodontic instrument used to cut ligature wire (*cortador de ligaduras*)

ligature director—orthodontic instrument used to direct the movement of the ligature (*director de ligature*)

ligature tucker—orthodontic instrument used to tuck or bend in the cut edges of the ligature wire

ligature tying plier—orthodontic plier used to tie off or twist ligature wire into a knot

line angle—junction of two tooth surfaces, such as mesial and incisal surfaces (*linea del ángulo*)

liner (**LINE**-er)—a thin coat of material that provides a barrier against chemical leakage into tooth structure; a ring lining placed inside the casting ring to allow for investment expansion

lingual (**LIN**-gwal)—surface of tooth or area touching the tongue (*de la lengua*)

litigation (lit-ah-**GAY**-shun)—a lawsuit (*litigiación*)

lobe (**LOWB**)—well-defined part of an organ that develops during tooth formation (*lóbulo*)

loop-forming plier—orthodontic instrument used to form loops in wires

lozenge (**LOZ**-enge)—solid mass of drug, flavored for holding in the mouth and dissolving slowly (*losange*)

Luer-loc syringe (**LU**-er-lock syringe)—barrel instrument with piston force plunger used to force or inject fluids

luting (**LOO**-ting)—holding together; binding two items (*vinculante, fijación*)

luxation (luck-**SAY**-shun)—movement; a loose tooth may be moved or loosened before extraction (*luxación*)

lymph (**LIMF**)—body alkaline fluid found in the lymphatic vessels (*linfa, linfáticos*)

lymphangioma (lim-fan-jee-**OH**-mah)—a tumor made up of lymphatic tissue

lymph node (**NO**-od)—mass of lymph cells forming a unit of lymphatic tissue (*los ganglios linfáticos*)

lymphocytes (**LIM**-foh-sites)—lymph cells that assist body defenses by attracting antigens (*linfocitos*)

lymphokine (**LIM**-foe-keen)—active lymph cell (*linfocina*)

lymphoma (lim-**FOH**-mah)—new tissue growth within the lymphatic system (*lymphoma*)

macrodontia (mack-roh-**DON**-she-ah)—abnormally large teeth (*dientes grandes*)

macrogenia (mack-roh-**JEE**-nee-ah)—large or excessive chin (*menton grande*)

macroglossia (mack-roh-**GLOSS**-ee-ah)—large tongue (*lengua grande*)

macrophage (**MACK**-roh-fayge)—large cell that ingests dead cells and tissues

magnum foramen (**MAG**-num **FORE**-ay-men)—large opening in the occipital bone for spinal cord passage (*foramen magnum*)

malady (**MAL**-ah-dee)—disease or disorder of the body (*enfermedad*)

malar (**MAY**-lar)—zygomatic bone; cheekbone (*pómulo*)

malignant (mah-**LIG**-nant)—harmful or growing worse; often used in connection with cancer (*malignas*)

malleability (mal-ee-ah-**BILL**-ih-tee)—ability of material to withstand deformation without fracture while undergoing maximum compression stress

mallet (**MAL**-ett)—surgical hammer (*mazo*)

malleus (**MAL**-ee-us)—largest of the three ossicles of the ear; serves as the ear mallet (*malleo*)

malocclusion (**mal**-oh-**CLUE**-shun)—disorder or improper occlusion (*malocelusión*)

malpractice—failure to provide proper care and treatment; lack of proper skill or ability (*negligencia professional*)

mamelon (**MAM**-eh-lon)—bump or scalloped edge on incisal area of new, anterior teeth

mandible (**MAN**-dih-bull)—strong, horseshoe-shaped bone forming the lower jaw (*mandibula*)

mandibular (man-**DIB**-you-lahr)—pertaining to the mandible or lower jaw

mandibular notch—located on the mandible's lower border; small notch or depression in jaw edge (*muesca mandibular*)

mandrel (**MAN**-drell)—rotary instrument that holds abrasive or treated wheels, disc, and items (*mandril*)

manipulation (mah-nip-you-**LAY**-shun)—the skillful operation or handling and use (*manipulación*)

marginal (mar-**JIN**-al)—pertaining to the margin; portion of gingiva that is unattached to underlying tissues

masseter (mass-**EE**-ter)—principal muscle of mastication that closes the mouth (*masetero*)

mastication (mass-tih-**KAY**-shun)—the act of chewing (*masticación*)

mastoid (**MASS**-toyd)—natural growth on temporal bone behind the ear; used for muscle attachment (*mastoid*)

matrix (**MAY**-tricks)—artificial wall material; may be metal or celluloid (*matriz*)

matrix holder—device used to hold a matrix band into place during use (*sósten de matriz*)

matrix wedge—small V-shaped wedge made of wood or plastic to support the matrix band and shape (*cuña de matriz*)

maxillary (**MACK**-sil-air-ee)—left and right bones that form the upper jaw (*maxilar superior*)

maxillofacial surgeon (mack-sill-oh-**FAY**-shul)—specialist who provides surgical care for the teeth, jaws, and related areas

maximum permissible dose (**MPD**) (radiation (**MPD**))—maximum X-ray exposure permissible for the exposed person (*dosis máximo permitido*)

meatus (mee-**AY**-tus)—opening in the temporal bone for auditory nerves and vessels to pass through (*meato*)

Medicaid—government provision for low-income and qualified persons to receive medical care

medicament (meh-**DICK**-a-ment)—medicine or remedy; agent used for treatment (*medicameto*)

Medicare—government program for the elderly (Part A for hospital care; Part B for physician care)

melanoma (mel-ah-**NO**-mah)—malignant, pigmented mole or tumor (*melanoma*)

memo—informal correspondence usually sent within the practice or in a group setting

meniscus (men-**ISS**-kus)—articular disc located between the mandibular joint bones (*disco articular*)

mental (**MEN**-tal)—chin (*barbilla*)

mentalis (men-**TAL**-iss)—chin muscle that moves the chin tissue and raises the lower lip

meperidine (**MEP**-er-ah-dine)—depresses the central nervous system (e.g., Demerol) (*meperidina*)

mepivacaine (mah-**PIV**-ah-kane)—anesthetic type of drug (e.g., Carbocaine, Polocaine)

mesenchyme (**MEZ**-en-kime)—connective tissue cells forming the mesoderm cells (*mesénquima*)

mesial (**MEE**-zee-ahl)—to the middle; side surface closest to the middle of the face

mesioclusion (me-zee-oh-**KLOO**-zhun)—Class III malocclusion, or a condition of a protruding lower jaw (*sobrésale la mandibula*)

mesoderm (**MESS**-oh-derm)—middle layer; development germ of middle cells (*capa media, mesodermo*)

metabolic shock (met-ah-**BAHL**-ick)—type of shock arising from a disorder of metabolism, as in diabetes (*metabólico shocke*)

metabolism (meh-**TAB**-oh-lizm)—the sum of all physical and chemical changes taking place in the body (*el metabolismo*)

metallic-oxide paste—two-paste impression system of zinc-oxide eugenol (**ZOE**) base (*óxido de zinc*)

metastasize (meh-**TASS**-tah-size)—move; movement of cancer throughout the body (*movimiento de cancer, metástasis*)

methadone (**METH**-ah-done)—depresses the central nervous system (e.g., Dolophine) (*metadona*)

microdontia (my-kroh-**DAHN**-shee-ah)—abnormally or unusually small teeth (*dientes peqgueños*)

microgenia (my-kroh-**JEE**-nee-ah)—small or undersized chin (*menton pequefia*)

micrognathia (my-kroh-**NAY**-thee-ah)—abnormal smallness of jaw; undersized mandible (*mandibula pequefia*)

microphage (**MY**-crow-fayge)—cell that ingests smaller matter, such as bacteria (*iliófagos*)

micropump (**MY**-crow-pump)—drug-releasing implanted device to release a sustained, timed dose (*microbomba*)

midline—imaginary vertical line bisecting the head at the middle of the face; determines right and left side (*linea media*)

milliampere (mill-ee-**AM**-peer)—one-thousandth of an ampere (electric current)

mobility (moh-**BIL**-ih-tee)—capable of movement; a diagnostic test in **RCT** (*la movilidad*)

modified block letter style—all parts of the letter are placed next to the left margin

modifier (**MAH**-dih-fye-er)—substance used to change the condition of a material

molar (**MOH**-lar)—large grinding tooth located in the posterior of the mouth (*molar, muela*)

molding (mol-**DING**)—shaping of an impression material over the edge of the tray for better adaption (*forma*)

molten metal/glass bead sterilization—method employed in endodontics to sterilize small tips

money order—similar to a check; a written order for funds (*orden de dinero, giro postal*)

morphine (more-**FEEN**)—depresses the central nervous system (*morfina*)

morphodifferentiation (more-foh-diff-er-en-she-**AY**-shun)—stage of tooth development that determines the shape and size of the tooth crown

mouth mirror—small hand instrument used to look into the oral cavity (*espejo de boca*)

mouth prop—device to maintain the mouth in an open position during dental procedures (*sósten de la boca*)

mucin (**MYOU**-sin)—slimy or sticky secretion that produces mucus (*muucosidad*)

mucocele (**MYOU**-koh-seal)—mucous cyst (*quiste mucosa*)

mucogingival (myou-koh-**JIN**-jih-vahl)—combination of mucous and gingival tissue (*mucogingival*)

mucogingival border (myou-koh-**JIN**-jih-vahl)—tissue junction evident by change of tissue color from pink gingival to red mucosal (*borde mucogingival*)

mucogingival excision—procedure used to correct defects in shape, position, or amount of a tooth's gingiva (*escisión mucogingival*)

mucoperiosteum (myou-koh-pear-ee-**AHS**-tee-um)—mucous lining covering tissues in the mouth

mucosa (**MU**-co-sah)—tissue lining an orifice (*mucosa*)

murmur (mur-**MUR**)—abnormal sound heard over the heart or the blood vessels (*murmullo*)

mutation effect (myou-**TAY**-shun)—abnormal growth or development resulting from radiation affecting a genetic change (*efecto de la mutación*)

Mylar (**MY**-lar)—heavy cellophane-type material that provides matrix support for anterior areas

mylohyoid ridge (my-loh-**HIGH**-oyd)—horizontal layered edge located on the mandible's lingual surface

myocardial infarction (my-oh-**KAR**-dee-ahl in-**FARK**-shun)—necrosis of the myocardium; heart attack

myocardium (my-oh-**KAR**-dee-um)—middle cardiac muscle layer (*miocardio*)

myotherapeutic (my-oh-ther-ah-**PYOU**-tick)—an exercise or treatment to correct misalignments (*terapia de los musculas*)

naproxen (nah-**PROX**-en)—nonsteroid, anti-inflammatory drug (e.g., Anapro, Naprasyn)

nasal (**NAY**-zal)—left and right bones that form the arch or bridge of the nose (*nasal*)

nasion (**NAY**-zhun)—point where the nasal, frontal suture crosses the skull midplain (*nasión*)

nasociliary (nay-zoh-**SIL**-ee-air-ee)—branch of the ophthalmic division of the trigeminal nerve (*nasociliar*)

nasopalatine (nay-zoh-**PAL**-ah-tine)—combined area of nose and palate; spot for tooth infiltration

neck—part of instrument situated between the working edge and the handle (*el cuella*)

necrotic (neh-**KRAH**-tick)—dead or nonvital tissue or organ (*tejido no vital*)

needle holder—device used to hold surgical needles for suturing

negative angulation (neg-ah-**TIVE** ang-u-**LAY**-shun)—angulation of positioning the **PID** upward; X-ray beam in minus angulation (*angluación negativa*)

negative reproduction (re-pro-**DUC**-shun)—an impression opposite of the condition; a cusp is a dent

negligence (neg-lah-**JENCE**)—lack of providing responsible skill, care, and judgment (e.g., improper sterilization) (*negligenciae*)

nematodes (**NEM**-ah-toads)—small parasitic worms, such as threadworms and roundworms

neoplasm (**NEE**-oh-plazm)—new tissue or growth (*nuevo tejido*)

neurofibroma (new-roh-fie-**BROH**-mah)—tumor of the connective tissue of a nerve

neurofibromatosis (new-roh-fie-broh-mah-**TOH**-sis)—condition of various size tumors of the peripheral nerves

neurogenic shock (new-row-**JEN**-ick)—type of shock arising from nervous impulses

neutroclusion (new-troh-**KLOO**-zhun)—Class I malocclusion, or teeth in normal occlusion with misaligned or tilted teeth

nitroglycerin (nigh-tro-**GLIS**-er-in)—medication for immediate relief of heart problems, angina pectoris (*nitroglicerina*)

noble metals—precious metals used in prostheses (e.g., gold, palladium, and platinum)

noise (**NOI**-se)—low-frequency and high-frequency components that hamper reception and computation of digital signals

nonexpendable supply—items used more than once and not of major cost

nosocomial (noh-soh-**KOH**-mee-ahl)—disease, such as staph, arising in care-giving situations

objective symptom—evidence observed by someone other than victim; also called a sign (*sintoma objetivo*)

obturation (ahb-too-**RAY**-shun)—to close or stop up; a procedural step in **RCT** (*rellernar*)

occipital (ock-**SIP**-ih-tal)—large bone in lower back of head forming the skull base (*occipital*)

occlude (oh-**KLUDE**)—jaw closing (*ocluir*)

occlusal (oh-**KLOO**-zahl)—chewing surface of posterior teeth (*occlusion*, *ochisal*)

occlusal film packet (oh-**KLOO**-zahl film **PACK**-et)—radiographic film used intraorally or extraorally for exposure of larger areas

occlusal guard—custom-formed acrylic night guard to prevent tooth grinding (*guardia oclusal*)

occlusal records—measurements of jaw relationships and articulation of teeth (*registros oclusales*)

occlusal rims—wax blocks placed on contoured baseplate wax in preparation for dentures (*bordes oclusales*)

oculomotor (ock-you-loh-**MOH**-ter)—(**III**) third cranial nerve (*oculomoter*)

odontoblasts (oh-**DAWN**-toh-blasts)—dentin-forming cells

odontoclasts (oh-**DAWN**-toh-clasts)—cells that break down tooth tissue, causing resorption

odontogenesis (oh-don-toh-**JEN**-eh-sis)—pertaining to tooth production

odontology (oh-dahn-**TAHL**-oh-jee)—study of the characteristics, shapes, and sizes of teeth (*odontologia*)

odontoma (oh-don-**TOH**-mah)—tumor of the tooth or dental tissue

-oid (**OYD**)—suffix meaning resembling or shaped like

ointment (**OINT**-ment)—medicine suspended in fatty substance, cream (*poamada*)

olfactory (ol-**FACK**-toh-ree)—(I) first cranial nerve

-ologist (**AH**-loh-jist)—suffix meaning *one who specializes in*

-ology (**AH**-loh-jee)—suffix meaning *the study of*

ondontalgia (oh-dahn-**TAL**-jee-ah)—toothache or tooth pain (*dolor de muelas*, *dientes*)

onlay (**ON**-lay)—milled or cast restoration to fit the preparation of proximal walls and most of occlusal surface

open bite—condition occurring when the anterior teeth do not contact with each other (*mordida abierta*)

operatory (**AH**-purr-ah-tore-ee)—dental room with chair, unit, and items needed for performing dental treatments (*sala de operación*)

operatory light—chairside light used to illuminate patient's oral cavity (*luz operatoria*)

ophthalmic (off-**THAL**-mick)—sensory nerve branch of the trigeminal nerve (*oftálmico*)

opioids (**OH**-pee-oyds)—narcotic drugs

opportunistic (ah-pore-too-**NISS**-tick)—an infection occurring when the body's resistance is low (*oportunistas*)

opposing arch (oh-**POSE**-ing **ARE**-ch)—the arch opposite the working arch; impression may be taken on the arch opposite of the worksite (*arco dental de oposición*)

oral maxillofacial (oral **MAX**-ill-oh-Fay-shall)—relating to the oral and facial areas

oral pathologist (oral path-**ALL**-oh-gist)—dentist who specializes in the nature, diagnosis, and treatment of dental disease (*patólogo oral*)

oral shield (oral shield)—vestibule device between the teeth and lip to train, correct, and maintain function (*protección oral*)

orbicularis oris (ore-bick-you-**LAIR**-iss **ORE**-iss)—circular muscle around the mouth; "kissing muscle"

oris (**ARE**-is)—inferius oris = lower lip; superius oris = upper lip (*labio superior*)

orthodontia (or-thoh-**DON**-shuh)—the specialty of preventing and correcting malocclusions

orthodontist (or-thoh-**DON**-tist)—dentist who straightens teeth and corrects malocclusions (*ortodoncista*)

orthognathic (ore-theg-**NATH**-ick)—manipulation of facial skeleton to restore esthetics

orthognathic surgery (or-thug-**NATH**-ic)—surgery of facial bones for improved function and esthetic purposes

orthopaedic (or-thoo-**PAY**-dic)—prevention or correction of deformities

osseointegration (oss-ee-oh-inn-teh-**GRAY**-shun)—union of bone with the implant device

osseous surgery (**OSS**-ee-us surge-**REE**)—surgery that involves alteration in the bony support of the teeth (*cirugia ósea*)

ossicle (**AHS**-ih-kul)—small bone of the ear (*pequeños hueso del oído*)

osteoblasts (**AHS**-tee-oh-blasts)—bone forming germ cell (*células formadoras de hueso*)

osteoclasts (**AHS**-tee-oh-clasts)—cells that destroy or cause absorption of bone tissue (*células destrocción ósea*)

osteogenic (oss-tee-oh-**JEN**-ick)—formation of bone in connective tissue and/or cartilage

osteomyelitis (oss-tee-oh-my-**LYE**-tiss)—an infection of the bone and bone marrow (*infección enelhueso*)

osteopenia (ahs-tee-oh-**PEE**-nee-ah)—lack of bone; bone thinning (*falta de huesos*)

osteoplasty (**OSS**-tee-oh-plas-tee)—surgery to form or recontour bones (*remolelación de huesos*)

osteotomy (oss-tee-**OT**-oh-me)—bone incision (*incision ósea*)

-otomy (**AH**-toh-mee)—suffix meaning the act of cutting into

out card—bright colored card indicating return place in file after use (*tarjeta de fuera*)

outgoing call—telephone call made or placed from a dental facility or station (*ilamada de fuera*)

outline form—stage of tooth preparation for the size, shape, and restoration placement (*forma de contorno*)

overdenture—prosthetic denture that is prepared to fit and be secured upon posts

overdose—undesirable effect from excessive drug dosage (*sobredosis*)

overjet—condition in which the anterior teeth overbite or improperly extend over the low incisor

overlapping—X-ray positioning error resulting in overlap of shadows on adjacent teeth (*solapamiento*)

oxygen flow meter—gauge device to adjust flow of oxygen gas (*medidor de fllujo de oxígeno*)

oxygen mask—device to be placed over the nose and mouth to administer gas to a patient (*mascara de oxígeno*)

palate (**PAL**-utt)—roof of mouth; composed of soft and hard palate (*palate, palador*)

palatine (**PAL**-ah-tine)—relating to the palate area (*palatino*)

palliative (**PAL**-ee-ah-tiv)—relieving or alleviating pain (*paliativos*)

Palmer numbering system—method for identifying teeth by using numbers and letters

palpation (pal-**PAY**-shun)—application of finger pressure to an area of concern (*palpación*)

pandemic (pan-**DEM**-ick)—all people; a disease in epidemic stages and occurring in many places (*pandemia*)

panoramic radiograph (pan-oh-**RAM**-ick)—special radiograph that exhibits the entire dentition area on one film

papilla (pah-**PILL**-ah)—tissue growth or bud (pl., papillae) (*papilla*)

papilloma (pap-ih-**LOH**-mah)—epithelial tumor of the skin or mucous membrane (*papiloma*)

papoose board—wrapping device for restraint of a child patient (*bordo de papoose*)

paralleling technique—method of exposing intraoral films at a parallel angle to the film surface

parenteral (pare-**EN**-ter-ahl)—not entering the body through the gastrointestinal system, such as an injection or needle-stick (*parenteral*)

paresthesia (pare-ah-**THEE**-zee-ah)—abnormal feeling that may occur after anesthesia has worn off (*parestesia*)

parietal (pair-**EYE**-eh-tahl)—bone that makes up the roof and side walls covering the brain (*parietal*)

parotid (pah-**ROT**-id)—largest salivary gland, located near the ear

participating provider—health-care provider who belongs to a specific organization's health-care plan and agrees to accept the benefits for the allowed care procedures

passive acquired immunity—immunity obtained from inoculation or vaccination to a disease (*immunidad pasiva alquirida*)

passive natural immunity—immunity that passes from mother to fetus; congenital (*immunidad pasiva natural*)

patch—medicated adhesive patch applied to skin for release (*parche*)

pathogenic (path-oh-**JEN**-ick)—a disease-producing substance (*patógenos*)

pathology (path-**AHL**-oh-jee)—study of disease (*estudio de enfermedad, patologia*)

patient file envelope—large file envelope used to gather and hold together patient's records (*sobre de archivos de paciente*)

patient health history—written and oral communication regarding the patient's health status (*historia de la salud de paciente*)

patient information chart—questionnaire filled out by the patient giving data for office records (*tabla de información de paciente*)

pediatric (pee-dee-**AT**-rick)—concerning child patients (*pediátrica*)

pedodontist (**PEE**-doh-don-tist)—dentist who cares for the teeth and oral tissues of children; also called a pediatric dentist

peg-board bookkeeping—method for recording the activities of the day on a ledger sheet (*contabilidad de bordo-peg*)

pellicle (**PELL**-ih-kul)—adhering film on the surface of the teeth (*pelicula*)

penicillin—a family of antibiotic drugs (*penicilina*)

pentazocine (pen-**TAZ**-oh-seen)—depresses the central nervous system (e.g., Talwin) (*pentazocaina*)

percussion (per-**KUSH**-un)—tapping on a body tissue; a diagnostic test in **RCT** (*percussión*)

peri- (**PEAR**-ee)—prefix meaning *around, about,* or *near*

periapical (pear-ee-**APE**-ih-kahl)—area around the apex of a tooth (*periapical*)

periapical film—most commonly used radiographic film for intraoral exposure (*pelicula periapical*)

pericardium (pair-ih-**KAR**-dee-um)—the sac encasing the heart (*periocardio*)

pericementitis (pear-ih-seh-men-**TIE**-tiss)—inflammation and necrosis of the tooth alveoli

pericoronitis (pear-ih-**KOR**-oh-**NIGH**-tiss)—inflammation around the crown of a tooth (*inflamación alrededor del diente corum*)

periodontal (pear-ee-oh-**DAHN**-tahl)—area around the tooth (*periodontal*)

periodontal abscess—abscess, collection of pus in the periodontal tissue; may be called pyorrhea (*abseso periodontal*)

periodontal flap surgery—surgical movement or treatment of the periosteum and pocket tissues (*cirugia periodontal*)

periodontal ligaments—fiber bundles located around the tooth; used to support and cushion tooth (*ligamentos periodontalales*)

periodontal pocket—abnormal open space between the tooth and the gingival; caused by gum recession or a loss of epithelial attachment

periodontist (pear-ee-oh-**DAHN**-tist)—dentist who specializes in treatment of the periosteum (*periodontista*)

periodontitis (**pear**-ee-oh-don-**TIE**-tiss)—inflammation of gingival and supporting tissues

periodontium (pear-ee-oh-**DAHNT**-shee-um)—tissue surrounding the tooth (*periodonto*)

periodontology (pear-ee-oh-dahn-**TAH**-loh-jee)—treatment of diseased tissues around the teeth (*periodoncia*)

periodontosis (pear-ee-oh-don-**TOH**-sis)—inflammation of the gingival and periodontal ligaments, accompanied by destruction of the alveolar bone

periosteal (pear-ee-**OSS**-tee-al)—pertaining to the area around the periosteum (*perió*)

periosteotome (pear-ee-**OSS**-tee-oh-tome)—instrument used for cutting around the bone

periosteum (pear-ee-**AHS**-tee-um)—fibrous membrane lining all oral mouth tissue surfaces (*periostio*)

periradicular (pear-ee-rah-**DICK**-you-lar)—around the root area; a cyst around the root apex

personal mail—mail meant for a specific person; private correspondence (*correo personal*)

petit mal (pah-**TEET MAL**)—smaller brain seizure consisting of possible momentary unconsciousness (*ataque de petit mal*)

petty cash—cash fund for minor or incidental necessities for office use (*dinero insignificante*)

phagocytes (**FAG**-oh-sites)—white blood cell that ingests and destroys antigens (*fagocite*)

phantom (**FAN**-tum)—device used for practice in learning radiation exposure techniques (*fantasma*)

pharmacokinetics (far-mah-koh-kih-**NEH**-ticks)—the study of drugs and their actions on the body

pharmacology (far-mah-**KAHL**-oh-jee)—the study of drugs and their effects (*farmacologia*)

pharyngopalatine (fare-in-goh-**PAL**-ah-tine)—a rear fauces between the pharynx and palate area

philtrum (**FILL**-trum)—median groove on the external surface of the upper lip (*filtrum*)

phosphors (phos-**FORE**)—a substance that emits light when excited by radiation

pickling solution—solution used to remove surface film from a cast restoration (*solución decapada*)

pit—pinpoint depression located at the junction of developed grooves or at the groove ends (*pozo*)

plaintiff (**PLANE**-tiff)—injured person or guardian in a lawsuit; one who initiates or files for a lawsuit (*demandante*)

plaque (**PLACK**)—buildup or plate; invisible film on tooth surface (*plaque*)

plastic filling instrument—hand instrument with flat blade; used to carry and smooth out materials when in a plastic (movable) shape

plasticizer (**PLAS**-tih-sigh-zer)—substance that causes softening effect upon polymerization

-plasty (**PLAS**-tee)—suffix meaning *surgical repair*

plexus (**PLECK**-sus)—network, grouping of vessels (*plexo*)

point angle—meeting of three surfaces of a tooth, such as mesial, distal, and occlusal (*ángulo de la punta*)

poly- (**PAHL**-ee)—prefix meaning *many* or *much*

polycarboxylate (pahl-ee-kare-**BOX**-ih-late)—permanent cementation for crowns, inlays, onlays, and bridges (*policarboxilato*)

polyether (pohl-ee-**EE**-thur)—elastic impression material (*poliéter*)

polymerization (pahl-ee-mare-ih-**ZAY**-shun)—changing of compound elements into another shape (*polimerización*)

polysulfide (pohl-ee-**SUL**-fide)—also known as mercaptan, rubber-based impression material (*polisulfuro*)

polytomography (poly-toe-**MAGH**-rah-fee)—several slices or sections of the tooth or body

polyvinyl siloxane (pohl-ee-vine-sil-ox-ain)—rubber-based impression material

pontic (**PON**-tick)—artificial tooth in bridgework that replaces a missing tooth (*póntico*)

porcelain (**POOR**-sih-lin)—hard, ceramic ware used in shells, veneers, facings, artificial teeth (*porcelana*)

porcelain fused to metal crown (**PFM**)—full metal crown with all surfaces covered with a porcelain veneer

porcelain jacket crown (PJC)—a thin metal and ceramic veneered crown for an anterior tooth (*corona de porcelana*)

porte polisher—instrument that holds wood; pointed tip used to hand-polish tooth surfaces (*pulidor de porte*)

positive angulation—angle achieved by positioning the **PID** downward for a plus radiation angle (*angulaciónpositivo*)

positive cast—reproduction of the patient's mouth

post and core crown—crown used for endodontically treated tooth with significant tooth loss (*corona de poste y corazona*)

postcard—small, heavy paper card to carry message on one side and address on the other side (*tarjeta postal*)

post dam—posterior edge of the maxillary denture that provides suction hold (*pospresa*)

posterior (pahs-**TEE**-ree-or)—toward the rear; area of mouth back from the corner of the lips (*posterior*)

posterior nasal spine—located in the upper arch between the nasal bone and the superio maxilla (*la espina de nasal posterior*)

post placement—insertion of a metal retention pin into the root canal or prepared area to provide stability to the restoration

postural shock (POSS-chew-rahl)—type of shock arising from sudden change in body position (*choque postural*)

potency (POH-ten-see)—strength of a drug (*potencia*)

preauthorization (pre-ah-thor-ah-**ZAY**-shun)—insurance approval for services requested in a pre-service claim form (*la authorización previa*)

preferred provider organization (PPO)—insurance—an employer, group, or organization makes a contract with a provider for lower than usual rates on dental services

prefix (PREE-fix)—word part added to the beginning of another word that qualifies the meaning of the word

premium (PREE-me-um)—payment amount required of the policyholder to keep the policy in force (*prima*)

premolar (pree-**MOH**-lar)—a bicuspid tooth; teeth between the canine and molars (*premolar*)

prescription (pre-**SCRIPT**-shun)—written order for a drug (*receta*)

preventive orthodontics—methods used to prevent or avoid future occurrences of malocclusion (*ortodoncia preventiva*)

prilocaine (PRIL-oh-kane)—anesthetic drug (e.g., Citanest) (*prilocaina*)

primary (PRY-mary)—first; first set of teeth, deciduous teeth, or "baby teeth" (*primario*)

primary radiation—the desired radiation beam during an X-ray exposure; radiation from the primary beam (*radiación primario*)

procaine (PRO-kane)—Novocain, an anesthetic drug (*procaina*)

procedural code—code system constructed to provide a specific number to each treatment (*código de procedimiento*)

process (PROS-cess)—a projection or an outgrowth of bone (*protuberancia*)

prognastic (prahg-**NAS**-tick)—position with the mandible forward

prognathia (prog-**NATH**-ee-ah)—protruding lower jaw

prognosis (prahg-**NO**-sis)—prediction of the course of a disease (*pronóstico*)

proliferation (pro-liff-er-**AY**-shun)—second stage of tooth development; causing reproduction of new parts (*profileración*)

prophy (PRO-fee)—short term for prophylaxis; a professional tooth cleaning (*profilaxis*)

prophylactic (proh-fih-**LACK**-tick)—warding off disease; anti-infective (*profilaxis*)

prophylaxis (pro-fih-**LACK**-sis)—professional cleaning and polishing of teeth

propoxucaine (pro-**POX**-ah-kane)—anesthetic drug (e.g., Ravocaine)

propoxyphene (pro-**POX**-ee-feen)—depresses the central nervous system (e.g., Darvocet)

proprietary drug name (pro-**PRY**-eh-tare-ee)—registered U.S. patented name of a drug (*nombre de propiedad de droga*)

prosthesis (prahs-**THEE**-sis)—an artificial appliance to replace a missing body part (pl., prostheses) (*prótesis*)

prosthodontist (prahs-thoh-**DAHN**-tist)—specialist who replaces missing teeth with artificial devices

protective (proh-**TECK**-tive)—shielding or caring for (*de protección*)

protocol (**PROH**-toe-kahl)—steps or method to follow (*protocolo*)

protozoa (proh-toh-**ZOH**-ah)—small animal parasites or organisms that live on another organism (*protozoos*)

protractor (pro-**TRACT**-or)—device used for triangular markings in cephalometric tracings

protrusion (proh-**TRUE**-zhun)—mandible thrust forward with lower jaw out (*salienta/ protuberancia*)

protuberance (proh-**TOO**-ber-anse)—projection, such as a chin (*protuberanci*)

provider (pro-**VIE**-der)—one who renders professional services (*proveedor*)

proximal (**PROX**-ah-mal)—side wall of tooth that meets with or touches side wall of another tooth (*proximidad, proximal*)

pseudocolor (**SUH**-doh-cull-or)—selection of a color shade to enhance a digital image

pseudo microgenia (soo-doh-mack-roh-**JEE**-nee-ah)—excess of soft tissue presenting a look of abnormal size, such as "witch's chin"

psychogenic shock (sigh-koh-**JEN**-ick)—shock arising from mental origins (*choque de psicógena*)

pterygoid (**TARE**-eh-goyd)—wing-shaped process; growth of sphenoid bone extending downward

ptosis (**TOE**-sis)—drooping or sagging of an organ

public health dentist—specializes in dental diseases among the community or general population (*dentista de salud pública*)

pulp—living tissue of the tooth, contains blood, lymph vessels, and nerve nedings (*pulpa*)

pulpalgia (puhl-**PAL**-jee-ah)—pain in the pulp or toothache from inflamed pulp (*dolor en la pulpa*)

pulp canal—small trench area in center of root, containing the pulpal vessels (*conducto de pulpa*)

pulp capping—placement of medication to sedate and treat an inflamed pulp

pulp chamber—open area in center of tooth, place for pulpal tissues; found in the crown area (*la cámara pulpar*)

pulp cyst (**SIST**)—closed fluid-filled sac in pulp tissues (*quiste de pulpa*)

pulpectomy (puhl-**PECK**-toh-mee)—surgical removal of the pulp tissue from the tooth; also known as root canal treatment (*pulpectomia*)

pulpitis (pul-**PIE**-tiss)—pulp inflammation; also called toothache

pulpotomy (puhl-**POT**-oh-mee)—partial excision of pulp tissue (*pulpotomia*)

pulp stone—small tooth growth in pulpal tissue; also called denticle

pulp tester—electric stimulation device used to detect pulp conditions

pulse—beating force of blood circulating through the arteries (*pulsación, pulso*)

purchase order (purr-**CHIS** or-**DER**)—printed request order for material and equipment (*orden de compra*)

purging (**PURR**-jing)—systematic process of review and removal of outdated file (*purga*)

putrefaction (pyou-trih-**FACK**-shun)—decaying animal matter (*putrefacción*)

pyorrhea (pie-oh-**REE**-ah)—pus discharge from periodontal pocket (*secreción de pus*)

quadrant (**KWAH**-drant)—one-fourth of the mouth; half of the maxillary or mandibular arch (*cuadrante*)

quaternary (KWAH-ter-nare-ee)—alloy composed of four metals (*cuatenario*)

quinary (KWIN-ar-ee)—alloy composed of five metals

R = (**Roentgen**)—the basic unit of exposure; the international unit is the coulomb per kilogram (C/kg) (*radiográfica*)

rad (**radiation absorbed dose**)—international unit is gray (Gy); calculated as equal to 100 ergs (energy units) per gram of tissue

radiant (RAY-dee-ant)—energy that is given off from a central source (*energía radiante*)

radicular (rah-DICK-you-lar)—area near the tooth root; site of root tip cysts

radiographic unit—X-ray device; may be single unit or have multiple heads with a single control board (*unidad radiográfica*)

radiology (ray-dee-AWL-oh-gee)—the study of the human body by use of X-ray technology

radiolucent (RAY-dee-oh-loo-sent)—radiograph that appears dark or the ability of a substance to permit passage of X-rays for film exposure

radiopaque (RAY-dee-oh-payk)—portion of the radiograph that appears light; the ability of a substance to resist radiation penetration resulting in light area on the film

rale (RAHL)—respiration sounds heard on the inhalation and expelling of air as noisy, bubbling sounds (*estertores*)

rampant caries (ram-PANT CARE-eeze)—widespread or growing tooth decay (*caries rampante*)

ramus (RAY-mus)—ascending part of mandible (*rama mandibular*)

ranula (RAN-you-lah)—cystic tumor found under the tongue or in sublingual ducts (*ránula*)

raphe (RAH-fay)—ridge or union between two bones or tissue halves (*rafe*)

reamer (REE-mer)—endodontic instrument used to scrape and enlarge the root canal (*escariador*)

reasonable fee—fee determined by the insurances from a survey of the providers of an area (*precio razonable*)

recall list—system of monitoring patients return; scheduling of patients for a future date (*lista de recuerdo*)

reconciliation (wreck-con-SIL-lee-aye-shun)—balancing of the checking account; agreement on balances of bank and account (*la reconciliación*)

rectal sedation—sedation administered by the placement of drugs in the rectum (*sedación rectal*)

recurrent caries (re-CUR-ent CARE-eeze)—decay occurring under or near previously repaired margins of a restoration (*caries recurrentes*)

reduction (ree-DUCT-shun)—lessening or reducing in size; restoration to normal position, as in a fracture (*reducción*)

reference initials (REF-er-ence AH-nich-els)—initials of person sending the letter and preparing the letter (*iniciales de referencia*)

refinement (re-FINE-ment)—to finish again; to make better (*refinamiento*)

refractory (ree-FRACK-tore-ee)—resistant to treatment; gingival tissue that will not heal (*refractario*)

release of information—form signed by a patient or guardian to permit confidential data release (*liberación*)

releasing—the process of identifying an item's readiness to be placed into the file system

rem (**roentgen equivalent measure**)—international unit is sievert (Sv), which is the unit of ionizing radiation needed to produce the same biological effect as one roentgen (R) of radiation

remission (ree-MISH-un)—a lessening or abating of a disease or condition (*remisión*)

remnant radiation (REM-nant RAY-dee-aye-shun)—radiation rays reaching the film target after passing through the subject (*la radiación remanente*)

reorder point—period of time when it is necessary to reorder a supply in order to have it on hand (***punto de reordenar***)

replantation (ree-plan-**TAY**-shun)—to replant or to replace a tooth that has been avulsed (***replantación***)

replenisher solution (ree-**PLEN**-ish-er)—super-concentrated chemical solution added to a tank to restore fluid level (***solución de reponer***)

resistance (ree-**SIS**-tence)—ability of a microorganism to be unaffected by a drug (***resistencia***)

resistance form (ree-sis-**TANCE** form)—preparation cuts to ensure that the restored natural tooth can withstand trauma

resorption (ree-**SORP**-shun)—removal of hard tooth surface and degeneration of the root tissues (***reabsorción***)

respiration (res-per-**AYE**-shun)—the inhaling or the taking in of oxygen and the exhaling of carbon dioxide (***la respiración***)

respiratory (res-per-uh-**TORE**-ee)—type of shock arising from insufficient breathing (***shock respiratorio***)

respondeat superior (Latin for "the master answers")—the employer is responsible for the actions of the employee

rest—small extension of removable prosthesis made to fit or seated atop the adjoining teeth (***soporte***)

restoration (res-**TOR**-aye-shun)—a repair that replaces an area; a tooth filling (***restauración***)

resuscitation (ree-**SUSS**-ih-tay-shun)—restoration of breathing (***resucitación***)

retainer (ree-**TAIN**-ur)—part of an appliance joining the abutting, natural tooth to the support (***retenedor***)

retention form—stage of tooth preparation for the undercut of walls to provide a mechanical hold (***retenció de forma***)

reticulation (reh-**tick**-you-**LAY**-shun)—cracked effect on X-ray film caused by extreme temperature changes (***reticulación***)

retraction cord (ree-**TRACT**-shun cord)—chemically treaded string or cord placed into the gingival sulcus to prepare the gingival for an impression

retractor (ree-**TRACK**-tore = *draw back*)—device used to hold back the cheek or muscle tissue from surgical area

retrieving (ree-**TREE**-ving)—the process of obtaining a file and return for that file (***recuperación***)

retro- (**REH**-troh)—prefix meaning behind or back

retrognathia (ret-tro-**NATH**-ee-ah)—receding lower jaw

retrograde (**REH**-troh-grade = *backward step*)—backward step in **RCT**; the restoration of a tooth from the root apex to the crown, instead of from the crown to the root

retromolar area (ret-trow-**MOLE**-ar)—located at the rear of the mouth distal to the molars (***área retromolar***)

retrusion (ree-**TRUE**-shun)—jaw position with the mandible drawn backward (***retrusión***)

rheostat (**REE**-oh-stat)—foot pedal or lever used to regulate the speed of the handpiece (***reóstato***)

rhinoplasty (**RINE**-oh-plas-tee)—plastic surgery of the nose

rhytidectomy (**rit**-oh-**DECK**-toe-mee)—excision of wrinkles by way of plastic surgery

rickettsia (rih-**KET**-see-ah)—microbes smaller than bacteria but larger than viruses

ridge—linear elevation that receives its name from its area or location (***cresta***)

right-angled bur (**RA**)—rotary bur that fits into right-angled handpiece (***pieza de mano de ángulo recto***)

right-angled handpiece—power-driven drill with head angled at 90 degrees

rinse—a washing out of the mouth; cleansing of the tooth surfaces by either water or rinses (***enjuague***)

rinsing (**in radiation**)—the water bath immersion between chemical exposures and the final water bath

rod (**enamel rod**)—prism-like rod that extends from the dentin-enamel junction to the outer tooth surface (*varilla (de esmalte)*)

rongeurs (**RON**-jeers = *bone cutting*)—a cutting instrument used to clip bony edges (*gubias, pinzas*)

root—bottom part of a tooth; may be single-, double-, or triple-rooted (*raiz*)

root amputation (**am**-pew-**TAY**-shun = *surgical removal of body part, root*)—surgical removal of a root (*la amputación de raiz*)

root canal condenser/plugger—long-necked instrument used to condense the gutta percha material placed in the canal (*condensador de canal de raiz*)

root canal spreader—instrument used to spread cement that has been placed in the root canal (*esparcidor de canal de raiz*)

root hemisection (**HEM**-ih-seck-shun = *cutting tissue or organ in half*)—cutting off of a tissue or a root part (*hemisection de raiz*)

root planing—removal of all detectable deposits and endotoxins on the root surfaces (*cepillado de raiz*)

rotary instrument—instrument that is placed into the handpiece for operation; includes bur, mandrels, diamonds, points, and stones

rotation (roh-**TAY**-shun = *turn around on an axis*)—movement of tooth; turn on the tooth axis; orthodontic movement (*la rotación*)

rugae (**RUE**-guy)—irregular folds on the surface of the palate (*rugas*)

saddle—that part of the removable prosthesis that strides or straddles the gingival crest (*silla de prótesis*)

safelight—device used to illuminate in a processing dark room (*luz de seguridad*)

sagittal plane (**SAJ**-ih-tol)—in radiation, an imaginary vertical line bisecting the face (*plano sagital*)

sagittal suture (**SAJ**-ih-tuhl)—union line between sutures on the top of the head (*suture sagital*)

salicylates (suh-**LIS**-uh-late)—analgesic, antipyretic, anti-inflammatory drug (e.g., aspirin, Empirin) (*salicilato, aspirina*)

saliva ejector tip—small tube-like device used to suction mouth fluids

salutation line (sal-you-**TAY**-shun line)—greeting part of letter, such as Dear Mrs. Horne (*linea de salutación*)

sanitation (san-ih-**TAY**-shun)—application of methods to promote favorable germ-free state (*saneamiento, sanidad*)

saprophytes (**SAP**-roh-fights)—organisms living on dead or decaying organic matter (*saprofito*)

sarcoma (sar-**KOH**-mah = *tumor of flesh/tissues*)—tumor of the flesh or tissues (*sarcoma*)

scaler (**SCALE**-er)—hand instrument with a sharp blade used to scrape or fleck off calculus

scalpel (**SKAL**-pell)—cutting instrument; may be one piece or have a handle and detachable blade (*bisturi, escalpelo*)

scattered radiation—radiation that is deflected from its path (*radiación diseminada*)

schedule of benefits—same as fee schedule; allowed benefits for a specific service or material (*programa de beneficios*)

scorbutic (skor-**BYOU**-tick = *lacking vitamin C*)—lacking vitamin C (*escorbútico*)

sealant (**SEE**-ah-lant)—clear or tinted acrylic substance painted on tooth surfaces to act as a decay preventive (*sellador*)

seating—process of placing and fitting an appliance into the oral cavity (*asiento*)

secondary effect—indirect effect or happening resulting from a drug action (*efecto secundario*)

secondary radiation—radiation given off from matter other than the area that is primarily exposed (*radiación secundaria*)

second-class mail—periodicals, magazines, and newspapers (*correo de segunda clase*)

sedation (see-**DAY**-shun)—process of allaying nervous anxiety (*sedación*)

selected removal—removal or smoothing of occlusal irregularities as a decay preventive measure (*eliminación seleccionada*)

semilunar valves—two heart valves: aortic and the pulmonary (*las válvulas semilunares*)

sensitivity (sen-ah-**TIV**-ah-tee)—ability of X-rays to penetrate and possibly ionize the body (*sensibilidad*)

separating medium—material placed on the die before wax is melted upon it, to ease separation

separator (**SEP**-ah-ray-tor = *device to set aside*)—device used to prepare tooth interproximal space to receive orthodontic bands (*separador*)

septic shock (**SEP**-tick)—shock caused by excessive microbial infection (*shock séptico*)

septoplasty (**SEPT**-toe-plas-tee)—plastic surgery of the nasal septum

sequestra (see-**KWESS**-trah)—small bone spicules working to the surface after surgery (singular is *sequestrum*)

serum (**SEAR**-um = *watery fluid*)—watery fluid produced by the body (*suero*)

setting time—period when material becomes as hard as it will be (*el tiempo de adjuste*)

shank—part of rotary bur that fits into the handpiece; may be plain or have a latch-notched end (*ceña*)

Sharpey's fibers—part of the periodontal ligaments that attach and hold the tooth (*fibras de Sharpey*)

sharps disposal unit—container designed to hold discarded, used needles and sharp items (*unidad/caja de disponer agudos*)

shelf life—period of time for the proper use or storage of a material before it expires (*la vida útil*)

shoulder (**SHOAL**-dur = *cut gingival margin edge*)—preparation of gingival margin edge to provide an appliance junction

sialoadenitis (**sigh**-ah-loh-**add**-eh-**NIGH**-tis; sial = *saliva*, aden = *gland*, itis = *inflammation*)—an inflamed condition of a salivary gland

side effect—reaction from a drug that is not the desired treatment outcome (*efect secundario*)

sigmoid notch—S-shaped curvature between the condyle and coronoid process

signature line—printed name of signature of person who is sending the letter (*linea de firma*)

silicone impression material (**SILL**-aih-kone)—putty base with a liquid accelerator or as a two-paste system (*materia silicona de impressión*)

silver point—endodontic restorative point that is cemented into the prepared canal (*punta de plata*)

simple cavity—a one-surface cavity or dental decayed area (*cavidad simple*)

sinus (**SIGH**-nus)—air pocket/cavity in a bone that lightens the bone and warms the air (*seno*)

slurry (**SLUR**-ee = *thin, watery mixture*)—thin, watery mixture; plaster slurry placed in the mix speeds up the set (*mezela*)

smile line—amount of tooth space viewed while the patient is smiling (*linea de sonrisa*)

solder (**SOD**-er)—process of uniting two metal objects by melting into a common alloy (*soldadura*)

solubility (**sahl**-you-**BILL**-ih-tee = *capability of being dissolved*)—ability to be dissolved (*solubilidad*)

solution—liquid containing a dissolved drug (*solución*)

somatic (soh-**MAT**-ick)—pertaining to the body (*somático*)

sorting—the process of arranging the files in preparation for the indexing or classifying act (*clasificación*)

space maintainer (space **MAIN**-tain-er)—device used to retain space acquired with a premature loss of tooth (*mantenedor de espacio*)

spacer—substance, usually wax, placed on a cast surface to allow impression material space

special delivery mail—post office delivers mail quickly when received at the local station (*separador*)

special handling of mail—delivers third-class and fourth-class mail by the fastest method but not by special delivery

spectrum (speck-**TRUM**)—range of a drug's activity in the body

sphenoid (**SFEE**-noyd)—skull bones; the occipital and ethmoid bones (*esférico*)

sphenopalatine (**sfee**-no-**PAL**-ah-tine)—sensory nerve branch ending for maxillary anterior mucosal and palatine tissues

spherical (**SFEAR**-ih-kul = *in the form of a sphere*)—in the form of a sphere (*esférico*)

sphygmomanometer (**sfig**-moh-man-**AHM**-eh-ter)—instrument used to determine blood pressure (*esfingomanómetro*)

spindle (**SPIN**-dul)—end area of union for odontoblasts and enamel rod endings

spirit—volatile drug substance solution in alcohol (*licor*)

spoon excavator (spoon ex-kah-**VAY**-tor)—instrument with spoon-like tip; used to scrape out decay and necrotic matter (*cuchara excavadora*)

spore—bacteria that encapsulates in protective covering when conditions are adverse (*espora*)

spot welding—electrical welding process of melting two metals together at a joint (*soldadura de sitio*)

spray-wipe-spray method—process of using a disinfectant substance to disinfect large areas (*método de regar y secar*)

sprue base (**SPROO**)—used to hold a wax pattern on a sprue pin during the investment process (*base de esprue*)

sprue pin (**SPROO**)—small plastic pin in the wax pattern to hold the wax during the investment process (*alfiler de esprue*)

squamous suture (**SKWAY**-mus)—also known as the temperoparieter suture (*sutura escamosa*)

stabilization (stay-bill-ih-**ZAY**-shun)—condition of being fixed, steady, or firm; to secure (*establización*)

stapes (**STAY**-peez)—ossicle in the middle ear; commonly called the stirrup (*estribo*)

statement—form requesting payment, which is sent to an individual or a responsible party (*declaración*)

statute of limitations—period of time during which a lawsuit or legal action may take place

sterilization (stare-ill-ih-**ZAY**-shun)—process of destroying all forms of microorganismsesterización (*esterilización*)

sternum (**STIR**-num)—the breastbone in the middle of the ribs (*esternón*)

stertorous respiration sounds (**STARE**-toe-rus)—rattling, bubbling sounds obscuring normal breaths; snoring (*esterotoso*)

stethoscope (**STETH**-oh-scope)—device employed to intensify body sounds (*estetoscopio*)

Stev plate—maxillary orthodontic bite plane covering the incisal edges of the anteriors (*plato de Stev*)

sticky wax—hard, brittle wax stick that is melted to hold dental units together (*cera pegajosa*)

Stim-U-Dent—flat, small wooden picks used to stimulate gingival tissue

stippling (**STIP**-ling = *spotting*)—natural spotting or pigmentation on the gingival (*punteado*)

stoma (**STOW**-mah = *mouth*)—mouth; small opening (*abertura, pequerña*)

stones, wheels, and discs—small abrasive items used to smooth, polish, and shine (*piedas*)

stool—seat for dentist or assistant; may be stationary, movable, or attached to dental chair (*silla, taburete*)

stop—indent or hole cut into the wax spacer to prevent the tray from being seated too deeply (*tope, bloqueador*)

strabismus (strah-**BIZ**-muss)—a condition in which the eyes are unable to fix on the same point (*estrabismo*)

stray radiation—radiation other than the useful beam; also called leakage radiation (*radiación dispersa*)

stress and tension gauge—orthodontic instrument used to test tension and internal forces (*caliber de cepa y tensión*)

stress breaker—connector applied in a stress-bearing location to provide a safe breakage area (*interruptor de la tension*)

stripes of Retzius (**RET**-zih-us)—brownish lines in enamel tissue (*tiras de Retzius*)

study model—gypsum reproduction of a patient's teeth and oral tissues (*modelo de estudio*)

styloid (**STY**-loyd)—growth from the temporal bone for attachment of some tongue muscles (*estiloides*)

subcutaneous (sub-kyou-**TAY**-nee-us = *under the skin*)—under the skin (*subcutánes*)

sublingual (sub-**LING**-gual)—under the tongue (*debajo de la lengua*)

subluxation (**sub**-lucks-**AY**-shun; sub = *under*, luxation = *displacement*)—partially loosened (*subluxación, parcialmente suelta*)

submandibular (sub-man-**DIB**-you-lar)—under the mandible (*en la mandibibula, submandibular*)

submucosal (sub-mew-**COH**-sul = *under the mucous membrane*)—under the mucous membrane (*submucosa*)

subperiosteal implant (sub-pear-ee-**AHS**-tee-uhl)—device placed under the peritoneum to provide a hold for attaching the prosthesis (*suscripción*)

subpoena (sah-**PEE**-nah)—a legal summons requiring a person to report to a trial or to provide testimony (*citación*)

subscriber—insured person, the policyholder (*suscripción*)

subscription—part of prescription containing the directions to the pharmacist

succedaneous (suck-seh-**DAY**-nee-us)—permanent teeth that replace deciduous teeth (*sucedáneo*)

suffix (**SUF**-icks)—word part added to the end of another word that qualifies the meaning of the word

sulcus (**SULL**-kus = *groove, depression*)—long depression between ridges and cusps; a valley on the tooth surface (*surco*)

superbill—preprinted form listing procedure numbers and services rendered to a patient; may be sent to insurance company in lieu of a claim form in some cases

supernumerary (sue-per-**NEW**-mer-air-ee)—extra; more than normal number of teeth (*supernumerario*)

superscription—part of the prescription that contains name, address, age, and the Rx symbol (*sobrescrito*)

suppository (sah-pause-ah-**TORY**)—medicated disc or cone-shaped form to be inserted into the rectum or vagina (*supositorio*)

suppurative (**SUP**-you-rah-tiv)—generating pus

supra- (**SOO**-prah)—prefix meaning *above*, *beyond*, or *over*

supraorbital (soo-prah-**OR**-bih-tal)—frontal bone opening above the orbit of the eye

supraperiosteal (soo-prah-pear-ee-**OSS**-tee-ahl)—about or above the periostium injection site

surgical bur—a rotary bur with a larger head to smooth off or score a tooth for bisectioning (*torno quirúrgico*)

suspension (sus-**PEN**-shun)—liquid drug obtained by mixing with but not dissolving in (*suspención*)

suture (**SOO**-chur = *closure*)—line where two or more bones unite; a surgical stitch (*suturae*)

symmetric (sim-**MEH**-trick; sym = *together*, metric = *measurement*)—balanced, evenly placed

symphysis (**SIM**-fih-sis)—center of the mandible or chin protuberance (*centro de la barbilla*)

symptom (**SIM**-tum)—perceptible change in body or body function (*sintoma*)

syncope (**SIN**-koh-pee = *fainting*)—fainting (*sincope*)

syndrome (**SIN**-drome = *running together*)—grouping of multiple signs/symptoms characterizing a disease (*el sindrome*)

synergism (**SIN**-er-jizm)—harmonious action of two drugs to produce the desired effect (*sinergia*)

synovial fluid (sin-**OH**-vee-al)—lubricating fluid in a joint (*liquido synovial*)

syrup (sear-**UP**)—drug mixed in a sugary solution (*jarabe*)

systolic pressure (sis-**TAHL**-ick)—pressure of the circulating blood while under pulsation (*presión sistólica*)

table of allowance—insurance company policy establishing a specific amount for a specific service (*tabla de autorización*)

tachycardia (**tack**-ee-**KAR**-dee-ah)—pulse rates over 100 beats per minute (*taquicardia*)

target film distance—in radiation, the distance between the film and the source of radiation (*distanceia del objecto y el obejetivo*)

target object distance—distance between the anode target and the object to be radiographed

teleradiography (tell-ih-**RAY**-dee-**aug**-rah-fee)—the ability to transfer the captured information to other sites and sources by computer

temperature (**TEM**-per-ah-ture)—balance of heat loss and production in the body (*temperaturae*)

template (**TEM**-plate = *guide or pattern*)—a pattern or design to follow (*plantilla*, *modelo*)

temporal (**TEM**-pore-al)—fan-shaped bone on each side of the skull

temporary coverage—protection for prepared tooth while awaiting permanent coverage; also called provisional coverage (*cobertura tempeoral*)

temporary crown—acrylic or composite crown prepared in the impression and provisionally cemented onto the prep for protection until the permanent crown is ready

temporomandibular (**tem**-poh-roh-man-**DIB**-you-lar)—pertaining to the mandible and temporal joint area

temporoparietal (**tem**-poe-roe-pah-**RYE**-eh-tal)—suture between the temporal and parietal bones (*sutura temporoparietal*)

tensile strength (**TEN**-sill)—capability of a material to be stretched (*resistencia a la tracción*)

teratogenic (**tare**-ah-toh-**JEN**-ick; terato = *monster*, genesis = *production*)—a drug that affects the fetus (e.g., thalidomide) (*teratogénicos*)

ternary (**TURN**-ah-ree)—alloy composed of three metals (*mezlca de metales*, *ternario*)

tertiary (**TERR**-shee-air-ee = *later stage*)—lower stage, such as a growth of reparative dentin (*terciario*)

testimony (tess-ta-**MOAN**-ee)—statement, given under oath, regarding details of an event or occurrence (*testimonia*)

tetracycline (teh-trah-**SIGH**-klean)—antibiotic-type drug (e.g., Achromycin V, Sumycin) (*tetraciclina*)

therapeutic (ther-ah-**PYOU**-tick)—healing agent (*therapeytico*)

thermal (**THER**-mahl = *pertaining to temperature*)—a heat measurement, condition, or diagnostic test in RCT (*conductividad térmica*)

thermoplastic (therm-oh-**PLAS**-tick)—material that softens and changes shapes when heated (*termoplástico*)

third-class mail—catalogs, circulars, books, and printed matter weighing less than 1 pound (*de tercera clase*)

third party—an organization making payment but is not part of the provider-patient contract (*tercero*)

three-prong plier—orthodontic plier used to close or adjust clasps (*alicates de tres puntas*)

thrombocyte (**THROM**-boh-site)—an old term for blood platelets (*plaquetas en sangre*)

thrombosis (throm-**BOE**-siss)—a blood clot (*trombosis*)

thrush—fungus infection of mouth and/or throat (*tordo*)

Tic Douloureux (tic-**DOO**-loo-roo)—degeneration or pressure on the trigeminal nerve causing pain

tincture (**TINK**-shur)—diluted alcoholic solution of a drug (***tincturae***)

tinnitus (tin-**EYE**-tuss)—ringing in the ears

title line—title of person sending a letter; title is placed below the printed signature line (***linea de titulo***)

TMJ—temporomandibular joint; union of the mandible and the temporal bones (***conjunto temporomandibular***)

tomogram (**TOE**-moe-gram = *image produce*)—the finished image in a tomography procedure

tomography (**toe**-MAGH-rah-fee)—the act of gathering and data measurement of a slice or section under view

tonsil (**TAHN**-sill)—lymphatic tissue mass found in the fauces (***amigdala***)

tooth stabilization—wiring or splinting of teeth to prevent movement (***establización de los dientes***)

topical (**TAH**-pih-kahl)—in a specific place

torque (**TORK**)—orthodontic movement of the tooth root without movement of the crown (***torque, torsión***)

torus (**TORE**-us = *rounded elevation*)—rounded, bony elevation (***toro***)

torus mandibularis (**TORE**-us man-dib-you-**LAIR**-us)—mandibular bony elevation growth under tissue in the lower jaw

torus palatinus (**TORE**-us pal-ah-**TEEN**-us; plural is *tori*)—bony elevation growth under tissue in the palate

tracheotomy (**tray**-kee-**AH**-toh-mee = *cutting into the trachea*)—cutting into the trachea to allow air to enter (***traquetomia***)

traction devices—orthodontic devices to be hooked onto the facebow and worn on the head (***depositivo de tracción***)

transferring—the process of movement of a file folder from one file system to another (***trasladar***)

transient ischemic attack (**TIA**)—local and temporary anemia due to circulation obstruction (***ataque isquémico transitorio***)

transillumination (trans-ah-**lum**-mah-**NAY**-shun = *passage of light through object/tissue*)—passage of light through an object; a diagnostic test in **RCT** (***transiluminación***)

translucency (trans-**LOU**-sen-cee)—ability to see through

transosteal (trans-**AHS**-tee-al)—through the bone implant (***a través del hueso, transóseo***)

transplantation (**trans**-plan-**TAY**-shun; trans = *across*, planta = *plant*)—the transfer of an object from one area to another (***transplante***)

traumatized (**TRAW**-mah-tized = *wounded*)—wounded or injured from an outside force (***traumatiza***)

traveler's check—bank or agency check sold to a patron; acceptable in many places (***cheques de viajero***)

Trendelenburg position—patient in supine position with feet placed higher than the head

trifurcation (try-fur-**KAY**-shun)—branching or separating into three roots (maxillary molar) (***trifurcación***)

trigeminal (try-**JEM**-in-al)—fifth cranial nerve

trismus (**TRIZ**-mus)—grating or tonic contracting of the jaws (***trismus, rejilla***)

trituration (**try**-ture-**AY**-shun = *pulverize*)—the mixing of mercury with an alloy to form an amalgam mix (***trituración***)

troche—soft, flavored medicinal mass of a drug, for holding in the mouth and dissolving (***trocisco, pastilla***)

trochlear (**TRAH**-klee-ur)—(**IV**) fourth cranial nerve

-trophy (**TROH**-fee)—suffix meaning *development* or *growth*

truncated (**TRUN**-kay-ted = *cut part off, lop off*)—cut part off, lop off, such as shortened burs (***truncado***)

tubercle (**TOO**-ber-kull)—small, knob-like prominence on a tooth's surface (***cortar la parte de tuberculo***)

tubule (**TOO**-bule)—small S-shaped tubes or channels extending from the enameo-dentin wall to the pulp chamber; also known as Tome's dentinal tubules

tuft—abnormal clump of rods; irregular grouping of undercalcified enamel (*copo, mata*)

tympanic (tim-**PAN**-ick = *pertaining to eardrum*)—pertaining to the eardrum (*tympani, timpano*)

ultrasonic cleaner—machine to clean instruments and items by cavitation (exploding of bubbles) (*limpiador ultrasónico*)

undercut—removal of tooth structure near the gingival edge to provide a seat or placement area (*para cortar en, inferiores*)

unilateral (you-nih-**LAT**-er-al)—one sided

unit (**YOU**-knit)—in prosthetics, a part or section of an appliance; unit is a section of appointment time (*unidad*)

universal charting method—procedure for numbering of teeth 1–32 (*método universal de gráficos*)

universal precaution—treating each case as if disease is present (*precauciones universales*)

urticaria (yur-tih-**CARE**-ee-ah = *vascular skin reaction*)—vascular skin reaction; hives

usual, customary, and reasonable fee (**UCR**)—benefits are percentages of the surveyed **UCR** fees (*precio, razonable, usual y acostumbrado*)

usual fee—average fee charged by provider for a specific service or material

utero (**YOU**-ter-oh)—during pregnancy (*intrauterine, útero*)

utility wax—soft, adhesive wax, supplied in stick or sheet form, used in mounting and adapt trays (*la cera de utilidad*)

uvula (**YOU**-view-lah)—small, fleshy growth in the back of throat, which descends from posterior of palate

vaccination (vack-sih-**NAY**-shun)—inoculation of serum or toxin to produce immunity (*vacunación*)

vaccine (**VAK**-seen)—solution of killed, weakened, or dead microbes (*vacuna*)

vacuum tube—X-radiation tube producer (*tubo de vacio*)

vagus (**VAY**-gus)—(X) tenth cranial nerve

vascular (**VAS**-kyou-lar = *small vessels*)—pertaining to the small blood vessels (*vascular*)

vasoconstrictor (vas-oh-kahn-**STRICK**-tore; vaso = *vessel*, constrictor = *tightener*)—chemical added to anesthetic to tighten blood vessels

vector (**VEK**-tors = *carriers that transmit disease*)—carrier that transmits disease (*vector*)

vector borne—diseased person with a natural immunity; one in an incubation period lacking signs

veneer (veh-**NEAR** = *tooth-shaped layer*)—thin, resin, tooth-shaped layer applied to tooth surface (*chapa*)

ventricle (**VEN**-trih-kul = *little belly*)—two lower chambers of the heart; one on each side (*ventriculo*)

vermilion border (ver-**MILL**-yon **BORE**-der)—area where the pink lip tissue meets facial skin (*vermellón*)

verruca vulgaris (ver-**OO**-kah, vul-**GAIR**-iss = *oral warts*)—oral wart (*verruga vulgar*)

vertical angulation—direction of the central X-ray beam moving in an up or down position (*angulación vertical*)

vertical overbite—amount of overlap of upper and lower central incisors while in occlusion (*sobremordida vertical*)

vertical window—placement position in a radiograph mount used for anterior films (*ventana vertical*)

vertigo (**VER**-tee-go)—dizziness (*mareos*)

vesicle (**VES**-ih-kuhl = *small blister*)—small blister (*vesicula*)

vestibule (**VES**-tih-byul)—open gum area between the teeth and the cheek (*vestibulo*)

vestibulocochlear (ves-**tib**-you-low-**COCK**-lee-ar)—(**VIII**) eighth cranial nerve

vestibuloplasty (ves-**TIB**-you-loh-**plas**-tee)—surgical alteration of gingival mucous membrane in the mouth vestibule

virulence (**VEER**-you-lense = *power*)—power of an organism to produce disease (*virulenia*)

virus (**VYE**-russ)—class of parasitic; tiny organisms that cause a variety of diseases (*virus*)

viscosity (viss-**KAHS**-ih-tee = *sticky or gummy*)—sticky or gummy ability or condition (*viscosidad*)

volumetric (vol-you-**MET**-rick)—addition of volume to an image to produce a more 3D quality image

vomer (**VOH**-mer)—bone forming lower and posterior part of the nasal septum (*vómer*)

voucher check—check with attached stub showing hours worked, deductions taken, yearly sums (*comprobante de verificación*)

voxel (**VOX**-el = *picture element giving image depth or volume*)—picture element giving depth and volume

wax elimination—burn out of wax pattern from investment material, leaving a shape void (*eliminación de la cera*)

wax pattern—exact replica of the prosthesis to be completed (*el diseño*)

welding—direct joining of two metals by a fusion process (*soldadura*)

workman's compensation—government policy covering employees injured at working site or on the job (*indemnización de las trabajadore*)

work order—written directions from the dentist to the laboratory completing the case (*orden de trabajo*)

xenograft (**ZEE**-no-graft)—bone graft taken from another species, such as a cow or pig (experimental) (*xenoinjertos, xenotrasplante*)

xerostomia (**zeer**-oh-**STOH**-me-ah; xeros = *dry*, stoma = *mouth*)—dry mouth (*sequedad en la boca*)

xiphoid (**ZIF**-oyd)—process or bones at the lowest part of the sternum (breastbone) (*esternón*)

X-ray—radiant energy produced from a vacuum tube (*rayo-X*)

zero angulation—position of X-ray source in a neutral angle, not up or down; zero-degree angle (*angulación cero*)

ZIP code—postal process used to sort and forward mail to a **ZIP** code location (*código postal*)

zygomatic (zye-goh-**MAT**-ick)—face bone under each eye; forms and gives shape to cheekbone (*cigomático*)

zygomaticofacial (zye-go-**MAT**-ee-coe-**fay**-shal)—foramen; opening in bone for nerve passage

GLOSSARY OF ACRONYMS

ALARA	as low as reasonably achievable
ADA	American Dental Association
	Americans with Disabilities Act
ADAA	American Dental Assistants Association
ADHA	American Dental Hygienists Association
AIDS	Acquired Immune Deficiency Syndrome
ANSI	American National Standards Institute
ANUG	acute necrotizing ulcerative gingivitis
ARC	AIDS-related complex
BIS-GMA	polymer used in pit and fissure sealants
BPM	beats per minute
CAHP	contra angle handpiece
CDA	Certified Dental Assistant
CDCP	Centers for Disease Control and Prevention
CDPMA	Certified Dental Practice Management Assistant
CDT	Certified Dental Technician
CERP	Continuing Education Recognition Program
CHF	congestive heart failure
CNS	central nervous system
COA	Certified Orthodontic Assistant
COMSA	Certified Oral Maxillofacial Surgery Assistant
CPR	cardiopulmonary resuscitation
CVA	cerebrovascular accident
DANB	Dental Assisting National Board
DB	direct bonding
DDS	Doctor of Dental Surgery
DEA	Drug Enforcement Agency
DHCW	Dental Health Care Worker
DMD	Doctor of Medical Dentistry
DNA	deoxyribonucleic acid
DR	digital radiography
EBA	ortho-ethoxybenzoic acid
EFDA	Expanded Function Dental Auxiliary
ELISA	Enzyme-Linked Immunosorbent Assay (HIV antibody test)
ENAP	excisional/new attachment procedure
EPA	Environmental Protection Agency

FDA	Food and Drug Administration
FDC	Federal Drug and Cosmetic Act
FDI	Federation Dentaire Internationale
FFD	film focus distance
FG	friction grip
HAV	Hepatitis A virus
HBIG	Hepatitis B immune globulin (plasma antibody for hepatitis)
HBV	Hepatitis B virus
HCV	Hepatitis C virus
HCW	health care worker
HIV	Human Immunodeficiency Virus
HIV+	positive serotest for HIV antibody
HVE	high-volume evacuator
IOR	interocclusal registration (bite registration)
IPA	Independent Practice Association
MMWR	Morbidity and Mortality Weekly Report
MPD	maximum permissible dose
MSDS	manufacturer's safety data sheet
NADL	National Association of Dental Laboratories
NIOSH	National Institute for Occupational Safety and Health
OPIM	other potentially infectious material
OSHA	Occupational Safety and Health Administration
PFI	plastic filling instrument
PFM	porcelain fused to metal
PID	position indicating device (radiology)
PIM	potential infectious material
PPE	personal protection equipment
PPO	preferred provider organization
RCT	root canal treatment
RDH	Registered Dental Hygienist
RPE	rapid palatal expander
SBDA	State Board of Dental Examiners
SDPA	State Dental Practice Act
SOP	standard operating procedure
TIA	transient ischemic attack
UCR	usual, customary, and reasonable (fees)
ZOE	zinc oxide eugenol

additional insured Any person not named under your plan who is not covered as insured in your documentation from the insurance company.

adjudication An administrative procedure used to process a claim for service according to the covered benefit of the plan.

administrative services only (ASO) An arrangement in which a licensed insurer provides administrative services to an employer's health benefits plan (such as processing claims), but doesn't insure the risk of paying benefits to enrollees. In an ASO arrangement, the employer pays for the health benefits.

adverse selection In a statistical estimate, a condition wherein a group has a greater demand for dental services and/or more services necessary than the average expected for that group.

allowable charge The maximum fee that a health plan insurance will reimburse a provider (dentist, doctor, facility) for a given service.

ancillary care Diagnostic and/or supportive services such as radiology, physical therapy, pharmacy, home health care, or laboratory work.

anniversary date The day after a coverage period ends under a health benefits plan. Usually, the month and day that a health benefits plan first goes into effect becomes its anniversary date each year.

annual out-of-pocket maximum The most a plan member will pay per year for covered health expenses before the plan pays 100% of covered health expenses for the rest of that year.

antireflection The tendency of persons with a poorer-than-average risk to apply for, or continue, insurance as compared with persons with average or better-than-average expectations of loss.

appeal A request to a dental plan to review a decision that denied or limited the treatment or proposed treatment to the beneficiary of the plan; usually made by the attending dentist on behalf of the plan beneficiary. Process is also available to the subscriber or agent appointed by the subscriber.

assignment of benefits An order from the subscriber to the plan to pay benefits from the procedure to the person designated as receiver of the benefit amount.

attending dentist's statement Also known as the ADA dental claim form; used to report dental procedures to a third-party payer. This claim form was developed by the American Dental Association.

audit An examination of records and accounts to check their accuracy. A post-treatment record review or clinical examination to verify information reported on claims may be performed.

balance billing Dentist fees that the enrollee is billed for amounts above the enrollee's portion of the coinsurance. Participating dentists agree to accept the plan's contracted fees and not to bill above that amount. Noncontracted dentists are under no obligation to limit the amount of their fees.

basic care Includes root canal therapy, extractions, and fillings (usually covered at 80%).

benefit booklet A booklet provided to the subscriber that contains a general explanation of the benefits and related provisions of the dental benefit program. Also known as a Summary Plan Description.

benefit year Usually begins on the month of the year that the employer purchased the plan.

birthday rule When a child is covered under the plans of both parents, the plan of the parent whose birthday (month and day, not year) falls earlier in the calendar year is billed first. (In cases of divorced or separated parents, there are other factors that must be considered.)

brush biopsy Brush biopsy is a painless procedure used to gather cells in the mouth. The dentist uses a small brush to take a tissue specimen, which is then sent to a laboratory for analysis to determine the presence of precancerous or early stage cancerous cells. Laboratory results are used to determine the need for further procedures.

cafeteria plan A benefit program in which an employer gives employees several different benefit plans to choose from (i.e., a selection of benefit plans).

calendar year deductible The dollar amount for covered services that must be paid during the calendar year (January 1–December 31) by members before any benefits are paid by the insurance company.

calendar year maximum benefit This is the maximum dollar amount that the insurance company or third party will pay per year for covered expenses for each covered member.

capitation plan A plan where the dentist is contracted with the administrator to provide dental services to persons covered under the program in return for payment on a per capita basis (per head).

care management A generic term that has been used in many different ways. Plan provided; an approach to medical and dental care from prevention through treatment and recovery.

carrier A term previously used for licensed insurance companies, although now is sometimes used to include both licensed insurers and HMOs.

carryover If the deductible was paid last year (usually the last quarter, Oct., Nov., or Dec.), the next year (or quarter, Jan., Feb., and March) the patient does not have to pay the deductible again.

case management Coordination of services to help meet a patient's health-care needs, usually when the patient has a condition that requires multiple services from multiple providers. This term is also used to refer to coordination of care during and after a hospital stay.

Centers for Medicaid and Medicare Services The federal agency responsible for administering Medicare and federal participation in Medicaid.

certificate holder The subscriber, usually the employee, who represents the family covered by

the dental benefit program; family members are referred to as "dependents."

certificate of coverage A printed description of the subscriber's benefits and coverage limits that forms a contract between the subscriber and the carrier. It states what will or will not be covered and the dollar maximums.

claimant Person who files a claim for benefits; may be the patient or the certificate holder.

closed panel This plan allows covered patients to receive care only from dentists who have signed a contract of participation with the insurance company. The third party contracts with a certain percentage of dentists within a particular geographic area.

COBRA The Consolidated Omnibus Budget Reconciliation Act of 1985 requires group health plans with 20 or more employees (in California, 2 to 19 employees for CAL-COBRA) to offer continued health coverage for employees and their dependents for 18 months after the employee leaves the job. Longer durations of continuance are available under certain circumstances. If a former employee opts to continue coverage under COBRA, the former employee must pay the entire premium, usually 110% of the cost of their group coverage.

coinsurance The portion of eligible expenses that plan members are responsible for paying, most often after the deductible is met. The copayment is usually determined as a percentage of the total cost.

complex rehabilitation The extensive dental restoration involving six or more units of crown and/or bridge in the same treatment plan or extensive procedures involved in complex rehabilitation requiring an extraordinary amount of time, effort, skill, and laboratory collaboration for a successful outcome.

contract An agreement between the dental insurance company and the applicant, including the enrollment and payment authorization form, the attached schedules, and any appendices, endorsements, or riders. This contract constitutes the *entire* agreement between the parties.

contract allowance The maximum amount allowed for a single procedure. It is the lesser of the dentist's submitted fee, and the scheduled maximum, if any, and the dentist's fee filed in the participating dentist agreement, if any, or the usual, customary or reasonable amounts (UCR).

contributory program A dental benefits program in which the employee shares in the monthly premium of the program with the program sponsor (usually the employer). Generally done through payroll deduction.

coordination of benefits A provision in a contract that applies when a person is covered under more than one group's health benefits program. It requires that payment of benefits be coordinated by all programs to eliminate overinsurance or duplication of benefits.

copayment (copay) Amount that a plan member must pay the provider at the time of service, usually after the deductible is met for eligible expenses. It is usually a set flat fee.

cosmetic (aesthetic) dentistry Any dental treatment or repair that is solely rendered to improve the appearance of the teeth or mouth.

deductible The portion of the patient's health care that the patient pays before insurance starts covering it; typically, the higher the deductible, the lower the premiums. Most insurance plans have a deductible of $50 to $100, pay only a specified percentage for each type of treatment, and have a yearly maximum amount of funds available for dental care.

dental service corporations Not-for-profit organizations that negotiate and administer contracts for dental care to individuals or specific groups of patients.

designated provider program (DPP) Each member chooses a designated care provider (network provider) but has the added convenience of going outside the network for care at any time. The benefits for out-of-network care are reduced and are subject to indemnity-style deductibles and coinsurance.

DMO (dental maintenance organization) A legal entity that accepts the responsibility of providing services at a fixed price. The enrollees

in these plans must have dental care provided through designated doctors. May also be known as *managed care*.

durable medical equipment Equipment that can withstand repeated use and is primarily and usually used to serve a medical purpose; generally, it is appropriate for use in the home.

enrollee An individual (member) who is enrolled and eligible for coverage under a health plan contract.

exclusions Specific conditions or services that are not covered under the benefit agreement.

exclusive provider organization (EPO) Patients receive dental care only from participating dentists. Although there may be some exceptions for emergency and out-of-area care, if a patient decides to see a dentist who is not listed on the EPO panel, charges for service will not be covered. An EPO contracts with a limited number of practitioners within a geographic area. The EPO also may limit the amount of services that a patient can receive in a given calendar year.

expiration date The date that insurance coverage expires. It is usually indicated in the insurance contract.

explanation of benefits (EOB) When a claim is filed, the patient will get an explanation of benefits (EOB) displaying what was submitted, what's been paid, and what balance is due.

family deductible Deductible that may be satisfied by the combined expenses of all covered family members.

fee for services A planned program in which the dentist is reimbursed for each service, rather than on a periodically paid fixed amount per patient. Fee-for-service allows the patient to go to the dentist of choice. The patient submits a claim and pays the invoice (to be reimbursed later) or authorizes the hospital or doctor to collect their fees directly from their insurance company Also termed *indemnity*.

flexible benefits A benefit program in which an employee may choose spending of entitled dollars for distribution among various benefit options, such as health and disability insurance, dental benefits, child care, or pension benefits; similar to cafeteria plan or a flexible savings account.

flexible spending accounts (FSA) An employer-sponsored benefit that allows employees to defer a portion of their paycheck into an account specifically intended to reimburse them for out-of-pocket costs. FSAs can be used for reimbursement of any medically related cost that is not covered by the health-care plan, such as deductibles and copays, birth control, dental, vision, and so on.

formulary A list of preferred, commonly prescribed prescription drugs. These drugs are chosen by a team of doctors and pharmacists; also called a drug list.

fraud A false representation of a matter of fact (whether by words or conduct, by false or misleading allegations, or by concealment of that which should have been disclosed) that deceives and is intended to deceive another to his or her legal injury. Insurance fraud is any act committed with the intent to fraudulently obtain payment from an insurer.

gatekeeper A primary care dentist in a managed care environment who is responsible for managing the patient's overall dental care. The gatekeeper must authorize all specialist referrals.

generic drug A prescription drug that has the same active-ingredient formula as a brand-name drug. A generic drug is known only by its formula name, and its formula is available to any pharmaceutical company. The Food and Drug Administration (FDA) rates the generic drugs to be as safe and as effective as brand-name drugs and are usually less costly.

group health coverage A health benefits plan that covers a group of people as permitted by state and federal law.

health maintenance services Any health-care service or program that helps maintain a person's good health. Health maintenance services include all standard preventive medical practices, such as immunizations and periodic examinations, as well as health education and special self-help programs.

396

HIPAA The Health Insurance Portability and Accountability Act of 1996 has several parts. The first part addresses health insurance portability and is designed to protect health insurance coverage for workers and their families when they change or lose their jobs. Another part of the law is designed to reduce the administrative costs of providing and paying for health care through standardization. The law also includes requirements of health plans, organizations, and providers to protect the private health information of individuals.

HMO (health maintenance organizations) Health organization that offers members an array of health benefits—usually including preventive care—for a set monthly premium.

incentive program A program that promotes prevention by increasing coverage from one benefit period to the next as long as you visit the dentist regularly. For instance, cleanings might be covered at 70% during the first year, 80% during the second year, and up to 100% as long as the program is used at least once a year.

indemnity plan This plan is commonly known as a fee-for-service or traditional plan. In this type of dental insurance plan, the patient has the option to visit any dentist or dental care professional or provider. The patient will need to pay a deductible on the indemnity dental insurance. After doing so, the insurance provider will cover a part of "usual and customary" dental costs. The amount the dental insurance will reimburse the patient will vary according to your provider plan. Many insurance providers offering this sort of plan will pay for 80% or even 100% of dental costs.

individual deductible Amount of eligible expense a covered person must pay each year before the dental plan will pay for eligible benefits.

in-network/out-of-network Plan services provided either by a contracted dentist or non-contracted dentist. In-network dentists have agreed to participate in a plan and to provide treatment according to certain administrative guidelines and to accept their contracted fee as payment in full.

LEAT Least expensive alternative treatment approach.

lifetime maximum benefit (maximum lifetime benefit) A cap on the benefits paid for the duration of a health insurance policy. Many policies have a lifetime limit of a specific amount, which means that the insurer agrees to cover up to that amount in covered services over the life of the policy. After the specific maximum is reached, no additional benefits are payable.

limitations Provisions stated in the dental plan coverage contract that explain limits on the coverage of certain benefits. Limitations are typically related to frequency (e.g., the number of treatments allowed), time (e.g., services covered within a given period), or age (e.g., orthodontic coverage for dependent children only).

limiting age of coverage The age at which a dependent covered by a dental plan is no longer eligible to receive benefits. Most dental plans offer an extension of benefits beyond the limiting age of coverage to students and handicapped dependents.

major care Includes crowns (caps), permanent bridgework, and full and partial dentures, as well as periodontal (gum) care. (These items are often covered at 50%.)

maximum benefit period Also known as the benefit duration; maximum length of time for which benefits are payable under the plan as long as the employee remains continuously disabled.

maximum monthly benefit The highest dollar amount an employee with a disability can receive on a monthly basis under the long-term disability plan.

Medicaid A joint state/federal health insurance program that is administered by the state. It provides health coverage for low-income individuals, especially pregnant women, children, and the disabled.

Medicare A federal government hospital expense and medical expense insurance plan primarily for elderly and disabled persons.

Medicare Part A Hospital insurance provided by Medicare that can help pay for in-patient hospital care, medically necessary in-patient care in a skilled nursing facility, home health care, hospice care, and end-stage renal disease treatment.

Medicare Part B Medicare-administered medical insurance that helps pay for certain medically necessary practitioner services, outpatient hospital services, and supplies not covered by Part A hospital insurance of Medicare coverage. Doctors' services are covered under Part B even if they're provided to a member in an inpatient setting. Part B can also pay for some home health services when the beneficiary doesn't qualify for Part A.

Medicare Part D A prescription drug benefit for Medicare-eligible seniors and disabled persons. It was established as part of the Medicare Prescription Drug, Improvement, and Modernization Act (MMA).

medigap A term used to describe health benefits coverage that supplements Medicare coverage.

member ID Unique identifying number for a member under the dental plan (sometimes their Social Security number).

National Committee on Quality Assurance (NCQA) An independent, nonprofit organization that assesses the quality of managed care plans, managed behavioral health-care organizations, and credentials-verification organizations.

nonduplication of benefits A term used to describe a method of coordination of benefits where the secondary plan will not pay any benefits if the primary plan paid the same or more than what the secondary plan allows as a fee for that dentist.

nonparticipating provider A dentist who has not contracted with a carrier to be a participating dentist for a plan.

open access A plan feature that allows enrollees to visit the dentists of their choice (freedom of choice). Also sometimes used to describe an enrollee's ability to seek treatment from a specialist without first obtaining a referral from the primary care provider.

open enrollment A period (usually a two-week or one-month period during the year) when qualified individuals (eligible employees) can enroll in or change their choice of coverage in group benefits plans.

out-of-plan This phrase usually refers to physicians, hospitals, or other health-care providers who are considered nonparticipants in an insurance plan (usually an HMO or PPO). Depending on an individual's health insurance plan, expenses incurred by services provided by out-of-plan health professionals may not be covered or may be covered at a reduced benefit level.

out-of-pocket costs Any amount for dental treatment that an enrollee is responsible for paying, for example, copayments, deductibles, and costs above the annual maximum.

out-of-pocket (OOP) maximum/limit Total dollar amount an insured will be required to pay for covered medical services during a specified period, such as one year. The OOP maximum may also be called the stop-loss limit or catastrophic expense limit.

palliative Treatment that relieves pain but is *not* curative.

participant A person who is eligible to receive health benefits under a health benefits plan. This term may refer to the employee, spouse, or other dependents.

participating provider A physician, hospital, pharmacy, laboratory, or other appropriately licensed facility or provider of health-care services or supplies that has entered into an agreement with a managed care entity to provide services or supplies to a patient enrolled in a health benefit plan.

pended claim Claims that require additional information prior to completing the adjudication process due to a specific reason code.

point-of-service (POS) plan A health plan allowing the member to choose to receive a service from a participating or nonparticipating provider, with different benefits levels associated with the use of participating providers.

policyholder The group or individual to whom an insurance contract is issued.

PPO (preferred provider organization) This type of plan allows a particular group of patients to receive dental care from a defined panel of dentists. The participating dentist agrees to charge less than usual fees to this specific patient base, providing savings for the plan purchaser. If the patient chooses to see a dentist who is not designated as a "preferred provider," that patient may be required to pay a greater share of the fee-for-service. Most PPO plans cover preventive care, cleanings, checkups, protective dental sealants, X-rays, and fluoride treatment at 80–100%.

preauthorization Statement by an insurance company or third-party payer indicating that a proposed treatment will be covered under the terms of the benefit contract.

precertification The process of obtaining certification from the health plan for routine hospital stays or health or dental outpatient procedures. The process involves reviewing criteria for benefit coverage determination.

predetermination An administrative procedure that may require the dentist to submit a treatment plan to the insurance company or third party before treatment is begun. The third party usually returns the treatment plan indicating one or more of the following: patient's eligibility, guarantee of eligibility period, covered services, benefit amounts payable, application of appropriate deductibles, copayment, and/or maximum limitation. Under some programs, predetermination by the third-party payer is required when covered charges are expected to exceed a certain amount.

preexisting condition A health condition (other than a pregnancy) or medical problem that was diagnosed or treated before enrollment in a new health plan or insurance policy.

preexisting condition limitations When an employee has a physical or mental condition that existed prior to the effective date of his or her insurance coverage, it is considered a preexisting condition. Most plans exclude or decrease disability benefits for an illness or injury for which an employee received medical treatment or consultation within a specified time period before becoming covered under the plan. The limitation generally expires after coverage has been in effect for a specified period of time.

premiums A prepaid payment or series of payments made to a dental plan by purchasers, and often plan members, for dental benefits.

prescription drug A drug that has been approved by the federal Food and Drug Administration, which can only be dispensed according to a physician's prescription order.

pretreatment estimate An estimate of how much of proposed treatment will be covered under an enrollee's dental plan as of a particular date. A pretreatment estimate is not a guarantee of payment. When the services are complete and a claim is received for payment, the company will calculate its payment based on the enrollee's current eligibility, amount remaining in the annual maximum, and any deductible requirements.

preventive care Includes regular checkups and cleanings; it is the basis of maintaining oral health.

provider directory Provider directories are listings of providers who have contracted with a managed care network to provide care to its participants. Participants may refer to the directory to select in-network providers.

reasonable and customary (R&C) charge A term used to refer to the commonly charged or prevailing fees for oral health services within a geographic area. A fee is generally considered to be reasonable if it falls within the parameters of the average or commonly charged fee for the particular service within that specific community.

reimbursement Payment made by an insurance company or third party to a beneficiary or to a dentist on behalf of the beneficiary, toward repayment of expenses incurred for services covered by the contractual arrangement.

single procedure A dental procedure that is assigned a separate procedure number, for example, a single X-ray file or a complete upper denture.

status change A lifestyle event that may cause a person to modify his or her health benefits coverage category. Examples include, but are not limited to, the birth of a child, divorce, or marriage.

submission date The date the claim was submitted and/or received by the insurance company or third party.

table program A dental plan where benefits are based on a specific table or schedule of allowances or fees. The table lists the maximum amount that a plan will pay for each procedure (covered amount). Enrollees are responsible for paying any difference between the amount the plan pays and the amount the dentist charges for the service.

usual, customary, or reasonable (UCR) The amount reimbursed to providers based on the prevailing fees in a specific area.

waiting period To become eligible for coverage under the policy, an employee must satisfy a certain number of continuous days of service as an active, full-time employee. This is known as the waiting period. In addition, a waiting period can also be the time period between when a disability occurs and when payments from the disability insurance policy begin.

waiver of premium When an individual becomes disabled and eligible for benefits, no further disability premium payments are required as long as benefits are being paid out.

yearly maximum Insurance or third-party organization's yearly maximum payment amount for services rendered. This amount does not accumulate from year to year.

INDEX

Forceps, 226, 227
Fordyce granules, 113
Forensic dentist, 62
Foreshortening (radiographic error), 159, 163
Fossa, 52
Fourth-class mail, 316
Fracture, 220
Fracture classification, 280
Fracture repair, 233
Frahms carver, 66
Framework, 199, 305
Frankfort plane, 158–159
Fraud, 332
Free margin gingiva, 259–260
Frena, 33
Frenectomy, 33, 188, 231, 278
Frenum, 33–35
Frequency of pulse, 96
Frequent respiration, 97
Friction grip (FG), 69, 71
Friction grip bur, 71
Frontal bones, 21
Frontal nerve, 27
Frontal process, 23
Frontal sinus, 22
FTC (Federal Trade Commission), 137
Full crown, 187, 198, 307
Full mouth denture set, 303
Full mouth extraction, 230
Full mouth reconstruction, 183
Full mouth survey (FMS/FMX), 160, 161
Fungi, 82
Fungiform papillae, 34
Furcation, 52, 268
Furnace, 302
Furrow, 52
Fusion, 43, 275

G

Galvanization, 295
Ganglion, 27
Gasserian, 27
Gastric distension, 99
Gates–Glidden drills, 216, 217
Gel application, 184–185
Gel state, 287

General anesthesia, 135–137
   equipment needed for, 136–137
   stages of sedation, 135–136
Generic name, 137
Genioplasty, 233
Geographic tongue, 114
Geographical filing system, 322
Germicide, 87
Germination, 43, 275
Gestational diabetes mellitus, 102
Gingiva, 47, 48–49
Gingival augmentation, 188–189
Gingival contouring, 188
Gingival disease, 259
Gingival isolation, 184
Gingival margin trimmer, 66, 67
Gingival recession, 188
Gingival reduction, 188
Gingival tissue, 259
Gingivectomy, 231, 264
Gingivitis, 113
Gingivoplasty, 231, 264
Glass bead heat, 85–86
Glenoid, 26
Glossa, 34
Glossitis, 114
Glossopalatine arch, 35
Glucose, 102
Gnarled enamel, enamel, 45
Gold alloy, 293
Gold foil, 176–177
Grand mal seizure, 103
Granuloma, 47, 115, 232, 276
Greater palatine foramina, 23, 24
Grit, 72
Groove, 52
Ground package service, 316
Group policy, 327
Group practice, 63
Guided tissue regeneration, 265
Gum abscess, 119
Gum tissue, 47, 48–49
Gummy smile, 188, 189
Gums. *See* Gingiva
Gutta-percha points, 218–219
Gypsum, 289
Gypsum mixing machine, 301

H

L